Language Disorders in Adults

Recent Advances

Editor in chief, Speech, Language, and Hearing Disorders Series
William H. Perkins, PhD

Language Disorders In Adults

Recent Advances

edited by
Audrey L. Holland, PhD
Speech and Hearing Center
University of Pittsburgh

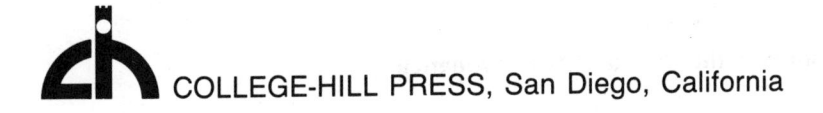

COLLEGE-HILL PRESS, San Diego, California

COLLEGE FOR HUMAN SERVICES
LIBRARY
345 HUDSON STREET
NEW YORK, N.Y. 10014

College-Hill Press
4284 41st Street
San Diego, California 92105

© 1984 by College-Hill Press, Inc.

All rights, including that of translation, reserved. No part of this publication may be reproduced, stored in a retrieval system, or transmitted in any form or by any means, electronic, mechanical, recording, or otherwise, without the prior written permission of the publisher.

Library of Congress Cataloging in Publication Data

Main entry under title:

Language disorders in adults.

Includes index.
1. Language disorders. I. Holland, Audrey L.
[DNLM: 1. Language disorders--In adulthood.
2. Aphasia--In adulthood. 3. Language disorders--In old age. WL 340 L28755]
RC423.L334 1983   616.85'5   83-7445
ISBN 0-933014-93-7

Printed in the United States of America

Publisher's Note

These volumes were developed under the supervision of a group of leading scientists charged with the responsibility of assessing the most critical book needs of the speech-language-hearing profession. In consultation with William H. Perkins and Raymond G. Daniloff, serving as editors in chief of the ensuing volumes on speech, language, and hearing disorders (Perkins) and speech, language, and hearing science (Daniloff), the publisher planned a series of nine mutually independent texts covering the entirety of state-of-the-art knowledge in these disciplines, with contributions by respected, productive, and current scholars known for their expertise as specialists in key areas.

Each contribution has been stringently refereed for content, pedagogy, and practical value for students and practitioners by the individual volume editors, Charles Berlin, Janis Costello, Raymond Daniloff, Audrey Holland, James Jerger, Rita Naremore, and their designated reviewers, in close consulation throughout with the editor in chief and the publisher. Users are thus assured that their needs for accurate, timely information, reflecting the highest standards of scholarship and professionalism, have been faithfully met.

On behalf of the speech-language-hearing profession, its researchers, teachers, practitioners, and students, present and future, the publisher thanks the more than 100 authors and editors who have given generously of their time and knowledge to produce this magnificent contribution to the literature.

Language Disorders in Adults, edited by Audrey Holland, is one of nine state-of-the-art volumes comprising the College-Hill Press series covering the current body of knowledge in speech, language, and hearing.

Volume Titles:	Editors:
Speech Disorders in Children	Janis Costello
Speech Disorders in Adults	Janis Costello
Speech Science	Raymond Daniloff
Language Disorders in Children	Audrey Holland
Language Disorders in Adults	Audrey Holland
Language Science	Rita Naremore
Pediatric Audiology	James Jerger
Hearing Disorders in Adults	James Jerger
Hearing Science	Charles Berlin

Editor in chief, Speech, Language, and Hearing Disorders Series: William H. Perkins

Editor in chief, Speech, Language, and Hearing Science Series: Raymond G. Daniloff

Contents

Contributors	viii
Foreword	ix
Preface	xi

Language Disorders in Adults:
State of the Clinical Art — 1
Robert T. Wertz

Effects of Aging on Normal Language — 79
G. Albyn Davis

Mild Aphasia — 113
Craig W. Linebaugh

Moderate Aphasia — 133
Jennifer Horner

Severe Aphasia — 159
Nancy Helm-Estabrooks

Right Hemisphere Impairment — 177
Penelope Starratt Myers

Language and Dementia — 209
Kathryn A. Bayles

Language Disorders in Head Trauma — 245
Chris Hagen

Nonspeech Language and Communication Systems — 283
Kathryn M. Yorkston, Patricia A. Dowden

Author Index — 313

Subject Index — 325

Contributors

Kathryn A. Bayles, PhD
Department of Speech and
Hearing Sciences
University of Arizona
Tucson, AZ 85721

G. Albyn Davis, PhD
Memphis Speech & Hearing
Center
807 Jefferson Ave.
Memphis, TN 38105

Patricia A. Dowden, MS
Department of Rehabilitation
Medicine
University of Washington
Seattle, WA 98195

Chris Hagen, PhD
Speech-Language Pathology
Department
Speech, Hearing &
Neurosensory Center
Children's Hospital and Health
Center
Sharp Rehabilitation Hospital
San Diego, CA 92123

Nancy Helm-Estabrooks, DSc
Audiology/Speech Pathology
Boston Veterans Administration
Medical Center
Neurology (Speech Pathology)
Boston University School of
Medicine
Boston, MA 02130

Jennifer Horner, PhD
Department of Surgery
Duke University Medical Center
Box 3887
Durham, NC 27710

Craig W. Linebaugh, PhD
Speech and Hearing Center
George Washington University
Washington, DC 20052

Penelope Starratt Myers
Speech & Hearing Center
George Washington University
Washington, DC 20052

Robert T. Wertz, PhD
Audiology and Speech Pathology
Veterans Administration Medical
Center
Martinez, CA 94553

Kathryn M. Yorkston, PhD
Speech Pathology Services
Department of Rehabilitation
Medicine
University of Washington
Seattle, WA 98195

Foreword

From 1977 to 1982, while editing the *Journal of Speech and Hearing Disorders,* I became increasingly aware of the rate at which information about communication disorders was expanding. Not only was it an information explosion, it was a conceptual explosion as well, particularly in the area of children's language. We are departing rapidly from a relatively insular profession in which clinical practice has been based largely on what we could learn from our own experience. What we are moving toward is a theory-based profession in which we are open to broad-ranging conceptions, most notably from linguistics, medicine, and psychology.

It was against this background that *Recent Advances: Speech, Language, and Hearing Pathology* was spawned. In accepting the responsibility of being editor in chief, I saw several opportunities. Above all, it offered a vehicle by which the profession could remain current. Some areas have moved so rapidly that they bear little resemblance to what they were even a decade ago. Not only has information proliferated, but so have the journals and texts in which it has been preserved. Here, then, in *Recent Advances,* was an opportunity to organize a coherent and comprehensive account of the current state of affairs in all clinical aspects of speech, language, and hearing.

A price paid for advancement of knowledge is not only inability to consume the increasing glut, but even to comprehend it. One must almost be a specialist to understand what other specialists are talking about. To chronicle the state of the art across all areas of communication disorders, and still make responsible statements, would require the best minds available in each area. To know who the experts in these areas are, and to obtain their participation, would require scholars of such stature as to attract them. Hence, my most important responsibility in this project was the selection of volume editors. I take great pride that Janis Costello, Audrey Holland, and James Jerger agreed to participate.

With their respective editorships established, my remaining responsibility was to consult with them in determining the chapters needed to report the state of the art in their areas, and in selecting authors most qualified to prepare the chapters. We sought authors who not only are established scholars, but who also write with clarity. We were as concerned that anyone in the profession be able to read and understand what is going on in any area as we were with assembling the best information available. Aside from nudging the project along occasionally and final editing, I can claim little credit for the sterling quality of these texts. That credit belongs to the editors.

William H. Perkins
Editor in chief

Preface

It has been a pleasure to edit this book. Part of the pleasure has come from having had the opportunity to share ideas and to interact with this enthusiastic and knowledgeable group of contributors. The major reason, however, is that it has been a significant learning experience for me. I regard this volume as a "state of the art" book about some major problems and issues concerning adult language disorders, and what can (or cannot) be done about a fair sampling of them. I have learned mightily in the process of working with these authors, and by virtue of it, catching up on new material, new research, new trends, and developing concepts about language and its disorders in adults.

The profession of Speech-Language Pathology and Audiology celebrated its 50th birthday a few years ago, and 1981 marked the occasion of 50 years of systematic treatment for aphasia by American speech-language pathologists. Nevertheless, most professions surely mature more slowly than do the people who practice them, and this one is no exception. In recent years, our still only dawning maturity has resulted in restructuring some of the methods that constitute clinical practice, some redefinition of the people and the problems we treat, some refocusing of clinical perspective generally, and even some returns to a few early beliefs that were discarded in the profession's brash adolescence. The content of this book reflects the profession's growth.

In this volume, some old problems such as aphasia are presented in a variety of new ways. Other problems, notably language disorders in dementia, closed head injury, and in patients with right-hemisphere damage, are singled out and emphasized as different from, and justifiably separated from, the aphasias that result from focal damage, usually to the left hemisphere. The coverage of non-speech language and communication in adults reflects a broadening of perspective in a field that used to be held in thrall by the spoken and written word and their respective forms of comprehension. Although the profession has long recognized the importance of understanding disordered language in children in the context of normal acquisition of language, this volume puts adult language disorders into their appropriate lifespan developmental context as well. Finally, throughout the book, concern for the patient-as-a-person is manifested.

Ideally, an introduction should simply set the stage, whet the readers' appetites, properly raise their levels of anticipation for the heady content to follow. So I will be brief in describing the topics and the authors, preferring to let them speak for themselves. Nonetheless, it is irresistible not to add my own perspective to what is covered in this volume, chapter-by-chapter.

Robert T. Wertz opens the book with a comprehensive overview of language disorders of adulthood, stressing recent trends in their study, diagnosis, and treatment. A crucial feature of Wertz' review is its breadth, and its inclusion of some new concerns, such as the language of schizophrenia, usually ignored by speech/language pathologists. My belief is that this chapter may well influence the direction of adult language pathology for some years to come.

G. Albyn Davis' chapter on normal adult language has the very difficult goal of summarizing a broad literature on language and normal aging, most of it coming from other disciplines, including geriatric psychology and sociology. His conclusion that surprisingly little of real substance is known about how language might change across the adult lifespan is a sobering one. Nevertheless, Davis has carefully described the crucial issues and has suggested many areas for future research, in addition to suggesting strategies for such study.

Three chapters are devoted specifically to the topic of aphasia. Aphasia has been split into mild, moderate, and severe forms of the disorder for consideration here. This split is a result of my belief that different treatment principles and goals for treatment derive from a consideration of the severity of the problem, as well as from the specific aphasic syndrome a patient is manifesting.

It is largely through the work of Nancy Helm-Estabrooks that aphasiologists are reconsidering the idea that severe aphasia, particularly global aphasia, is hopeless. She has been responsible for the development of techniques specifically directed to such patients and has been careful to quantify their effectiveness. In her chapter on severe aphasia in this book, she shares not only her approaches to such patients, but also her unique way of thinking about them.

Jennifer Horner has taken the territory about which aphasiologists appear to have known the most for the longest, the problems of the moderately impaired patient. She has fitted these problems with a new suit of clothes, partly fashioned by her own clinical experience, but also influenced by her understanding of neuropsychology and its potential for contributing to aphasia rehabilitation in very direct ways.

Craig Linebaugh has filled a very tough assignment, describing the treatment of aphasic patients whose impairments are mild. The importance of developing keener insight into the mildly impaired aphasic patient is great, for not only are they virtually ignored in clinical texts, but they are the patients with the highest likelihood of returning to their pre-aphasia lifestyles and vocations.

Before leaving the subject of aphasia, it is pertinent to add that medical advances themselves have led us to consider more explicitly those patients whose aphasias are at the poles of severity. Better medical management of stroke has resulted in more survivors who might previously have died, and possibly thereby has forced the more severely impaired upon our consciousness. Better medical management has also lessened the likelihood of severe stroke, and similarly left the aphasiologist with a significantly larger number of mildly impaired patients. The example aptly illustrates that not only self-contemplation but medical, social, and philosophic concerns interact to bring about advances in the profession.

In a related field, Penelope Meyers has broken new ground with her comprehensive chapter on the problems of patients who have incurred right-hemisphere deficits. Few students of aphasia rehabilitation have been required to study right-hemisphere problems, yet speech-language pathologists are increasingly being called on to work with the visuospatial, language, and cognitive deficits that occur as a result of damage to the formerly "minor hemisphere." Meyers' chapter breaches this void.

Kathryn Bayles has filled a similar need with her broad overview of dementia. Dementia is another problem that has recently begun to attract the attention of speech-language pathologists who work with adults. As aging generally has become the focus of national concern, professional interest in one of its major disorders has also increased. Yet, few speech-language pathology curricula are prepared to teach the clinician about dementia, and few clinicians are prepared to develop a principled stance about their role in working with dementia, either as it occurs in pure form, or as it might accompany aphasias and other disorders of aging. At the same time, speech-language pathologists increasingly find employment in chronic care facilities, nursing homes, and institutions for the aging and infirm. Bayles' chapter provides the background against which the speech-language pathologist can develop his or her own principled beliefs.

As the nation's largest killer of people under the age of 35, closed-head injury is increasingly recognized as a major American problem. And those who survive head injury have rapidly swelled the clinical caseloads of aphasiologists, who, in working with these patients, are beginning to recognize the limitations of the well-known treatments for aphasia. Chris Hagen, whose work with the head-injured has considerably influenced most of the systematic treatment programs for the problem, has provided for this volume a meticulously detailed, comprehensive approach.

No volume purporting to discuss recent advances in language disorders could avoid having a chapter on nonspeech language and communication if it chose to be worthy of the title. And this book's final chapter by Kathryn Yorkston and Patricia Dowden serves simultaneously to educate the speech-language pathologist about the importance of understanding nonspeech language advances and to give a very current overview of this, probably the profession's most rapidly advancing topic.

It is past time to stop my own enthusiasm and let readers get down to the business of stirring up their own. In closing, allow me to share a final rumination and speculation. As this volume was planned and as it has developed over the past year, I became fascinated with trying to imagine what I would have expected of it, had I been planning it 20, or even 10, years ago. I do not think I would have come close to what every reader will recognize as the new directions, new problems, and new solutions presented here. And it is also fascinating to think what might be encountered in a *Recent Advances* 10 or 20 years in the future. I expect that it will be at least as unpredictable. The great satisfaction of this profession is the surprises it holds and the constancy of its change.

Audrey L. Holland
Editor

Robert T. Wertz

Language Disorders in Adults: State of the Clinical Art

On February 26, 1885, William Osler began his "State of the Art" Gulstonian Lectures on malignant endocarditis. He summarized the past, defined his present purposes, and predicted the future.

> Mr. President and gentlemen—It is of use, from time to time, to take stock, so to speak, of our knowledge of a particular disease, to see exactly where we stand in regard to it, to inquire to what conclusions the accumulated facts seem to point, and to ascertain in what direction we may look for fruitful investigations in the future. (Osler, 1885, p.1)

Fair enough! But, Osler's task was, for him, an easy one. First, he knew what he was talking about. Much of what was known about malignant endocarditis had resulted from his labors. Second, the etiological, clinical, and anatomical characteristics of the disease had been fairly well ascertained. And, third, he was ready with a review of over two hundred cases he had seen in the General Hospital in Montreal.

A similar attempt to present the clinical state of the art on language disorders in adults can agree with the utility of Osler's purpose. It is of use to take stock—to determine where we are, what we know, and where we might go. However, the task is exceedingly more difficult. First, even though all language disorders in adults are frequently collapsed into one, aphasia, there are others. Second, no single individual is sufficiently knowledgeable to complete the task. Third, each chapter in this volume

©College-Hill Press, Inc. All rights, including that of translation, reserved. No part of this publication may be reproduced without the written permission of the publisher.

represents a "state of the art" on a specific language disorder, or a portion of a specific language disorder, and, therefore, may render what follows superficial and redundant. And, fourth, any attempt to state "the state of the art" is historical before it reaches print.

Even though one may not succeed, one can try. So, what follows is one person's "state of the art" filtered through his information, his misinformation, and his biases. My purpose is to examine what I think we know today about managing language disorders in adults that I am not certain we knew ten or more years ago. Specifically, I will discuss six conditions in which adult language may go awry—normal, older individuals who may find themselves in an abnormal environment; confusion; schizophrenia; right hemisphere involvement; dementia; and aphasia. Because this is an attempt to state the "state of the *clinical* art," each condition will be considered under what I believe are the four steps in clinical management—appraisal, diagnosis, prognosis, and treatment. I will attempt to determine whether our science has influenced our service, if research has reached reality, whether our data are reflected in our deeds.

The Disorders

Any attempt to list, lacks. One person's pathologies include another's "no problems." One person's exclusions contain another's emphasis. Conversely, while some societies have no name for "it," others have several. So, while my list of potential language disorders in adults may be limited, I will attempt to describe each in order for others to identify that which they label differently. These are the language disorders that find their way to our clinical door.

Environmental Influence on the Normal Aged

Getting old affects more than the bladder. Davis, in this volume and elsewhere (Beasley & Davis, 1981), tells us what can go wrong with communication as one migrates through life's later decades. Certain performances decline as the organism ages, and older folk venture into the period when the nervous system is attacked more frequently by disease. For example, the incidence of cerebral vascular accident is greater after 65 than before 45. Some carry their communication problems with them as they travel further into life. All of these conditions exist, and they coexist. The individual whose stuttering began at 6 and accompanied him or her through life can be battered by a stroke in his 60s, a time when he or she is beleaguered by presbycusis and the physiologic decline that comes with years lived. Attempts to study aging make the strongest scientists weep.

Another complication in any attempt to bring order to aging is the variability in performance among older individuals. Forty-year-old nervous systems seem to reside in some who are 80, and 90-year-old nervous systems are housed in some who are 60. Set out to collect "normative" data on the elderly and you are certain to return with a sack full of extremely large standard deviations.

But, some do survive the rigors of living with their faculties in fine fettle. They function until they find themselves in an environment that erodes their intact skills. Holland (1978) and Lubinski (1981) have documented the disastrous effects an abnormal environment can have on a normal older person's communicative ability. We see these individuals in our clinics. They may have entered our medical centers with down-stream problems— an ornery prostate or arthritis, but after a few weeks, a consult is sent by the ward physician to please evaluate Mr. Boomis' confusion, or "this 80-year-old male's dementia." Similarly, social circumstances that dictate the elderly leave the stimulating environment of their familiar neighborhood and take up residence in a nursing home, or other extended care facility may lead, eventually, to language deficit. Holland (1980) reports that normal older individuals in institutionalized settings achieve lower scores on her measure, *Communicative Abilities in Daily Living* (CADL), than normal older individuals who reside in noninstitutionalized environments.

Thus, custody appears to confound cortex, at least the cortex utilized for communication. I list this condition as a potential language disorder in adults, and label it as language deficit in a normal older person residing in an abnormal environment. Lubinski (1981) uses the phrase "a communication-impaired environment" to describe a setting where there is reduced opportunity for successful, meaningful communication. This typifies some, not all, of our acute and chronic care facilities, where at least one in five of our nation's elderly will spend time prior to demise.

A specific set of symptoms to identify the normal older person whose language has eroded as a result of residing in a communication-impairing environment is difficult to list. Obler and Albert (1981) have provided some clues for identification. They indicate that the expected ravages of age affect naming skills and auditory comprehension in the healthy elderly. To cope, the healthy oldster utilizes strategies—syntax to cue naming ability and context to improve comprehension. Dropped into an unfavorable environment where few listen or speak, the healthy elderly find their strategies no longer result in solutions, and they abandon them. They cease attempting to convey and seek information when faced with misinformation or no information. Because communication is a "use it or lose it" phenomenon, the lack of use results in loss.

So, impaired language in the normal aged exists and it confronts the speech pathologist. It needs to be identified, to be differentiated from disorders—confusion, aphasia, dementia—it may masquerade as, and it needs to be managed appropriately.

Language of Confusion

Observe a group of medical residents being quizzed for a diagnosis by a senior physician and you hear an interesting dialogue. "What is your diagnosis young doctors?" asks the senior staff member. "Pneumonoultramicroscopicsilicovolcanoconiosis," replies the first-year resident. "Yes," responds the mentor, "there is one case reported in the entire history of medicine. Do you believe we have another?" We ignore the most probable and remember the odd, the bizarre, the interesting.

Similarly, the language of confusion is rare, but, if we have seen it, we remember it by its bizarre characteristics. And, like the young doctors, our memory may tempt application when the term is inappropriate. Darley, in a paper presented to the American Speech and Hearing Association (1969), has defined the language of confusion as:

> Impairment of language accompanying neurologic conditions; often traumatically induced; characterized by reduced recognition and understanding of and responsiveness to the environment, faulty memory, unclear thinking, and disorientation in time and space. Structured language events are usually normal and responses utilize correct syntax; open-ended language situations elicit irrelevance, confabulation.

Neurologists (Mayo Clinic, 1976) identify this condition as "confused state" or "confusion." Speech Pathologists (Halpern, Darley, & Brown, 1973) use Darley's term, the "language of confusion." Though rare, usually less than five percent of the language disorders we see in our clinic, it exists and requires our attention. These patients are not aphasic, and they are not demented. They need to be identified and to be managed appropriately.

Schizophrenia

Jaffe (1981) asked if a schizophrenic patient suffered a left hemisphere CVA with subsequent Wernicke's aphasia, would anyone notice? A partial answer to Jaffe's question is, probably, the speech pathologist would not. We know language deficit in aphasia, but I am not certain we know language deficit in schizophrenia. We see few patients who demonstrate the language of confusion because it is rare. We see few schizophrenic patients. Less than 1% of the referrals sent to our clinic are from the psychiatric wards. Consult a list of references in schizophrenia or, more specifically, references on the language of schizophrenic patients, and you will find few contributions by speech pathologists. Yet, language is disrupted in schizophrenic patients, and should it come to our attention, we need to identify it and differentiate it from other language disorders.

DiSimoni, Darley, and Aronson (1977) have reviewed language involvement in schizophrenia. They tell us schizophrenic patients may not use language for informational purposes, their prosody may be abnormal, they may dwell on certain themes and perseverate in their ideas, their performance may vary with the mode of stimulus presentation, they may display disrupted syntax, they may be disoriented, they may confabulate, and their verbal and written responses may be paraphasic.

As is true with most language disorders, language disturbance in schizophrenia varies with severity, and, specifically in schizophrenia, severity is linked with time postonset. Darley (1982) reports that as duration of the illness increases, performance declines. Deterioration of language in schizophrenic patients may migrate through the language performance displayed by a confused patient to, eventually, the language performance displayed by a demented patient.

Some (Chapman, 1966) suggest that an aphasia exists in schizophrenia. Others (Benson, 1973) do not. Some (Elmore & Gorham, 1957) do not differentiate the language of schizophrenic patients from the language of chronic brain syndrome patients, who are usually classified as demented. Whether the same as or different from, most agree language is not normal in schizophrenia. Therefore, it qualifies as a language disorder one may see in adults.

Right Hemisphere Involvement

Myers (1978, 1979), as she does in this volume, directs our attention to a communication deficit that may be present following right hemisphere damage. For years, we have suspected that the right hemisphere did something, that it was more than a spare if the left was damaged. Joynt and Goldstein (1975) have listed what may go wrong when the right hemisphere is damaged. The problems include: spatial perception and body image disorders, visual perception disorders, constructional disabilities, auditory perception disorders, somatosensory disorders, speech disorders, and motor impersistence. These have been studied by neurologists and psychologists. One wonders, what is left for the speech pathologist in the right hemisphere patient? A lot, Myers and West (1978) tell us.

Patients who suffer damage to the right hemisphere may have few overt language deficits, but they have difficulty communicating. Myers (1978) suggests that to communicate means more than just to impart. It also means to take part. While the right hemisphere patient's ability to impart may approach normality, his or her ability to participate is abnormal.

Historically, damage to the right hemisphere is reported to result in a variety of language deficits. Eisenson (1962) believes the right hemisphere patient has difficulty with high level language functions. Critchley (1962) reports difficulty in auditory and visual identification of language. Swisher and Sarno (1969) note difficulty in comprehending lengthy auditory stimuli. Weinstein (1964) observed naming errors. Archibald and Wepman (1968) reported aphasic-like responses on the *Language Modalities Test for Aphasia* (LMTA) (Wepman & Jones, 1961). And, several (Denny-Brown, Meyers, & Horenstein, 1952; Hecaen & Marcie, 1974; Metzler & Jelinek, 1977) have observed writing disturbance.

So, right hemisphere involvement appears to result in both nonverbal and verbal deficits. To these, Myers (1978, 1979) adds a disruption in cognitive style. The symptoms are inability to use visual imagery, inability to understand figurative language, altered affect, and an abnormal sense of humor. Together, they influence the way patients look at the world, the way they integrate what they see and hear, and the way they respond. Abnormal cognitive style has been described by Gardner (1975):

> The right hemisphere patient appears unconcerned about his message, insensitive to his situation or to the environment. He resembles a langauge machine, a talking computer that decodes literally, gives the most immediate response, insensitive to the ideas behind the question or the implications of the questioner. (p. 296)

Myers (1978) adds that the right hemisphere patient misses nuances and subtleties. His or her sense of humor, if present, is caustic. These patients are verbally dependent. They ignore context. They cannot, or do not, do what normals and aphasic patients do—fill in what is not present in the words.

Until recently, right hemisphere patients were not referred to the speech pathologist, or were referred "for our interest." More and more, they are being referred for evaluation and for treatment. Their problems and what we may be able to do about them classify them for inclusion in a list of language disorders in adults.

Dementia

"Mind! Mind!" one of my aphasic friends used to say when his brain and tongue failed to connect. His "mind" was fine. He was aphasic. Not so, for many who suffer dementia, more accurately, the dementias. Literally, the term means "deprived of mind." Estimates indicate 5% of our fellow citizens over 65 are severly demented. Another 10% are reported to be mildly to moderately demented.

The dementias result from brain diseases that erode mental abilities. Memory slips as does attention, judgment, and ability to learn. A few dementias are treatable. Most are not. Bayles, in this volume and elsewhere (Bayles, 1982b), tells us dementia is the chronic, progressive deterioration of intellect due to changes in the central nervous system. The culprits include Alzheimer's disease, now considered the same as senile dementia or senile brain disease; multiple infarcts; ideopathic Parkinson's disease; Huntington's disease; Creutzfeldt-Jakob disease; Pick's disease, and Korsakoff's disease. Causes of dementia with a brighter future, in that they may respond to treatment, are intoxication, poor nutrition, subdural hematoma, depression, tumor, metabolic disorders, and occult hydrocephalus (Foley, 1972).

Speech pathologists are attracted to dementia by its language symptoms. The intellectual loss is measured and documented by psychologists. The language deficits are measured and documented in the speech clinic. Darley (1969, 1982) has classified these as the language of generalized intellectual impairment. His definition is:

> Deterioration of performance on more difficult language tasks; reduced efficiency in all modes; greater impairment evident in language tasks requiring better retention, closer attention, and powers of abstraction and generalization; degree of impairment roughly proportionate to deterioration of other mental functions. (in a paper presented to the American Speech & Hearing Assn., 1969)

We see these patients, and our task is to separate them from patients with other language disorders. Our contribution transcends deciding that this patient is less intelligent than he sounds, hence, demented, and that patient is more intelligent than he sounds, hence, aphasic. We can step beyond diagnosis and document change over time, and we can manage demented patients as well as our tools and talents permit.

Aphasia

If neurologists, neuropsychologists, neurolinguists, and speech pathologists know anything, they know aphasia. In fact, they know enough to disagree on its definition and the words to be used in talking about it. Most agree that aphasic patients have difficulty in auditory comprehension, reading, oral-expressive use of language, and writing. However, confusion can arise, as Rosenbek (1983) points out, when books are titled *Aphasia, Alexia, and Agraphia* (Benson, 1979a). This might imply that aphasia involves listening and speaking, but not reading and writing. One must read the text to discover that all four are impaired in aphasia. Further, some have narrowed aphasia's boundaries to relate exclusively to "a disturbance in verbal language as opposed to other forms of language, for example, the language of gestures or of facial expression " (Damasio, 1981, p. 52).

The tendency to limit aphasia or to subdivide it into the aphasias can be contrasted with Darley's (1982) general definition of it as:

> Impairment, as a result of brain damage, of the capacity for interpretation and formulation of language symbols; multimodality loss or reduction in efficiency of the ability to decode and encode conventional meaningful linguistic elements (morphemes and larger syntactic units); disproportionate to impairment of other intellective functions; not attributable to dementia, confusion, sensory loss, or motor dysfunction; and manifested in reduced availability of vocabulary, reduced efficiency in application of syntactic rules, reduced auditory retention span, and impaired efficiency in input and output channel selection. (p. 42)

Darley prefers his aphasia lean, without adjectives. He draws support for his point of view from the Schuell, Jenkins, and Carroll (1962) factor analysis of results obtained on the *Minnesota Test for Differential Diagnosis of Aphasia* (Schuell, 1965a). The failure to find several dimensions led Schuell et al. to conclude that aphasia is a general language deficit that is not modality specific. This lack of evidence for a taxonomy or a dichotomy—sensory-motor, receptive-expressive, input-output—is amplified by Darley. Differences among aphasic patients, he believes, may not indicate different types of aphasia, but the presence of two disorders, for example, aphasia and apraxia of speech. Further, severity of aphasia confounds taxonomy and does not justify the conclusion that there are differrent aphasic types. Finally, Darley points out that time postonset erodes severity and differences. There is a migration among aphasic types as time postonset increases and severity decreases (Kertesz & McCabe, 1977; Wertz, Kitselman, & Deal, 1981). Thus, unlike a rose, a Wernicke's not always is a Wernicke's is a Wernicke's.

This "aphasia is one" point of view coexists in the literature and the clinic with the position that stresses classification. Classification of the aphasias is a core course in the curriculum of most neurologists, neuropsychologists, neurolinguists, and some speech pathologists. The systems popularized by Benson (1979a), Kertesz (1979), and Goodglass and Kaplan (1972) are used, and when clinicians with differing points of view meet to discuss a patient, confusion can result. And, the terminological debate is bound to become more complex. As we learn more about the contribution of subcortical structures to speech and language (Ojemann, 1975), subcortical aphasic syndromes find their way into the literature (Benson, 1979a; Alexander & Lo Verme, 1980).

While one may not agree, one can become bilingual. Rosenbek (1983) suggests settling on the best available definition of aphasia and the most clinically useful classification of people with it, because our failure to do so may affect our clinical practice. So, while we may not agree on what to call it, we seem to recognize it when we see it. This is fortunate, because we see a lot of it.

The State of the Art

These are the disorders that fill our literature and find their way to our clinic. The list is not exclusive, and little attention has been given to the possibility of coexisting disorders. Further, the literature contains debate on whether the language deficits in one disorder really represent another disorder.

Recently, we reviewed the percentages of different neurogenic speech and language disorders referred to our clinic during a one-year period. The figures were: aphasia, 28%; language of confusion, 6%; language of generalized intellectual impairment, 8%; dysarthria, 38%; apraxia of speech, 9%; and undetermined, 11%. The exercise told us more than we wanted to know, but it did not tell us enough about what we need to know. For example, disorders coexist. All of the apraxia of speech patients demonstrated coexisting aphasia. Apraxia of speech was just the most salient symptom. What was represented under the undetermined label? Here we put the right hemisphere patient, the rare schizophrenic patient, the patient with bilateral head trauma, and the ones we just could not label.

So, our list lacks. If it matters what you call it, and I believe it does, we need to find some names and apply them appropriately. For example, referrals from psychiatry, though few, are not all schizophrenic. Some have affective disorders, and not all schizophrenic patients demonstrate a thought disorder. Further, where do we put the bilateral head trauma patient with brain stem involvement? If the latter affects speech, dysarthria is an appropriate label, but what about the patient's language deficits? Are they aphasic? Holland (1982a) argues they are not, really. Or, at least, they differ from aphasia subsequent to a left hemisphere cerebral vascular accident. But what if both hemispheres are injured? Do these patients behave the way right hemisphere patients do? Somewhat, but not totally. Damage both sides of the brain and behavior differs from that seen following lateralized damage. Porch (1973) presents percentiles on his test, the *Porch Index of Communicative Ability* (PICA), for patients who have bilateral damage. The percentiles differ from those he presents for patients with left hemisphere damage. Is it useful to label the bilateral patients aphasic? I am not certain it is. But, is the language of generalized intellectual impairment more appropriate? Yes and no. And, what about the language disorder in dementia? Is it aphasic? Appell, Kertesz, and Fishman (1981) argue that it is. I (Wertz, 1982) have rebutted this—it is not.

Not long ago, I ran across a review of a book that was titled *Progress in Anatomy* (Harrison & Holmes, 1981). I wondered, how can there be progress in anatomy? Anatomy is. One studies it; not about it. Yet, some are studying about it. Similarly, we can make my error when we think language disorders in adults *are*; that we have compiled and completed the list. The state of the art in the labels we use is not etched. It is evolving. Two disorders appear in this chapter—environmental influence on the normal aged and schizophrenia—that did not appear in a survey I did five years ago (Wertz, 1978).

Appraisal

One way to test the validity of a list of language disorders is to pass it through a sieve of clinical scrutiny. Do patients find a place to abide on the list? Are there leftovers? Clinical scrutiny is another way of saying appraisal.

Appraisal, I believe, is a process of collecting data—biographical, medical, and behavioral. The purpose of appraisal is to find out what a patient has to tell you about his or her problem. Its ends are to make a diagnosis, formulate a prognosis, and either focus treatment or justify a decision not to treat.

There have been several influences on appraisal of language disorders in adults in recent years. First, available tests, at least for aphasia, abound. Second, neuropsychology has come out of the laboratory into life. Third, speech pathologists are beginning to realize that tests for aphasia are not the only—or best—tools for appraising other language disorders. Fourth, neurology has evolved from safety pin and mallet to some highly sophisticated neuroradiological techniques.

In 1979, 14 tests for appraising acquired language dysfunction were reviewed (Darley, 1979a). These included: the *Aphasia Language Performance Scales* (ALPS) (Keenan & Brassell, 1975); the *Appraisal of*

Language Disorders in Adults: State of the Clinical Art

Language Disturbance (ALD) (Emerick, 1971); *Boston Diagnostic Aphasia Examination* (BDAE) (Goodglass & Kaplan, 1972); *Examining for Aphasia* (Eisenson, 1954); *Functional Communication Profile* (FCP) (Sarno, 1969); *Halstead Aphasia Test, Form M* (Halstead, Wepman, Reitan, & Heimburger 1949); *The Language Modalities Test for Aphasia* (LMTA) (Wepman & Jones, 1961); *The Minnesota Test for Differential Diagnosis of Aphasia* (MTDDA) (Schuell, 1965a); the *Neurosensory Center Comprehensive Examination for Aphasia* (NCCEA) (Spreen & Benton, 1969); the *Orzeck Aphasia Evaluation* (AE) (Orzeck, 1964); the *Porch Index of Communicative Ability* (PICA) (Porch, 1973); the *Sklar Aphasia Scale* (SAS) (Sklar, 1966); the *Token Test* (TT) (DeRenzi & Vignolo, 1962); and the *Word Fluency Measure* (WF) (Borkowski, Benton & Spreen, 1967). Additional measures that have appeared subsequently are: the *Communicative Abilities in Daily Living* (CADL) (Holland, 1980); the *Revised Token Test* (RTT) (McNeil & Prescott, 1978); and the *Western Aphasia Battery* (WAB) (Kertesz, 1982). While most of these tests were designed to appraise aphasia, they have been applied with other langauge disorders.

More and more, neuropsychologists are involved in the clinical management of language-disordered adults, and their primary involvement has been in appraisal. Certainly, the contribution of neuropsychology to clinical management is not new in some settings. For example, there is a rich history in the Boston Veterans Administration Medical Center on the clinical contributions of neuropsychology, and the *Boston Diagnostic Aphasia Examination* (Goodglass & Kaplan, 1972) is a significant part of the testimony. Other medical settings have been slower to add clinical neuropsychologists, but, today, most psychology services contain both psychologists and neuropsychologists.

One product of the clinical growth in neuropsychology has been the development of tests. And, a significant representative in this development was the standardization of Luria's (1970) clinical tools into the *Luria-Nebraska Neuropsychological Battery* (Golden, Hammeke, & Purisch, 1980). Like any new test, the Luria-Nebraska has attracted converts and controversy. Criticism has ranged from the general to the specific. Crosson and Warren (1982) suggest the test may not be valid for patients with language disturbance. Their use of it failed to distinguish between patients with language disturbance and patients with other deficits, and they were unable to differentiate among types of language disturbance. Spiers (1981) believes the test is not capable of providing a comprehensive assessment of neuropsychological functioning in its present form. Delis and Kaplan (1982) reported an aphasic patient whose performance on the Luria-Nebraska was not consistent with his language behavior, or with the localization of his lesion. Holland (1982b) suggests that the problem with the language sections in the Luria-Nebraska is the language. Her analysis of the 269 items in the test revealed that 139 required speech as a response. She recommends not using the test in its present form with language problems if one hopes to measure anything other than language contamination. She concludes that the battery may also penalize, inappropriately, the demented patient and the less well educated, and that it does not indicate where, or how, to focus treatment. Parsons (1982) has pointed out that part of the problem, and the reactions to the Luria-Nebraska, may be cultural. He suggests that Luria's techniques were qualitative and flexible. Conversely, the Luria-Nebraska is quantitative and standardized. This clash of two cultures, Parsons concludes, results in what happens whenever two cultures clash—conflict. Whatever the state or the fate of the Luria-Nebraska, it represents the clinical activity (perhaps storm) and active involvement neuropsychology has with language disorders in adults.

Speech pathologists have had the tendency to use old tools to appraise problems that are new to them. We have taken our trusted tests for aphasia and attempted to measure language deficits in dementia, confusion, and the right hemisphere patient. Some—for example, Halpern, Darley, and Brown's (1973) use of an adaptation of Schuell's (1957) short examination for aphasia to differentiate among four different disorders—have been more successful than others. Our use (Deal, Deal, Wertz, Kitselmann, & Dwyer, 1979) of the PICA to evaluate language deficits in right hemisphere patients led to the conclusion that there must be a more appropriate measure for that population. Fortunately, there is a growing trend to leave aphasia tests to the evaluation of aphasic patients and select or develop other measures for the other language disorders. Myers (1979) is refining a battery to appraise the right hemisphere patient, and Bayles (1982b) has developed a battery for appraising language deficits in dementia.

Finally, advances in neuroradiologic techniques have changed our previous practice, where neurologists localized lesions by observing language behaviors and compared their results with neuropsychology's localization, which was also based on observing language behavior. This circular approach has been shattered by transmission computerized tomography (CT) to localize the site of structutral lesions and positron emission tomography (PET) to reveal the functional locus of lesions.

Environmental Influence on the Normal Aged

If the normal aged person's communication is influenced by his or her environment, adequate appraisal requires a look at both the individual and the individual's environment. The task is to determine whether the environment is the culprit, or whether the real villain is some other cause that may erode communication.

Lubinski (1981) discusses what to look for in order to detect a communication impairing environment. One problem is that there may be no one looking. Surveys by Mueller (1978) and Mueller and Peters (1981) indicate that many institutionalized environments do not provide speech and language services. Therefore, in the absence of a communication specialist, the influence of the environment on communication is not appraised.

But, if one does look, what does one look for? Lubinski (1981) recommends appraising opportunities for successful, meaningful communication; places within the setting to have a private conversation; administration and staff attitudes about the value of communication and their communicative behavior with patients; patients' values and attitudes about communication; rules that govern communication in the setting; and the influence of the physical design of the setting on communication. Her suggestions come from observation of institutional environments and interviews (Lubinski, Morrison, & Rigrodsky, 1981) with residents living in institutions.

If 15% of our nation's elderly are demented, 85% are aphasic, confused, schizophrenic, or normal. The task of appraisal is to find out who is who. Unfortunately, as Lubinski (1981) points out, none of the popular tests is designed to sort the normal aged suffering communication deficit arising out of environmental influences from those with other language deficits. None focuses on the communication needs of the institutionalized person—ability to communicate health care and personal needs, interaction with the staff or fellow residents or family. The measure that comes the closest is the CADL (Holland, 1980), and its use tells us older persons perform worse than younger persons, and institutionalized persons perform worse than noninstitutionalized persons (Holland, 1978). So, age itself, as well as being old in an institutionalized environment, can have an effect on useful communication.

Appraisal of the aged, like all appraisal, requires collecting biographic, medical, and behavioral data. One seeks explanations. For example, sensory deficits may erode mental abilities. Snyder, Pyrek, and Smith (1976) found a relationship between vision and mental status in their elderly subjects. Performance on the *Mental Status Questionnaire* (Kahn, Goldfarb, Pollack, & Peck, 1960) dropped as visual acuity became worse. A similar case can be made for hearing (Beasley & Davis, 1981). Further, one wants to rule out drug effects. Although the elderly make up only 10% of the population, they use 25% of all prescription drugs sold. Finlayson and Martin (1982) suggest age-related changes alter drug absorption. A therapeutic dose for an older person may be 50% less than that for a younger person.

The appraisal tools we have are many, but appropriate ones for the aged may be few. The use of the CADL to tap environmental influences was documented above. Duffy and Keith (1980) provide data about normal performance on the PICA (Porch, 1973). Their results indicate PICA test scores drop and test time increases as age increases. However, they were able to differentiate 92% of their normal sample from aphasic patients.

Others have devised measures to meet their needs. Keenan (1979) uses conversation with elderly patients in a custodial facility to rate: hearing, comprehension, and alertness; voice and articulation; rate, prosody, and fluency; vocabulary and grammar; talkativeness; and content and relevance. He begins with how the patient talks and whether the patient believes he has a problem. Keenan combines his observations of behavior with an assessment of physical, psychological, and environmental influences. To this he adds the patient's willingness to work on the problem, if one is present. Brandt, Rose, and Lucas (in press) have devised a similar approach for use in nursing homes.

Another appraisal technique we have used with other disorders is diagnostic treatment. We let the patient tell us what he or she has by the response to what we do with him or her. While environmental influence on communication may not be distinguishable from other disorders when appraised, it should change if its causes are removed or manipulated. Folsom (1968) has used reality orientation to change a diagnosis from dementia to normal aging. Diagnostic therapy might employ similar methods to make a diagnosis in patients whose communication is influenced by where they reside.

Language of Confusion

Appraisal of confusion seeks answers to four questions posed by Darley (1964). First, is the patient oriented in place and time? The confused patient is not. Second, does the patient stay in contact with the examiner? The confused patient does not if given the opportunity to wander. Third, how aware is the patient of the inappropriateness of his or her responses? The confused patient is not aware he or she is inappropriate. Fourth, how well structured are the patient's responses? The confused patient has normal sentence structure and decent vocabulary.

Answers to the above questions come from behavioral measures. Also, there are some useful signs in the patient's biographical and medical data. For example, an accurate biography is needed to determine if the patient confabulates when queried about himself or herself and his or her past.

Medical signs have been provided by Halpern, Darley, and Brown (1973). Eighty percent of their patients had a rapid onset, less than 10 days. All of their patients were less than 3 months postonset when evaluated. All patients displayed either diffuse or disseminated lesions. Half of the sample suffered trauma, and 30% suffered hemorrhage of hematoma.

Behavioral appraisal requires presenting tasks that flush the confused language. Chedru and Geschwind (1972) studied patients in an acute confusional state and compared their performance with control subjects. Tests that differentiated the confused from the nonconfused were temporal-spatial orientation tasks, digit span, writing, word fluency, and imitation of movements. Tests that did not differentiate were comprehension tasks, oral spelling, praxis tasks, visual recognition tasks, proverb interpretation, and spontaneous speech. Geschwind (1974a) has elaborated on the use of writing tasks, particularly copying, writing words from dictation, and writing sentences on a specific topic. He reports confused patients' writing is not very legible, letters and words are spaced poorly, and it contains syntactic and spelling errors.

Halpern, Darley, and Brown's (1973) results run contrary to those of Chedru and Geschwind (1972). Both observed disturbance in writing from dictation, but that is where the similarity ends. Halpern et al. found confused patients were deficient in arithmetic, reading comprehension, relevance, adequacy, and auditory comprehension. Syntax; naming; auditory retention, measured partially by digit span; and fluency were less impaired. The primary measure that differentiated confused patients from those with aphasia, dementia, and apraxia of speech was relevance, tapped primarily by proverb interpretation and spontaneous speech. Mills and Drummond (1980) have contested the naming results of Halpern et al. by suggesting the need for more detailed analysis. Comparing naming errors on high uncertainty and low uncertainty stimuli, response time, and semantic analysis of errors, Mills and Drummond differentiated confused patients from aphasic patients.

While the reports on language behavior in confusion do not agree, they do suggest appraisal tasks. Apparently, confused patients will identify themselves when asked to write and when asked to speak with few constraints imposed by the examiner. In confusion, we look for irrelevance and confabulation.

Schizophrenia

Most agree that the schizophrenic patient has a problem, but few agree on what constitutes the problem. Darby (1981) describes schizophrenia as a group of diseases with a symptom complex that produces massive disruption in thinking, mood, and behavior. Not all symptoms are present in every patient, and symptoms vary with time—from time to time, and as time postonset increases.

Debate rages on whether the schizophrenic patient has a language disorder. Benson (1975) holds that schizophrenia is characterized by abnormality in thinking, and this is mirrored in the patient's speech. He suggests it is unusual for the patient to have a breakdown in language. The schizophrenic patients he sees demonstrate intact speech and language, a sizable vocabulary, and corrrect use of grammar and syntax. It is the bizarre content of the patient's language that characterizes what is called "schizophrenic language." Brown (1972) agrees. Schizophrenic patients do not reveal a breakdown in language; they reveal a breakdown in thought. So, he suggests, there is not schizophrenic speech or language, there is schizophrenic thought that may be reflected in the patient's speech and language. Chaika (1974) disagrees and lists six features that characterize schizophrenic speech: disrupted phonological rules, disruption in matching semantic features, preoccupation with too many semantic features, influence by previously uttered words rather than the topic, disrupted syntax, and failure to self-monitor. But, Fromkin (1975) disagrees with Chaika. Except for problems in sequencing ideas, Fromkin points out that Chaika's features are prevalent in normal speech.

Whether the problem is one of thought or one of language, or both, language is used to identify schizophrenia. Chapman (1966) observed three features in schizophrenic verbal behavior: intermittent episodes of word-finding difficulty, inability to "screen out" unwanted words, and involuntary echoing of what is heard. Ostwold (1963) found prosodic abnormality in the speech of a sample of schizophrenic patients. Similarly, Todt and Howell (1980) found schizophrenic patients could be differentiated from normals on the basis of vocal qualities—less inflection, poorer enunciation, more repetitions and substitutions, and a significantly slower oral reading rate. Using a type-token ratio analysis to measure vocabulary diversity, Fairbanks (1944) found schizophrenic patients used fewer different words in speaking and writing than normals. A replication of Fairbank's effort by Feldstein and Jaffe (1962), however, showed no significant differences between schizophrenic patients and normals. Rochester, Martin, and Thurston (1977) observed that their schizophrenic patients were adequate communicators; however, the schizophrenic speech samples could be distinguished from nonschizophrenic samples with 75% accuracy. They relate that the schizophrenic speaker makes the listener's task difficult by requiring him to search for information which is never clearly given and by providing few conjunctive links between clauses.

Several investigations have compared schizophrenic patients with aphasic patients or used aphasia tests to seek language disturbance in schizophrenia. Taylor, Greenspan, and Abrams, (1979) administered an aphasia screening test to schizophrenic patients, patients with affective disorders, and normals. Their schizophrenic group made significantly more total errors and demonstrated temporoparietal signs including anomia, neologisms, and letter and number agnosias. Farber and Reichstein (1981) compared schizophrenic patients with "formal thought disorders," manic and depressed patients, and normals on the BDAE (Goodglass & Kaplan, 1972) and the Token Test (DeRenzi & Vignolo, 1962). The schizophrenic patients displayed significantly more errors on the Token Test and on the repetition of phrases BDAE subtest. The authors suggest that there is a subgroup of schizophrenic patients that could be labelled schizophasic schizophrenia. Conversely, Strohner, Cohen, Kelter, and Woll (1978) found no significant differences between schizophrenic patients, aphasic patients, and normals on a task of matching familiar environmental sounds with pictures. Horsfall (1972), using the PICA (Porch, 1973), observed his sample of schizophrenic patients were less severe than a sample of aphasic patients and a sample of bilateral brain-injured patients; however, the test profiles did not reveal useful differences among groups. Rausch, Prescott, and De Wolfe (1980) compared schizophrenic patients, aphasic patients, and normals on a word-ordering task. The aphasic group made significantly more errors and took longer to complete the task than the other two groups, and schizophrenic patients did not differ from normals except on items that required rearranging words to make sentences containing direct and indirect objects. Finally, Gerson, Benson, and Frazier (1977) found six differentiating characteristics when they compared schizophrenic patients with aphasic patients who had posterior lesions. First, the schizophrenic patients' responses were longer. Second, the aphasic patients were aware of their language deficit and disturbed by it, but the schizophrenic patients were not. Third, the aphasic patients used nonverbal substitutes or pauses to enlist the aid of the examiner. The schizophrenic patients did not. Fourth, the aphasic patients substituted letters, words, or neologisms. The schizophrenic patients did not. Fifth, vagueness in the aphasic patients' responses resulted from shifts in subject matter. And, sixth, aphasic patients displayed no persisting themes in their responses, but the schizophrenic patients produced bizarre themes and repeated them throughout their responses.

Benson (1973) suggests using six tasks to differentiate schizophrenic patients from aphasic patients: conversation, comprehension of spoken language, repetition, confrontation naming, reading, and writing. Di Simoni, Darley, and Aronson (1977) report that schizophrenic patients can be differentiated from aphasic patients on the measure used by Halpern, Darley and Brown (1973). In addition, they used Part V of the Token Test (DeRenzi & Vignolo, 1962); the Word Fluency Measure (Borkowski, Benton, & Spreen, 1967); a general information test; and a Temporal Orientation Test (Benton, Van Allen, & Fogel, 1964) to obtain a comprehensive sample of schizophrenic language. They observed that their sample had the most difficulty with relevance, arithmetic, and reading comprehension. Best performance was in syntax, adequacy, and naming. Only two of 27 patients displayed any articulatory deficits. Seventy percent of the sample performed within normal limits on Part V of the Token Test. Conversely, 75% fell below 80% correct on the general information test. The authors conclude that language disturbance in their sample was mild. The patients had no difficulty in making their wishes known. Performance on open-ended questions was much worse than on short-answer, specific questions. On the former, the patients displayed a wealth of extraneous conversation and irrelevant responses.

So, what does one use to appraise language in schizophrenic patients? If the tasks are to determine the presence or absence of deficits and to differentiate schizophrenia from other language disorders, the methods suggested by Benson (1973) and those employed by Di Simoni, Darley, and Aronson (1977) seem appropriate. One needs to include tasks that permit the schizophrenic patient to reveal his primary disorder—irrelevance. Conversation and open-ended questions should suffice. Appraisal may not answer the question of whether the patient's communication disorder results from disrupted thought or disrupted language. But, appraisal must determine whether a deficit is present and whether it differs from other language disorders.

Right Hemisphere Involvement

Appraisal of patients who have suffered a right hemisphere lesion presents similar problems to those encountered in appraising the schizophrenic patient. First, the problem is not clear. Is it disrupted language, or is it disrupted communication in patients with fairly intact language? Second, no ready-made tests or test batteries are available, so the appraiser must roll his own. Third, speech pathologists do not have a lengthy history of contact with the right hemisphere patient and are just beginning to learn what to look for.

Earlier, I suggested that the right hemisphere patient may have one or more of three problems—disrupted speech and language, disrupted nonverbal communication, or disrupted cognitive style. The speech has been described as "copious and inappropriate; as confabulatory, irrelevant, literal, and occasionally bizarre" (Myers, 1979, p. 38). Appraisal's task is to find out which, why and whether anything can be done about it.

We (Deal et al., 1979) followed tradition and used a measure—the PICA (Porch, 1973), traditionally used with aphasic patients—to look at behavior in right hemisphere patients. Using a discriminant function analysis (Porch, Friden, & Porec, 1976), 62% of our sample could not be distinguished from aphasia, 31% could, and 7% fell in a grey area—not aphasia, but not not aphasia. The PICA subtests that differentiated right hemisphere patients from aphasic patients were VIII, matching pictures with objects; XI, matching identical objects; A, writing the function of objects; and F, copying geometric shapes. Right hemisphere patients displayed relative difficulty on subtests VIII, XI, and F. Aphasic patients displayed relative success on these tasks. Right hemisphere patients did fairly well on subtest A. Aphasic patients found this task the most difficult one in the battery. We presented percentiles for right hemisphere performance to provide a measure of severity, but we concluded that there are probably more appropriate measures for detecting communication deficit in right hemisphere patients.

Myers (1979) reported her initial results with a battery she is developing to appraise right hemisphere patients. It includes the BDAE (Goodglass & Kaplan, 1972); the Hooper Test of Visual Organization (Hooper, 1958); a retelling-a-story task that presents the same information in three contexts—one emphasizing spatial context, one emotional context, and one noncanonical context—and an intensive interview with the patient and a family member. Initial results indicate that performance on the BDAE was within normal limits. However, verbal performance on the Cookie Theft picture, when filtered through the Yorkston and Beukelman (1977) analysis, contained mostly itemized responses and very few inferences. Right hemisphere performance on the Hooper was significantly lower than normal performance. Myers concluded that the right hemisphere patient has difficulty integrating information on a formal and a perceptual level. The deficit is represented in verbal expression. If the patient is irrelevant, Myers suggests investigating the reasons for it. Is it truly confabulatory and bizarre, or does it consist of related but unintegrated bits of information? The reason for irrelevance may surface when one compares responses on highly structured questions to responses on open-ended questions.

Myers and Linebaugh (1981) have appraised one aspect of cognitive style in right hemisphere patients, the ability to comprehend figurative language. Their right hemisphere patients gave literal responses indicating a lack of comprehension. Even though they demonstrated decent language skills, they were unable to use context to gain meaning, the way many aphasic patients and normals do.

Adamovich and Brooks (1981), recognizing that language batteries appropriate for left hemisphere patients do not provide a sufficient evaluation of communication deficits in right hemisphere patients, combined several measures to compare right hemisphere patients with normals. Their measures included: the BDAE (Goodglass & Kaplan, 1972); the Revised Token Test (McNeil & Prescott, 1978); the Hooper Test of Visual Organization (Hooper, 1958); the Detroit Test of Learning Aptitude (Baker & Leland, 1967); the Word Fluency Measure (Borkowski, Benton, & Spreen, 1967); and the Boston Naming Test (Kaplan, Goodglass, & Weintraub, 1976). They observed that right hemisphere patients had significant deficits in auditory comprehension, verbal expression, and reading, when performance was compared with their normal sample. They concluded that the deficits appeared to result from cognitive and linguistic lack rather than problems in visual perception, organization, or memory.

Given our present knowledge and our present ability to appraise the right hemisphere patient, Myers' (1979) suggestion to look at three areas appears wise. We need to tap speech and language ability to determine the presence or absence of specific or general problems, evaluate nonverbal communication, and appraise cognitive style. Some of our existing measures are appropriate for the first. Tools for the latter two are being developed and await refinement.

Dementia

Appraisal of the demented patient requires a look at biographical, medical, and behavioral data. Knowing a patient's biography may indicate how far the dementia has progressed, how far the patient has fallen. Knowing the medical history may assist in determining whether one is dealing with a true dementia or, perhaps, a pseudodementia resulting from depression. And, even if the dementia is real, the medical record may indicate whether it is one that may respond to treatment. Further, information about rapidity of onset, hemispheric localization, and whether the lesion is focal, diffuse, or disseminated may assist in differentiating dementia from aphasia.

Behavioral data on language abilities in demented patients come from two sources: the use of tests developed to appraise other disorders and the use of tests specifically designed to appraise dementia. Halpern, Darley, and Brown (1973) studied demented patients with their adaptation of

Schuell's (1957) short examination for aphasia. They found demented patients made more errors on tasks of adequacy, reading comprehension, arithmetic, and auditory comprehension, and fewer errors on tasks of fluency, writing to dictation, relevance, and syntax. Our replication (Deal, Wertz, & Spring, 1981) of their effort resulted in only somewhat similar results. While we agreed on the difficulty of tasks of adequacy and arithmetic and the ease of tasks of fluency, relevance, and syntax for demented subjects, we disagreed on writing to dictation and auditory retention tasks. Both were among the most difficult for our patients, but both were among the easiest for Halpern and colleagues' patients.

Appell, Kertesz, and Fishman (1981) used the WAB (Kertesz, 1982) to evaluate a group of patients with Alzheimer's disease. They report the patients' performance was aphasic. Patients were classified as global, Wernicke's, transcortical sensory, or anomic types. In addition, the sample showed severe deficits on other subtests—reading, writing, praxis, and construction—not used to measure aphasia on the WAB.

Watson and Records (1978) gave the PICA (Porch, 1973) to a sample of demented patients and a sample of aphasic patients. While the aphasic group was more severe, the demented group showed marked language deficit (60th percentile overall) on the PICA. Watson and Records suggest performance on specific subtests discriminated between aphasic and demented patients. The demented group had relatively more difficulty with primarily visual subtests—VIII, XI, E, and F—and relatively less difficulty with auditory subtests—VI, X, B, and C. The aphasic sample showed opposite performance, more difficulty with auditory than visual subtests.

Schwartz, Marin, and Saffran (1979) and Bayles and Boone (1982) report that semantic knowledge deteriorates in dementia, but there is relative preservation of syntactic and phonologic abilities. Horner and Heyman (1982) agree, but they suggest that as severity increases, demented patients begin to show syntax and phonologic errors, as well as semantic errors.

Some have attempted to develop measures for appraising language deficit in dementia. For example, Nelson and O'Connell (1978) developed the New Adult Reading Test (NART), a measure that assesses familiarity with words rather than the ability to decode unfamiliar words phonetically. Demented patients had no significant difficulty reading NART words; therefore, Nelson and O'Connell suggest performance will provide an estimate of premorbid intelligence.

Hughes, Berg, Danziger, Coben, and Martin (1982) have developed a clinical scale to determine the severity of dementia. Their Clinical Dementia Rating (CDR) uses a patient interview and tasks from a variety of tests to rate performance in six areas: memory, orientation, judgment + problem solving, community affairs, home + hobbies, and personal care. Ratings range from CDR 0, healthy; through CDR 0.5, questionable dementia; CDR 1, mild dementia; CDR 2, moderate dementia; to CDR 3, severe dementia.

Bayles (1982b) has developed a battery of measures to detect the presence and to rate the severity of dementia. Discriminant function analyses (Bayles, 1982a; Bayles & Boone, 1982) indicate that language tests are extremely sensitive in detecting dementia. Patients are classified as mild, moderate, or advanced on the following measures: receptive pragmatics, vocabulary, sentence error correction, visual/spatial, verbal reasoning, mental status, story retelling, sentence disambiguation, verbal description, and picture naming.

While we no longer rely exclusively on tests for aphasia to detect the presence and severity of dementia, our tools to evaluate the language of generalized intellectual deficit are few. Bayles (1982b) has demonstrated that language measures are as good as, if not better than, other psychometric measures for evaluating demented patients. Thus, the utility of appraising language deficits in demented patients has been established and justifies additional effort.

Aphasia

Each of the 17 tests listed at the beginning of this section were, primarily, designed to appraise aphasia. So, the problem in appraising aphasic patients is not a paucity of tools, but a problem in selecting among existing tools. Each of the existing measures has its strengths and its weaknesses. None constitute an adequate appraisal by itself. Typically, clinicians combine several measures into a battery and supplement the battery with additional measures if the patient's behavior dictates. This has been the approach with individual patients and with large, controlled studies of aphasia (Ludlow, 1983; Wertz et al., 1981). Unfortunately, the controlled studies are that, controlled, and do not have the flexibility of day-to-day patient management. Nevertheless, what is used to appraise a patient in a large, controlled study probably represents the state of the art, or at least one version of it, at the time the study is being conducted.

Table 1-1 shows the measures we are using in the current Veterans Administration Cooperative Study, "A Comparison of Clinic, Home, and Deferred Treatment for Aphasia." It differs from the battery we used in the first VA Cooperative Study (Wertz et al., 1981), and it differs from the battery employed in the Viet Nam Head Injury Study (Ludlow, 1983). It is more extensive than most clinicians employ with individual patients,

TABLE 1-1
Measures used to appraise aphasic patients in the Veterans Administration Cooperative Study, "A Comparison of Clinic, Home, and Deferred Treatment for Aphasia."

MEASURE	PURPOSE
Porch Index of Communicative Ability (Porch, 1973)	Quantified measure of communicative ability
Boston Diagnostic Aphasia Examination (Goodglass & Kaplan, 1972)	Provides type of aphasia and extends language sampled on the PICA
Communicative Abilities in Daily Living (Holland, 1980)	Measures "functional" communicative ability
Token Test (Spreen & Benton adaptation, 1969)	Extends measures of auditory comprehension
Reading Comprehension Battery for Aphasia (LaPointe Horner, 1979)	Extends measures of reading comprehension
Motor Speech Evaluation (Wertz & Rosenbek, 1971)	Determines the presence and severity of apraxia of speech and/or dysarthria
Coloured Progressive Matrices (Raven, 1962)	Estimate of nonverbal intelligence

but certain patients, in some clinics, may receive all of the measures listed at some time during the course of their management. The measures listed in Table 1-1 are not prescriptive. They are descriptive. They represent the "best" available tools, our biases; the most comprehensive, our needs; and economy, our limitations.

Probably, the most identifiable activity in appraising aphasia during the past 10 years has been the emphasis placed on "functional" communicative ability. The previous 10 years, 1965 through 1975, had seen the development of several standardized tests. The past ten years have seen a move to determine whether behavior on these standardized tests reflects what a patient does or does not do in nontest environments. Holland's CADL (1980) represents an organized means of evaluating functional language skills. Other measures include speech samples; for example, conversation on the BDAE (Goodglass & Kaplan, 1972) and WAB (Kertesz, 1982), or the length and complexity analysis suggested by Keenan and Brassell (1974).

Holland (1982c) cautions that the best measure of functional ability is to observe a patient communicating without prompts in the right environment.

So, the state of the art in appraising aphasic patients is characterized not by poverty but by preference. There are sufficient measures to select among, and the selection is influenced by the clinician's bias. Those who modify aphasia with adjectives select the BDAE or the WAB. Those who do not, pick a PICA or the MTDDA. Usually, patient performance, not clinician perference, dictates the measures used to supplement the primary measure or measures. This is as things should be.

The State of the Art

We have a wealth of measures for some disorders and few measures for other disorders. This prompts borrowing from the rich to appraise the poor. Recent experience indicates it may be better to develop appropriate measures for disorders that lack them, rather than apply tests designed for other disorders. When we use an aphasia test to appraise disorders other than aphasia, there is a good chance of finding aphasia in confusion, aphasia following a right hemisphere lesion, aphasia in dementia, etc. Not only do we need to develop appropriate measures for the environmental influences on the normal aged, for the language of confusion, and for schizophrenia, we also need to refine the batteries being developed by Myers (1979) for the right hemisphere patient and by Bayles (1982b) for the demented patient.

The purposes of appraisal, I believe, are to collect sufficient data to make a diagnosis, state a prognosis, and, if appropriate, focus therapy. I am not certain we are very efficient or reliable on any of these, especially on differentiating among disorders. Darley (1979b) seemed to agree. He suggested constructing tests trimmed down to those components that allow precise differentiation among disorders. An example of this type of appraisal measure might resemble Buschke's (1975) proposed method for evaluating language competence that is shown in Table 1-2. While Buschke intended his measure for aphasic patients, it may be useful in differentiating among language disorders. For example, if the required response eliminates the need for elaborate verbal, gestural, or written output, the aphasic patient may have the opportunity to display linguistic competence. Similarly, the demented patient may be identified by a lack of cognitive competence, the confused patient by irrelevance, etc. Thus, not only do we need measures to tell us that a disorder is present, we need measures to tell us that a disorder differs from other disorders.

TABLE 1-2
Method for evaluating language competence. (Adapted from Buschke, 1975)

PURPOSE	TASK	STIMULI	RESPONSE
Lexical Competence	Distinguishing real English words from paralogs	Hotel Vumac	Yes = real No = not real
Semantic Competence	Distinguishing meaningful sentences from nonsensical but grammatical strings of words	"Black clouds mean sudden storms." "Rich clouds have important persons."	Yes = makes sense No = does not make sense
Syntactic Competence	Distinguishing grammatical strings from random word strings	"Wild gentlemen mean clear battles." "Animal skies famous sudden buy."	Yes = right order No = wrong order
Cognitive Competence	Distinguishing true from false sentences	"Some dogs have short tails." "Snow is soft and warm."	Yes = true No = false

Finally, we need to become better at playing the game of appraisal. The appraisal room is an abode of boredom, confusion, and fear; fear of being found out, fear of failure. Our appraisal story is uneven. We are better at the middle, the testing, than we are at the beginning, preparing the patient for testing, and at the end, explaining to the patient how he or she did. Wheelchairs can become tumbrels as they roll to the place of appraisal. We can execute a patient with abundance. We have added new measures, but we have discarded few of the old measures. Our tests may corrode what a patient can do. There is a need for ecological evaluation, one that avoids erosion of what the patient brings with him to the appraisal session.

Diagnosis

Diagnosis involves putting a label on what one observes. We match the appraisal data—biographical, medical, behavioral—with our definitions and look for a best fit. Some signs have diagnostic significance and indicate the presence of one disorder, but not others. For example, Geschwind (1974b) suggests mutism is uncommon even in the most severe aphasia. Certain psychotic syndromes, however, may present with mutism. In dementia, mutism indicates the dementing process has progressed to the point where the patient has nothing more to say. Diagnosis, therefore, is the use of appraisal data to determine who is who.

Environmental Influence on the Normal Aged

The label "environmental influence" is applied when the person's environment is the culprit and there is no evidence of an organic or psychiatric cause of the communication deficit. Therefore, we must rule out the language of confusion, schizophrenia, a right hemisphere lesion, dementia, and aphasia. And, we must provide evidence that the person's environment has eroded communication skills that were intact until the environment worked its influence.

Biographical data should certify that the normal aged person was, indeed, normal. We look for evidence that indicates communication skills were appropriate for the person's age until entering his or her present environment. We seek intellectual and educational information from the person's past to estimate "premorbid"—in this case, prior to entering the present environment—abilities. We seek to avoid false accusation of the environment when potential causes may be lifelong low intelligence or illiteracy. And, we seek information on how communicative the person was prior to being institutionalized. A taciturn nontalker probably will not become verbose after entry into a nursing home.

Medical data are essential. We look for a clean bill of neurologic health. If we do not have a neurologic evaluation that concludes there is no evidence of CVA, trauma, degeneration, etc., we request that an evaluation be conducted. Confusion, aphasia, and right hemisphere signs erupt. Dementia and schizophrenia may creep. So, we look at performance and change in performance over time. Similarly, we look for sensory deficits—hearing, visual—that may interfere with communication and explain some of the patient's deficit. And, finally, the patient's medication—types, dosage—need to be explored to determine their possible influence on communication. The medical data, therefore, tell us that the normal aged person's communicative deficits cannot be explained by an organic cause, a psychiatric problem, sensory deficit, or medications. The lack of these prompt us to probe the environment for an explanation.

If we confuse environmental influences on communication with one of the other disorders being discussed here, we are likely to confuse it with dementia. The lack of an abrupt onset usually rules out confusion, aphasia, and right hemisphere involvement. Schizophrenia often can be ruled out because it leaves a trail. Seldom does it occur abruptly simply because the person's living environment has been changed. Schizophrenia, typically, has its onset in adolescence or early adulthood. Its onset in an elderly person would be considered a psychiatric curiosity.

Differentiating environmental influence on communication from dementia is more difficult. Bayles' (1982b) mildly demented patients differed from her normal age-matched controls, but not markedly. Holland's (1980) CADL data on institutionalized older persons show deficits, but they are not marked. Could they represent the early stages of dementia? Possibly. Our behavioral data may show deficits, but these data must be expanded to show not only what the patient can do, but also what he or she could do if environmental conditions were more favorable. Thus, we may need to manipulate our measures and probe areas of deficit by indicating that we are really interested in what the patient has to say and whether he or she understands what is said to him or her. We may need to suggest that a patient use coping strategies; for example, the use of context to improve comprehension and word finding, to determine whether skills are just rusty and not eroded. Sometimes, a final decision must await observation of change in the patient's communication after the environment is manipulated.

Some of the normal aged person's communication deficit may result from depression. Blazer and Williams (1980) report that 5 to 44% of the elderly are depressed. If severe, depression may masquerade as dementia. Finlayson and Martin (1982) label this condition pseudodementia. It shares similar signs with dementia, including lack of self care, restlessness, irritability, loss of creativity, somatic complaints, disorientation, and memory and concentration difficulties. Table 1-3 contrasts pseudodementia resulting from depression with true dementia. There are significant differences betweeen the two, and correct diagnosis requires that we look for these differences.

Finally, even after organic and psychiatric causes have been ruled out, diagnosis of environmental influence on communication requires documenting the presence of detrimental environmental influences. We look for the conditions listed earlier—a lack of opportunity for successful communication; no place to have a private conversation; low priority on communication by administration, staff, and patients; rules that restrict communication; and physical barriers that prevent communication.

TABLE 1-3
Comparison of pseudodementia and dementia. (After Finlayson & Martin, 1982)

PSEUDODEMENTIA	*DEMENTIA*
Onset quite abrupt	Onset insidious
Progression usually rapid	Progression usually slow
Patient aware of deficits	Patient not as aware
Complaint of memory loss	Patient tries to hide loss (confabulates)
Global responses ("I don't know.")	Near-miss answers
Patient gives evidence of deficits	Patient emphasizes accomplishments
Impairment not usually worse at night	Usually worse at night
Mood depressed	Patient is typically "happy"
History of psychiatric disturbance common	Psychiatric history not common
Suicide risk considerable	Suicide risk much lower

Language of Confusion

Confused language fascinates. It must be differentiated from the bizarre responses and preoccupation with specific themes seen in the schizophrenic patient, the sometimes irrelevant responses made by the patient with a right hemisphere lesion, and the irrelevant respones that may flow from the aphasic patient with a severe auditory comprehension deficit that prevents him from understanding what was requested. Similarly, the normal aged in an impoverished communication environment, or the demented patient, any appear confused, because he or she is not oriented to date, to place, or to his or her condition. But, unlike the patient with the language of confusion, neither confabulate.

Biographical information provides data to identify the confused patient's confabulation. Knowing that a patient parked cars for a living assists in identifying a tale of being a fish farmer as confabulation. Biographical information provides an accurate data base.

Medical data confirm the presence of bilateral brain injury, often traumatically induced, as a cause of confused language. The absence of brain damage or the presence of unilateral damage lead us to look elsewhere for a diagnosis, perhaps schizophrenia or environmental influence, when there is no evidence of brain damage, and, perhaps, right hemisphere deficits or aphasia, when there is a unilateral lesion.

The behavioral data, however, pull the confused patient's covers. The absence of word-finding deficits and the good syntax, coupled with irrelevance and confabulation, signify confusion. Halpern, Darley, and Brown (1973) report that the confused patient may show the specific deficits seen in aphasia and dementia—reading and writing deficits and a lack of adequacy—but the patient's lack of relevance differentiates confusion from those with aphasia or dementia.

Schizophrenia

Schizophrenic patients may masquerade as demonstrating another disorder. Sometimes, their bizarre responses are difficult to differentiate from the irrelevance and confabulation seen in the language of confusion. Their "word-salad" composed of real words, phonemic substitutions, verbal substitutions, and neologisms may make their speech unintelligible and similar to that seen in some aphasic patients. What Kleist (1960) has called "ethical flattening" and "affective blunting" in schizophrenia may be difficult to differentiate from similar behavior in a patient with a right hemisphere lesion. Again, one turns to the appraisal data to determine who is who.

Biographical information should indicate that a schizophrenic patient's history was influenced by the onset of psychiatric disturbance some time in late adolescence or early adulthood. His or her educational and work history may reveal how schizophrenia has influenced his or her life. Medical data should indicate the history of psychiatric disturbance and the lack of focal or diffuse cerebral pathology as an explanation for past and present behavior. Kitselman (1981) suggests that when an adequate history is available, differentiating schizophrenia from aphasia is not difficult. Similarly, the history coupled with behavioral data should permit differentiating schizophrenia from other disorders.

Di Simoni, Darley, and Aronson (1977) report that both relevance and reading comprehension are impaired in schizophrenia. Halpern, Darley, and Brown (1973) report similar results for confused patients. However, examination of both sets of data indicates relevance is more impaired than reading comprehension in schizophrenia, and the reverse is seen in confusion. Further, schizophrenic patients make more fluency errors, relative to their performance on other tasks, and fluency errors were the least frequently occurring problem—relative to their performance on other tasks—in confused patients. Finally, a comparison of the two reports indicates schizophrenic patients make about 50% fewer total errors than are made by confused patients. Nevertheless, Di Simoni et al. found schizophrenic patients deteriorate as time postonset increases. At some point in time, the schizophrenic patient may be difficult to differentiate from the confused patient. One must look at the medical data. The presence or absence of demonstrable brain injury will tip the diagnostic decision.

Differentiating schizophrenia from aphasia, according to Benson (1975), should not be difficult. He suggests schizophrenic "word-salad" is seen only in chronic, severe schizophrenia and, therefore, if present, usually represents a true aphasia when there is no history of mental problems. When in doubt, Benson recommends using a test of auditory comprehension to differentiate aphasia from schizophrenia. Horsfall's (1972) PICA data indicate that his sample of schizophrenic patients showed they were less severe than a sample of aphasic patients and a sample of bilaterally damaged patients. These results are shown in Figure 1-1. His schizophrenic sample performed at approximately the 85th percentile overall on left hemisphere norms and at the 95th percentile overall on bilateral norms. Because a difference in severity may imply differences in the pattern of performance that do not exist, I have equated performance among the three samples by using 85th percentile left hemisphere and 95th percentile bilateral norms from the PICA manual. This manipulation is shown in Figure 1-2. When performance is equated for severity with aphasia and bilateral brain injury, there is little in the test profiles that differentiates schizophrenic patients from the other two groups.

Di Simoni et al. (1977) report that impaired relevance and relatively intact writing, reading, and listening abilities differentiate the schizophrenic patient from the aphasic patient. Even the older, long-time postonset schizophrenic patient in their sample was more likely to resemble dementia than aphasia. Thus, diagnosis of schizophrenia can be made by noting the presence of a high degree of irrelevance, an absence of signs that indicate central-language impairment, and an absence of brain injury.

Right Hemisphere Involvement

To diagnose right hemisphere involvement, one looks for information in the biographical data indicating that the patient was a normal communicator prior to suffering a right hemisphere lesion. We check education to rule out illiteracy. The medical data should show the presence of

FIGURE 1-1
PICA Ranked Response Summary comparing performance by schizophrenic, aphasic, and bilateral brain-injured patients. (After Horsfall, 1972).

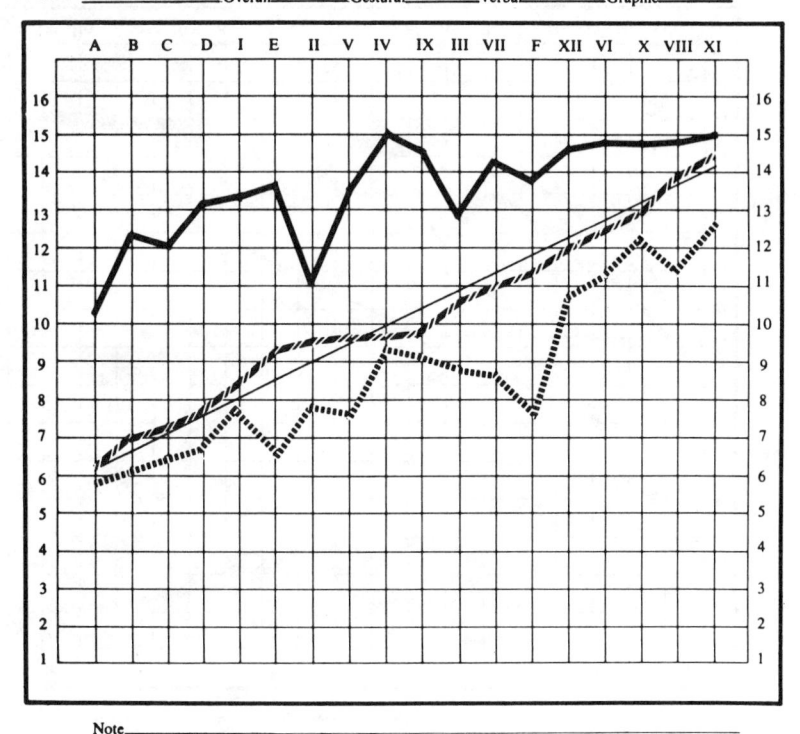

FIGURE 1-2
PICA Ranked Response Summary comparing performance by schizophrenic patients with aphasic and bilateral brain-injured patients who have been equated for severity. (After Horsfall, 1972)

Porch Index of Communicative Ability

RANKED RESPONSE SUMMARY

Name_____ Case No._____

Age_____ Birthdate_____ Sex____ Race_____ Handedness_____

Diagnosis_____ Onset_____

— x̄ SCHIZOPHRENIA Overall 13.49 Gestural 13.89 Verbal 14.27 Graphic 12.45

⋯⋯ 95 %ile BILATERAL Overall 13.50 Gestural 14.13 Verbal 14.55 Graphic 11.97

▰▰ 85 %ile APHASIA Overall 13.32 Gestural 14.15 Verbal 14.20 Graphic 11.63

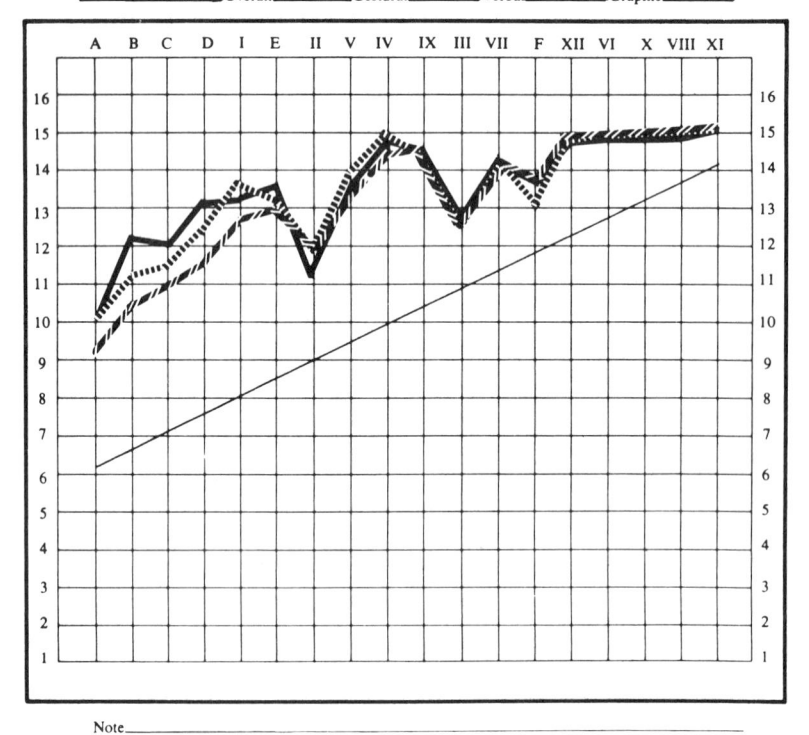

Note_____

Published by
CONSULTING PSYCHOLOGISTS PRESS
577 College Avenue   Palo Alto, California

a right hemisphere lesion and its suspected cause. In the behavioral data provided by other disciplines, we look for the presence of other disorders—spatial perception and body image disorders, visual perception disorders, constructional disabilities, auditory perception disorders, somatosensory disorders, motor impersistence—which suggest right hemisphere involvement. In our language data, we look for behavior that differentiates the patient from those who are aphasic, demented, and schizophrenic.

Though rare, some individuals demonstrate "crossed aphasia." This condition, today, refers to aphasia in a right-handed person following damage to the right hemisphere (Hecaen & Albert, 1978). Estimates of incidence range from 0.4% (Hecaen, Magurs, Remier, et al., 1971) to 10% (Branch, Milner, & Rasmussen, 1964). These patients appear to be aphasic and should be diagnosed as such. They are not the patients being discussed here who demonstrate communicative deficits subsequent to a right hemisphere lesion. Nevertheless, the latter group have been described as displaying "aphasia-like" behavior (Archibald & Wepman, 1968), and 62% of our right hemisphere sample resembled aphasia on the PICA (Deal et al., 1979). So, they may create a diagnostic dilemma.

The general sign that differentiates the patient with right hemisphere communication impairment from the left hemisphere aphasic patient is the former's relatively good language, which contrasts sharply with his impaired communication. Myers' (1979) specific signs—failure to integrate information on a perceptual level, tendency to itemize rather than interpret information, irrelevance, better performance on structured tasks than on open-ended tasks, lack of affect, caustic sense of humor—tend to help separate right hemisphere communication deficit from aphasia.

Medical data differentiate the right hemisphere patient from the demented patient. The former has a unilateral, usually focal, lesion, and the latter has bilateral, diffuse, disseminated, or multifocal lesions. Similarly, the presence of a unilateral, right hemisphere lesion differentiates the right hemisphere patient from the schizophrenic patient who has no evidence of brain injury.

Dementia

Wells (1982) discusses two types of errors that can be made in diagnosing dementia. The first is a failure to recognize dementia, thus labeling the patient's problem as functional. The second is the reverse of the first; diagnosing dementia when the problem is functional, and not organic. Usually, either error occurs when dementia and depression coexist, as they frequently do. The main source of error, Wells believes, is to assume that cognitive loss automatically indicates organicity. While cognitive deficit is a primary sign of an organic syndrome, Wells does not believe it is diagnostic of it. He does not think any neuropsychological measure of cognition can be devised to differentiate dementia from functional disorders that resemble it. He suggests a diagnosis of dementia is appropriate only when there is approximately the same amount of impairment in cognition, behavior, and affect. Diagnosing dementia, therefore, may be more difficult than one might expect.

Certainly, environmental influence on the communication of the normal aged can be considered functional. It is necessary to differentiate them from demented patients. The influence of depression on behavior in older persons was discussed earlier, and differential diagnostic signs provided by Finlayson and Martin (1982) were listed. Nevertheless, Bayles (1982b) relates that misdiagnosis occurs in approximately 15% of demented patients. Her cluster analyses (Bayles, 1982a) identified 83% of her demented sample and 77% of her normal sample correctly. Bollinger (1970) reported little difficulty in differentiating normals from demented patients on the PICA. His normal sample performed significantly faster than his demented patients, and the latter identified themselves by writing performance that was significantly worse than their gestural and verbal performance. Thus, utilization of data in the three areas requested by Wells (1982)—cognition, behavior (for our purposes, language behavior), and affect—plus medical evidence of bilateral brain injury, should be sufficient to differentiate the normal aged in a communication-impairing environment from the demented person.

The patient with the language of confusion may masquerade as a demented patient. Halpern et al. (1973) have demonstrated that the key diagnostic sign to differentiate between the two disorders is relevance. In their samples, the confused group made 40% relevance errors and the demented group made only 10% relevance errors. Reading was similar in the two groups, but writing to dictation differed. Confused patients made 44% writing errors and demented patients only 10%. The presence of bilateral brain injury does not tell who is who. Both of Halpern and associates' groups tended to be bilateral. However, rapidity of onset and duration of symptoms differed. Eighty percent of the confused patients had a rapid onset—less than 10 days—and 90% of the demented group had a slow onset. Similarly, 100% of the confused patients had a duration of symptoms of less than 3 months. Conversely, 90% of the demented patients had a duration of symptoms of over 3 months. Combined medical and language data, therefore, assist in differentiating dementia from confusion.

Language Disorders in Adults: State of the Clinical Art 35

A similar approach can be used to differentiate dementia from schizophrenia. Di Simoni et al. (1977) have shown relevance errors abound in schizophrenic patients, 45%, and Halpern et al. (1973) have demonstrated they are rare in dementia, 10%. Fluency errors were the fourth most frequent type in the Di Simoni et al. schizophrenic sample. Fluency errors were the least frequent type in the Halpern et al. demented sample. Di Simoni et al. do note that the older, long-time postonset schizophrenic patient may, eventually, resemble the demented patient. However, for most, comparing the language behavior of the two groups and the presence of bilateral injury in dementia, and its absence in schizophrenia, should sort out dementia from schizophrenia. If one is still puzzled, a look at the age of onset may make the decision. Dementia is a problem that occurs in later life, and schizophrenia, typically, has its onset in late adolescence or early adulthood.

Demented, or aphasic, or both? This question plagues clinicians, and, gradually, they are beginning to line up behind one of the three possibilities. I stand in the queue that differentiates the language deficit in dementia from that seen in aphasia. While some of the language behavior in the demented patient resembles that seen in aphasia, I see no useful purpose served by talking about aphasia in dementia. Yet, some do.

Ernst, Dalby, and Dalby (1970) reported "aphasic symptoms" in dementia. Watson and Heilman (1974) believe aphasia may be seen in degenerative diseases, such as Alzheimer's and Pick's. Hecaen and Albert (1978) report that aphasia may suddenly appear in a previously demented patient. Appell et al. (1981) administered the WAB (Kertesz, 1982) to a sample of Alzheimer's patients and concluded that all were aphasic. And, Horner and Heyman (1982) differentiate between focal aphasia and dementia, but they label the language deficits in the latter, Alzheimer's aphasia.

Conversely, Rochford (1971) has demonstrated that the naming deficit in dementia results from visual misrecognition of the stimulus and not the linguistic anomic deficit seen in aphasia. Halpern et al. (1973) observed that reading comprehension was the second most frequent error in their demented patients, and it was the third least frequent error in their aphasic sample. In addition, their aphasic patients had severe auditory retention deficits, but their demented patients had only moderate difficulty on auditory retention tasks. Finally, fluency errors were frequent in the aphasic patients, 33%, but they were rare, 9%, in their demented sample. They concluded that the language of intellectual impairment seen in their demented patients could be differentiated from aphasia by comparison of each group's profile of deficits on a battery of language tests. Our replication (Deal, Wertz, & Spring, 1981) of their effort, including the use of Q-correlations to provide an index of similarity between profiles, tended to pick out the aphasic patients, 17 of 21, but was less than adequate for classifying the demented patients, only 8 of 15. Nevertheless, when we used all data—biographical, medical, and behavioral—all patients, aphasic and demented, were diagnosed correctly. Thus, Well's (1982) requirement for more data than that provided by a neuropsychologic measure, appears sage. When combined data are used, typically, one can differentiate dementia from aphasia and from other disorders.

Aphasia

Because diagnosis of aphasia is being discussed last, there appears to be little left to say about differentiating it from other disorders. But, for a patient to be labeled aphasic, he or she must meet one's definition of aphasia. And, as was true with the other disorders, we scan the biographical, medical, and behavioral data for evidence.

Information about premorbid literacy and intelligence should be obtained. Diagnosis of aphasia may be complicated in patients who lacked education or had diminished intelligence at onset. Sensory deficits—vision, hearing—if present must be identified and weighed in the diagnostic decision. We must have evidence of unilateral, typically left hemisphere, brain damage. And, we must see a general language deficit that crosses all communicative modalities—auditory comprehension, reading, oral expressive language, and writing. Deficits in all areas need not be, and usually are not, equal, but to be aphasic, one must show deficits in all areas.

The latter requirement creates an interesting difference in the identification of aphasia between those who do and those who do not use adjectives to modify it. The former group, generally, utilize the BDAE or WAB to detect the presence, severity, and type of aphasia. Neither instrument requires the examiner to use reading and writing performance to diagnose aphasia. Both utilize conversation, picture description, verbal repetition, naming, and auditory comprehension to make the diagnosis, estimate severity, and determine type. The latter group, those who do not type, typically include reading and writing performance along with auditory comprehension and oral expressive performance to make a diagnosis and determine severity. I do not imply that those who type aphasia would do so if the patient displayed no deficits in reading or writing. But, it is interesting to note that even though the BDAE and the WAB contain excellent means for appraising reading and writing, performance in these areas is not required to make a diagnosis of aphasia.

As with several other disorders, Halpern et al. (1973) provide a profile for aphasia. The most salient subtests in their battery were tasks of auditory retention, auditory comprehension, and fluency. Deficits in these areas tended to differentiate their aphasic patients from their demented and confused groups. In addition, their aphasic sample displayed more total language deficit than the other groups studied. Our use (Deal et al., 1981) of the Halpern et al. profile for aphasia successfully classified 17 of 21 aphasic patients. When we combined language performance with medical data—all aphasic patients had a rapid onset, less than 10 days; all had a left hemisphere lesion; and all had a focal lesion—we had no difficulty in differentiating aphasia from dementia.

A persisting problem in the diagnosis of aphasia is not necessarily its identification but whether it is present in the other disorders being discussed here. For example, is aphasia the communicative deficit in the normal aged person, the schizophrenic patient, the confused patient, the patient with a right hemisphere lesion, and the demented patient? I believe it is not very useful to say it is. While we seem to know more about aphasia than we do about the other disorders, calling the language deficit in the other disorders aphasia does not add to our knowledge; it complicates it.

However, disorders can, and do, coexist. We talk about apraxia of speech coexisting with aphasia (Darley, 1982; Wertz, 1978). Why not aphasia coexisting with dementia? If we can tease out evidence for the presence of two disorders in coexisting aphasia and apraxia of speech, for example, articulatory errors indicating apraxia of speech and semantic and syntax errors indicating aphasia, we might be able to identify aphasia coexisting with dementia. Some (Appell et al., 1981) argue that the language deficit in dementia is aphasia. Others (Hecaen and Albert, 1978) suggest that the two coexist. I believe neither position is correct or, at least, very useful. Unlike coexisting aphasia and apraxia of speech, where the former is a language disorder and the latter is a motor speech disorder, both aphasia and the demented patient's language of generalized intellectual impairment are language disorders. Calling one the other or indicating the coexistence of two language disorders in the same patient does not assist in patient management.

I (1982) have utilized Watson and Records' (1978) PICA data to demonstrate that the langauge deficits in aphasia and dementia differ. Figure 1-3 shows PICA performance by their aphasic and demented samples. Performance in the aphasic sample has been equated for severity with the demented sample. The demented patients do better on more difficult writing tasks—Subtest A, B, and C; worse on most verbal tasks—Subtests IV, IX, and XII; worse on auditory tasks—Subtests VI and X; and worse on visual tasks—Subtests VIII and XI. If one compares PICA Subtest percentiles, as shown in Figure 1-4., the profiles of the two groups differ even more markedly. Finally, use of the Porch et al. (1976) discriminate function analysis, which requires multiplying selected subtest

FIGURE 1-3
PICA Ranked Response Summary comparing performance by aphasic patients with performance by demented patients. The samples have been equated for severity. (After Watson & Records, 1978)

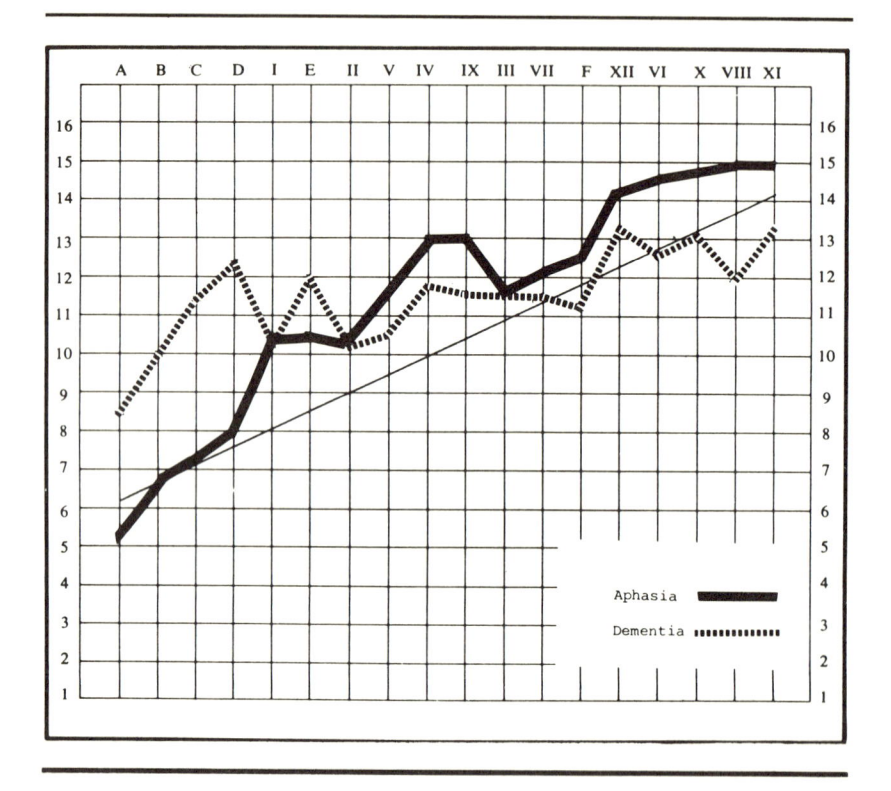

percentiles by an appropriate weight to obtain a discriminate score, indicates that the demented sample is not aphasic. Scores larger than −.211 represent aphasia, and scores less than −.279 are considered nonaphasic. My calculations for Watson and Records' demented sample yield a score of −.612, clearly nonaphasic.

A final problem in the diagnosis of aphasia is determining when a patient is no longer aphasic. Some suffer a mild aphasia, others improve to a point where they no longer are aphasic on the measures we use. Duffy (1981) has discussed this "grey area" between mild aphasia and normal language ability. His PICA data (Duffy & Keith, 1980) show that scores achieved by left brain-injured patients above the 90th percentile overlap with scores achieved by normal subjects. Other tests for aphasia—Token

FIGURE 1-4
Comparison of PICA subtest percentile performance by demented and aphasic patients. (After Watson & Records, 1978)

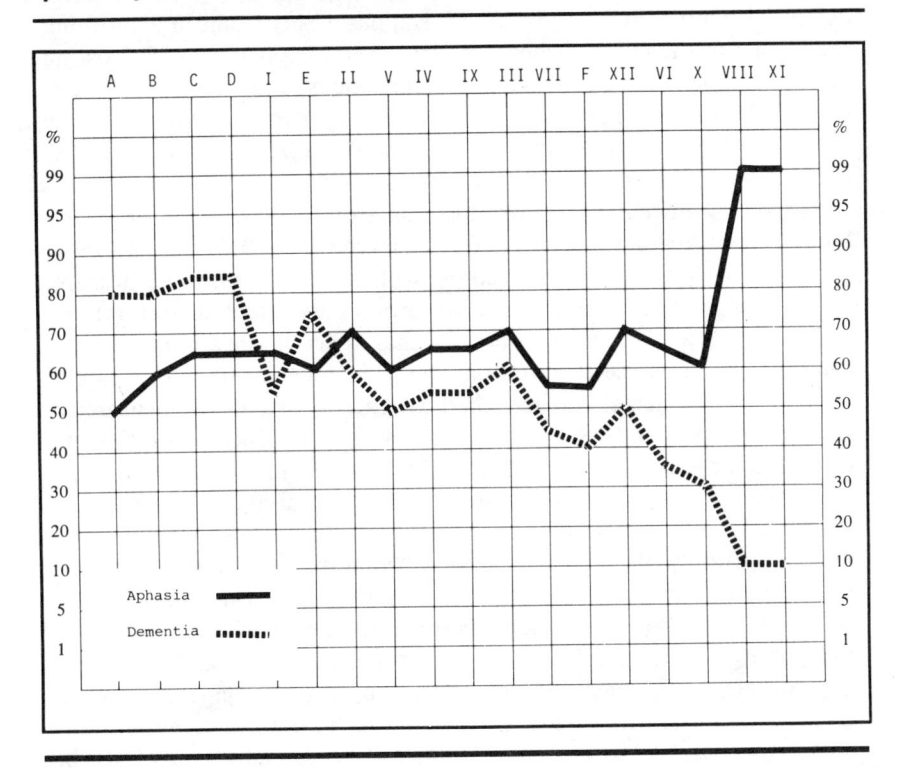

Test, Word Fluency Measure, BDAE—contain similar problems in differentiating mild aphasia from no aphasia. Presently, one of the best solutions to the dilemma is to ask the patient, "Is your language as good as it was before your stroke?" The sanity of this approach is well documented in Moss's (1972) account of his own aphasia.

State of the Art

As we mature, we become more and more adroit at differentiating among language disorders and less and less prone to abet mislabeling. However, problems persist. Only recently have we discovered some disorders, for example, communication deficit in the normal aged brought on by environmental influence; and only recently have we probed problems we have known exist, for example, communication deficits in schizophrenia and following a right hemisphere lesion. We lack measures to explore the new, and we tend to apply measures for the new that may be appropriate only for the old. For example, appraising right hemisphere deficit with a measure appropriate for aphasia may result in identifying the former as the latter. We have not resolved the dilemma of coexisting disorders. Does a patient display more than one type of language disorder, or does the way we appraise problems dictate a "two for" when only one exists? Finally, time postonset confounds. What begins as one disorder may gradually assume the characteristics of another.

Progress in differentiating one disorder from another has been steady but not rapid. Efforts akin to those of Halpern et al. (1973) and Di Simoni et al. (1977), that compare one disorder with another on the same measure, are marked by their rarity. Table 1-4 shows data adapted from reports by Halpern et al., and Di Simoni et al. that differentiate among aphasia, dementia, the language of confusion, and schizophrenia. Absent are similar data for environmental influence on the normal aged and right hemisphere involvement. When the state of the art is written on diagnosis in 5 years, one would hope that the missing data will have been provided, or, perhaps, a new measure that tells who is who will have replaced our current tools.

I believe what you call it is important; that determining who is who is useful. Certainly, the words are not important, but what the words imply should make a difference. Diagnosis is more than arranging phonemes to create labels that differ one from the other. Diagnosis carries implications that transcend the labels. It implies prognosis, and it dictates appropriate management. Sometimes, we suffer the same fate as our patients whose ideas, like most of their ideas, pass through their minds without words, and any attempt to form the ideas into words fails, indeed may chase the ideas from their minds. Clinicians, like their patients, continue to seek the right words to label what they observe.

Prognosis

Attempts to prognose are exercises in augury. We utilize what the patient brings with him or her—a biography, medical data—and combine these with what he or she has to tell us about his or her problems—behavioral data—and the diagnosis to predict his or her future. Nothing is more important to the patient, and unfortunately, this is what we do less well than anything else.

Usually our prognostic statements are a best guess, and the precision we are capable of is restricted to predicting change on a specific language measure. What we can do may have little to say about what the patient will

TABLE 1-4
Salient speech and language behaviors for four language disorders.

	APHASIA	*DEMENTIA*	*CONFUSION*	*SCHIZOPHRENIA*
M O S T I M P A I R E D	Adequacy Auditory Retention Fluency	Adequacy Reading Comprehension Auditory Retention	Reading Comprehension Writing to Dictation Relevance Adequacy	Relevance Reading Comprehension Fluency
L E A S T I M P A I R E D	Reading Comprehension Writing to Dictation Relevance	Relevance Writing to Dictation Fluency	Auditory Retention Fluency	Auditory Retention Writing to Dictation Adequacy

Generally, "most impaired" indicates percent of error is above the mean percent of total errors for each disorder, and "least impaired" indicates percent of error is below the mean percent of total errors for each group. **(Adapted from Di Simoni, Darley, & Aronson, 1977)**

---

be able to do. We are not very good at stating prognosis for "What." Dresser, Meirowsky, Weiss, McNeel, Simon, and Caveness (1973) indicated that 75% of their sample of Korean War veterans with head trauma were involved in some kind of employment 15 years after onset. Such reports are very rare.

Frequently, prognosis must be filtered through whether the patient will or will not receive treatment. Jellinek and Harvey (1982) report 73% of their brain-injured sample were considered appropriate for vocational and/or educational rehabilitation, but only 51% of these received a rehabilitation program. None of the patients who did not receive rehabilitation returned to work or school, whereas 78% of those who were treated did. Thus, treatment appears to influence prognosis.

Finally, our ability to state a patient's future is better for some language disorders than it is for others. For example, we are better at prognosticating for the aphasic patient than we are for the normal aged in a communication-impairing environment. The following is what I think we know, but mostly, what I think we do not know about prognosis for the different language disorders being discussed here.

Environmental Influence on the Normal Aged

I find no empirical evidence to indicate that the normal aged person in a communication-impairing environment has a bright or a bleak future. By definition, we might assume that the patient's future depends upon modification of the environment. If it can be changed to promote a favorable climate for communication, the patient's future should be promising. If it cannot, lack of change or additional erosion should be the result. But, we do not know. Only a few treatment studies, to be discussed later, imply that patients in a custodial setting improve if given appropriate stimulation. However, it is not clear whether these patients are those whose communication deficits result from environmental influence, or whether they should be placed in another diagnostic group.

Thus, we can say little about the normal aged person's potential for regaining environmentally eroded communication skills. Can what has been lost be regained? Are there variables which may predict who is most resistent to environmental influences? Will improvement result if the environment becomes more favorable? We do not know. Of course, we could find out. Comparison of language behavior pre- and post-environmental manipulation appears to be a first step.

Language of Confusion

One might expect the patient with the language of confusion to have a favorable prognosis. Chedru and Geschwind (1972) used the adjective "acute" to modify confusional state. So, change is expected. But, in what direction? Brosin (1967) suggests confusion is a disorder caused by reversible, temporary, diffuse disturbance in brain function. He believes it is usually brief, but he cautions it may persist up to 1 month or longer and may end in health and cure, death, or chronic disease. Pick a prognosis from this description. Reversible, temporary, brief, health and cure imply a favorable future for the confused patient. Death or chronic disease forecast something else. Again, I have found no empirical evidence to predict who can expect what.

My clinical experience indicates that patients who are correctly diagnosed as demonstrating the language of confusion can expect to improve rapidly and markedly. One returned to his previous position as a high school mathematics teacher within a year postonset. Another went back to parking cars. My clinical experience also indicates that the confused patient who does not make marked and rapid improvement may receive a change in his or her diagnosis. Lack of positive change may shift the confused patient's diagnosis to dementia or language disturbance undetermined. Because the language of confusion is rare, few clinicians see enough of it to build a data base for prediction.

Perhaps what causes the confusion may hold an answer. For example, the acute cases studied by Chedru and Geschwind (1972) included patients with acute alcoholic intoxication, barbituate intoxication, those undergoing electro-convulsive therapy, and those undergoing general anesthesia. All of these conditions could be expected to improve, and Chedru and Geschwind report they did. However, we know little about the future for the tumor, trauma, infection, and hematoma cases studied by Halpern et al. (1973).

Schizophrenia

A few pieces of information are beginning to emerge to assist in predicting the schizophrenic patient's future. However, none are specifically applicable for predicting change in the schizophrenic patient's language behavior.

Negative prognostic signs include age, duration, and intelligence. Di Simoni et al. (1977) report older schizophrenic patients and those who are a long time postonset have more severe language deficits, often resembling the language of confusion or dementia. Rioch and Lubin (1959) have observed that schizophrenic patients with IQs below 90 do not respond favorably to long-term intensive psychotherapy. However, their patients with IQs at, or above, 110 varied in their response to treatment and did not permit prediction. Pollack, Levenstein, and Klein (1968) suggest that patients with higher IQs do better in treatment than those with lower IQs.

A positive prognostic sign appears to be the patient's social milieu. Klonoff, Fibiger, and Hutton (1970) observed that ambulatory outpatients performed better than nonambulatory inpatients on the Halstead-Reitan battery. Caton (1982) found that the quality of a patient's living environment and the relationship with significant others are critical in determining whether he or she will require hospitalization. Interestingly, Caton also observed that the patient's length of hospitalization bore no relationship with subsequent hospitalization, treatment compliance, or social functioning in the community.

Thus, older, long-time postonset, low intelligence schizophrenic patients with unfavorable living environments and poor relationships with significant others appear to have a poor prognosis for improvement. Conversely, younger, close-to-onset schizophrenic patients, with favorable living environments, and good relationships with significant others have a brighter future. That is not much on which to hang a prognosis. But, it is a beginning.

Right Hemisphere Involvement

What we know about prognosis for the right hemisphere patient is sparse, but what we do know indicates the prognosis is not very good. Prognostic information comes from two sources, examination of variables that may predict whether the patient will return to work, and comparison of improvement in patients with right hemisphere lesions to improvement made by patients with left hemisphere lesions.

Weisbroth, Esibill, and Zuger (1971) examined the influence of seven variables on the probability of the right hemisphere patient returning to work. They found no predictive information in age and education. Gender; ambulation; use of the affected upper extremity; and cognition, measured by performance on a block design task, all had prognostic significance. More females in their right hemisphere sample returned to work than males. More patients who could walk, and who had some use of their affected upper extremity, returned to work than those who were nonambulatory, and/or had minimal use of their affected upper extremity. Those with better cognition were more likely to return to work. In the Weisbroth et al. sample of 28 patients, only 11 returned to work. The average time postonset when they re-entered the world of work was 19 months. All who returned to work had received an average of 10 months of vocational rehabilitation.

Right hemisphere patients make less gain in developing self-care activities than left hemisphere patients, even though they receive longer inpatient rehabilitation (Gordon, Drenth, Jarvis, Johnson, & Wright 1978). Even after discharge, Forer and Miller (1980) and Lorenze and Canero (1962) report that the right hemisphere patient demonstrates greater impairment in activities of daily living than the left hemisphere patient. Golper (1980) compared right and left hemisphere patients on a verbal picture description task at 1 week and 1 month postonset. The left hemisphere patients improved the efficiency of their verbal communication. The right hemisphere patients continued to give redundant statements and irrelevant remarks, indicating that their recovery of language was characterized by less efficiency than the left hemisphere patients.

Based on the minimal information available, the patient with a right hemisphere lesion, therefore, has a guarded prognosis. Less than half return to work. Their ability to walk, their use of their involved upper extremity, and their cognitive ability appear to predict whether they will become employed. Even though they have less language deficit than the left hemisphere patient, their communication skills continue to be impaired.

Dementia

Causes of dementia can be divided into those that are treatable and those for which there is no treatment. Prognosis is, of course, better for patients with a treatable cause than for those with an untreatable cause. Prognosis is best for those who have been misdiagnosed—for example, pseudodementia resulting from depression.

The most frequent cause of dementia is Alzheimer's disease. It strikes, typically, in the 4th or 5th decade of life, and the downhill course may continue for up to 10 years before death intervenes. Older Alzheimer's patients may survive only a few years. Thus, dementia resulting from Alzheimer's disease has a poor prognosis for improvement. Prognosis, like diagnosis, is complicated in Alzheimer's disease, because its presence is usually verifiable only at autopsy (Friedland, 1982). Thus the patient is typically labeled as demonstrating Alzheimer's "type" dementia. Nevertheless, these patients constitute the overwhelming majority of demented patients, and their future is bleak.

Treatable dementias are few. Freeman and Rudd (1982) found only 16 patients with a potentially reversible cause in a sample of 110 who had progressive intellectual deterioration. Twelve of the 16 responded favorably to medical, surgical, and psychiatric treatment. Their underlying illnesses included normal-pressure hydrocephalus, subdural hematoma, depression, hempatic encephalopathy, and chronic drug overdose. The intellectual deterioration in this group was of short duration, and all patients showed less cortical atrophy on their computed tomographic scans than patients with idiopathic dementia. The average age of the treatable patients did not differ significantly from the average age of the patients with idiopathic dementia.

Aphasia

We have used three methods to predict the aphasic patient's future: prognostic variables, behavioral profiles on language measures, and statistical prediction. The first approach utilizes biographical, medical, and behavioral characteristics to predict change or the lack of it. The second involves evaluating a patient, constructing a profile of performance, and comparing this with change made by previous patients with a similar profile. The third employs multiple regression techniques to predict performance on a measure of aphasia at different points in time postonset. Use of prognostic variables and the behavioral profile are limited to forecasting with an adjective—good, fair, guarded, poor. Unfortunately, prognostic variables coexist, and a patient may have both favorable and unfavorable signs. We do not know how positive and negative signs interact to influence change. The behavioral profile approach is hampered by inability to classify some patients into a specific prognostic group. Finally, statistical prediction has promise, but it is not sufficiently developed for use with individual patients.

Over the years, we have observed the influence of specific variables on change in aphasia. Some have withstood the test of time. Others have not. Table 1-5 shows the conclusions I reached in a recent review (Wertz, 1983a) regarding the influence of selected variables on improvement in aphasia. Age, formerly believed to have prognostic importance, has not held up as a significant sign in recent reports. Education, premorbid intelligence, and occupational status have always been debatable as prognostic indicants, and they remain so today. Etiology has an influence on the patient's future. Aphasia resulting from closed head trauma improves more than aphasia resulting from CVA (Alajouanine, Castaigne, L'Hermitte, Escourolle, & De Ribancourt, 1957; Eisenson, 1964; Kertesz & McCabe, 1977; Luria, 1963). The size of the lesion and its localization influence recovery. Yarnell, Monroe, and Sobel (1976) and Rubens (1975) are consistent in their observations that patients with small lesions, a single lesion, and lesions that avoid the temporal-parietal region have a better prognosis than those with large lesions, multiple or bilateral lesions, and damage in the temporal-parietal cortex. Health, severity, and time postonset have held up as useful prognostic signs. Patients in good health postonset improve more than those in poor health (Anderson, Bourestom,

TABLE 1-5
Selected variables suggested to have an influence on improvement in aphasia. + = agreement, ? = conflicting reports.

VARIABLE	STATUS
Age	?
Education	?
Premorbid Intelligence	?
Occupational Status	?
Etiology	+
Size of Lesion	+
Localization	+
Health	+
Severity	+
Time Post onset	+
Type of Aphasia	?

& Greenberg, 1970; Eisenson, 1949, 1964). Almost everyone who has looked suggests that less severe patients at onset have a better future than those with more severe aphasia (Basso, Capitani, & Vignolo, 1979; Hartman, 1981; Kertesz & McCabe, 1977; Sarno & Levita, 1979; Schuell, Jenkins, & Jimenez-Pabon, 1964). The closer to onset, the more improvement a patient can expect (Basso et al., 1979; Deal & Deal, 1978; Kertesz & McCabe, 1977; Vignolo, 1964; Wertz et al, 1981). Finally, the influence of type of aphasia is debatable. Kertesz and McCabe (1977) and Lomas and Kertesz (1978) report anomic and conduction types have the best prognosis. Prins, Snow, and Wagenaar (1978) found no influence of type of aphasia on improvement.

Therefore, the prognostic variable approach for stating an aphasic patient's prognosis indicates that a patient who suffered closed head trauma resulting in one small lesion that does not involve temporal-parietal cortex, who is in good health, mildly aphasic, and less than a month postonset has an excellent prognosis for improvement. Unfortunately, most of our patients do not display this kind of syzygy. Positive and negative signs coexist, and coexistence complicates prediction.

Schuell (1965b) and Keenan and Brassell (1974) have popularized the behavioral profile approach. Language data are used to construct the profile, and the profile is compared with previous patients' profiles. Schuell developed five major prognostic groups and two minor syndromes based on her retrospective look at initial MTDDA performance by patients whose improvement or lack of it was documented. Initial profiles for patients who showed marked improvement were used to forecast a positive prognosis, and initial profiles for patients who displayed limited recovery were used to predict a poor prognosis. This approach permits making an early, data-based prediction. Problems arise when a patient's performance cannot be classified in one of Schuell's prognostic groups. Keenan and Brassell were interested in predicting improvement in verbal performance. They observed that auditory comprehension and verbal performance could be used to forecast a patient's future behavior. Initial reading and writing performance had little predictive use. If a patient can be classified, the behavioral profile is useful for stating prognosis. However, even if a patient can be classified, the prognostic statement is limited to an adjective and may not indicate prognosis for what.

Statistical prediction is promising but not, as yet, practical. Multiple regression analysis and two-group discriminant analysis have been used in medicine to predict mortality from coronary and from shock. Meehl (1965) believes that statistical techniques result in more precise prediction than that obtained from clinical judgment. Porch and his colleagues (1973, 1974, 1980) have used a step-wise multiple regression analysis to predict change in aphasia as measured by the PICA. Patients were tested at various times postonset, followed, and retested at a later date. A retrospective analysis was done using performance in the early test to determine whether performance on the later test could have been predicted. When predicted performance was correlated with performance actually obtained, correlations ranged from 0.74 to 0.94. All were significant, indicating the multiple regression formula was a reasonably accurate means of predicting change in aphasia. Deal et al. (1979) used the multiple regression formula developed by Porch, Collins, Wertz, and Friden (1980) to test its clinical application. The group results were significant, indicating that patients obtained PICA scores close to those predicted. However, analysis of individual data indicated less than two thirds of the sample obtained scores that fell within a -5 to $+5$ percentile range of the score predicted. Thus, the Deal et al. results lend credence to the caution counselled by Porch et al. (1980). The multiple regression formula they generated is not ready for clinical application.

So, while there has been a good deal of activity in developing prognostic tools for predicting the aphasic patient's future, we are yet to devise methods that permit us to tell the patient and his or her family, with any precision, how much improvement can be expected, when that improvement will occur, and what it will permit the patient to do.

The State of the Art

We know far less than we need to know about predicting change in the language disorders being discussed here. Whether the communicative deficit suffered by the normal aged in a communication-impairing environment will improve, remain the same, or get worse is unknown. Heuristically, we might expect change if the environment is manipulated to foster communication rather than impede it. But, we do not know if things are that simple. Can what has been depressed be elevated? We do not know. Clinical experience indicates that the patient with the language of confusion will improve. But, we play a questionable game. If he or she does improve, we assume our diagnosis was correct. If the patient does not, we may change the diagnosis, typically to dementia. There is little to tell us about the schizophrenic patient's future. Age, duration of symptoms, and social milieu are believed to influence improvement or the lack of it. But, what we know does not permit us to predict with much precision. The patient with the right hemisphere lesion may not demonstrate the severe language deficits seen in other brain-injured patients, but his or her communicative ability may be severely impaired and remain so. The meager data to date indicate that the right hemisphere patient does not make the gains made by left hemisphere patients in self-care abilities or communicative efficiency. The demented patient has a poor prognosis. The course is downhill unless he or she suffers one of the few cases that respond to treatment, and these make up less than 20% of the demented propulation. We know more about predicting change in aphasia than we do about predicting change for the other language disorders. But, our abilities are not very precise, or they are limited to predicting change on a specific language measure.

Because prognosis is so important to the patient and his or her family, and because it may justify whether to intervene with treatment, emphasis on improving our predictive ability should rise to the top of a need hierarchy in the management of language disorders in adults. To date, we have employed retrospective approaches that seek predictive variables, performance profiles on measures early postonset, and statistical prediction to forecast the future.

Perhaps the methods we have been using require ablution, or perhaps they require rejection. A possible alternative to what we have done includes looking at the patient's ability to learn. For example, regardless of our philosphy of therapy, we expect our patients to learn to do whatever it is they could not do when they came to our attention. Perhaps a brief battery of learning tasks, administered early postonset, would tell us which patient will learn and which will not. Those who do learn may have a brighter future than those who do not. Finally, we need to focus on predicting prognosis for what. For example, improved PICA performance may or may not relate to potential for returning to work, for participation in a dinner conversation, for finding enjoyable activities to fill the day.

Unfortunately, the path to improving our ability to prognose wanders through the land of the natural history study. We need to identify and follow large samples of patients over a long period of time to determine what they have to tell us about their problems and how those problems change. At the end of the path, we can take a retrospective view of what we missed along the way. Utilization of these data should assist us in predicting for future patients. The natural history study appears to be the tool for doing the task, but the natural history study has the lowest probability of attracting funding.

Treatment

LaPointe (1983) observed that the idea of shattered language being mended (that is, it can be darned instead of damned) is all too recent. He was talking about aphasia where, today, treatments abound. For many disorders—environmental influence on the normal aged, the language of confusion, schizophrenia, right hemisphere involvement—we continue to search for the proper egg, the right gauge needle, the proficient seamstress. And, frequently, we continue to fill the air with vituperative maledictions rather than proficient patches.

Two points of view have developed about treating language disorders in adults. In one, there is a leap to treat. If a problem exists, it must be treated. In the other, there is a reluctance to intervene. Because a problem exists does not mean there is a treatment for it. The former attempts to assuage symptoms. The latter awaits knowledge of the cause and evidence that a treatment is efficacious. Probably, more of the former exists than the latter. Certainly, successful treatments have not always awaited finding a cause. Quinine was given for malaria prior to the malarial parasite being identified. The cause of Parkinson's disease remains obscure, but observation of a deficit in dopamine has resulted in administration of L-dopa. In aphasia, we know the cause, but that knowledge does not assist, greatly, in treating the symptoms.

Today, many treatments exist, but many have not been demonstrated to be efficacious. In fact, the existence of a treatment often prevents research designed to test its efficacy. Because it exists, some believe it is unethical to withhold it in a treatment trial. In what follows, I will discuss what has been, is being, and is not being done to treat language disorders in adults.

Environmental Influence on the Normal Aged

Elimination of environmentally influenced deficits in the normal aged has taken two approaches. One is modification of the environment to remove the suspected cause of the problem. The second is direct treatment through individual or group therapy. The latter is, typically, reality orientation therapy which, in a sense, is a manipulation of the environment.

Manipulation of the environment begins with the premise that normal aging is normal, not pathological (Holland, 1983), however the environment may be pathology producing. Lubinski (1981) suggests that the speech pathologist has a role in refurbishing a communication impairing environment that transcends staff education and appraisal, diagnosis, and treatment of individual patients. She suggests that the speech pathologist become a patient advocate. Her intensive (Lubinski, Morrison, & Rigrodsky, 1981) interviews with aged residents in an institutional setting lead her to suggest avoidance of individual treatment in favor of treating the patient and the environment as a single unit. Labouvice-Vief, Hoyer, Baltes, and Baltes (1974), Rebok and Hoyer (1977), and Solomon (1982) also advocate combining behavioral treatment and behavioral ecology techniques to produce behavior change. MacDonald (1976) reports that this approach will increase the rate of verbalization in elderly nursing home patients, and that it is not necessary to add new resources, but simply to rearrange existing resources.

Lubinski's (1981) specific techniques include: creating a need for residents to communicate, providing places where communication can occur, teaching staff and patients that the act of communicating is in itself treatment, reducing rules that inhibit communication, showing staff and patients what they can do and how to do it, identifying and matching communication partners, and supplementing enviromental changes with sensory training and reality orientation. Solomon (1982) adds the need to demythologize concepts about aging for staff members, use model staff members to train others by precept, and give residents autonomy by teaching them to master their environment.

Adelson, Nasti, Sprafkin, Marinelli, Primavera, and Gorman (1982) have developed a behavioral rating scale to quantify health professional's interaction with geriatric patients. They took 15 traits from the literature that are believed to affect staff and patient relationships. These were tested with two groups of staff, one group supervisors judged to have good relatioships with patients and one group supervisors judged to have poor relationships with patients. Ten of the traits correlated significantly with the supervisors' ratings. These are listed in Table 1-6. The traits that were most predictive of good relationships were banter, engaging patients in

TABLE 1-6
Behavioral traits for rating health professional's interaction with geriatric patients. (After Adelson, Nasti, Sprafkin, Marinelli, & Primavera, 1982)

* Uses patient's name by whatever title patient wishes to be called.
* Banter: Engages patient in conversation.
* Asks for feedback: Gives choices, develops options for the patient, asks if something hurts or how it feels.
* Gives procedural information: Warns patient of upcoming sensation, touch, taste, or smell.
* Compensates for disabilities: Adapts to patient's impairment, for example, loss of hearing, sight, or other physical disabilities.
* Social touches: Uses physical contact that is an expression of affection, comfort, reassurance, or concern, and not considered procedural.
* Attends to patient comfort: Expresses concern for the patient's ease and is sensitive to the patient's needs.

  Amount of appropriate smiling: Too little, adequate, very good.

  Pacing of procedure: Poor, adequate, very good; if poor, too slow or too fast.

  Pacing of speech: Poor, adequate, very good; if poor, too slow or too fast.

NOTE: * Rated in total number of occurrences and whether occurred or not.

---

conversation, giving procedural information; smiling appropriately; asking for feedback; and using the patient's name. The value of the Adelson et al. scale is that it permits rating what staff do and do not do and provides specific behaviors to be developed and modified in staff members. Thus, it is a means for rating how the patient's environment is influenced by staff, what to change, and how to change.

Several suggest individual and group reality orientation for the normal aged in an institutional setting. Brandt, Rose, and Lucas (in press) used the terms "remotivation and resocialization" and "reality orientation." These imply involving the patient in social activities, including group discussion, and bombarding the patient with who he or she is, who the staff are, the date, the place, his or her schedule, etc. And, they require participation by everyone in the environment, from custodians to administrators. Individual and group sessions are supplemented with a reality orientation board which is individualized for the patient. Citrin and

Dixon (1977) have reported results from a clinical trial with treated and untreated groups. The treated patients received "24-hour" reality orientation supplemented by group sessions. Change was measured by a reality orientation sheet. Their treated group displayed significantly better orientation than their untreated group at the end of the program.

Some have offered an alternative to institutionalization. The premise is that if an institutional environment erodes abilities, keeping the patient out of an institution should be attempted. Rathbone-McCuan (1976) reported the positive effects of a geriatric day care center. The service lessened the family's physical burden of daily care by providing a daily supervised environment for the aged person, psychological support for the aged person and his or her family, and gave the aged person some interaction with peers. Rathbone-McCuan suggested that the day care center permits the family to keep the aged individual at home for as long as possible and is a "last ditch" effort to avoid an institutionalized environment. Steinhauer (1982) has discussed the use of geriatric foster care as an alternative to institutionalization for the elderly who have no family. Private family residences are found to house and care for those without relatives.

Direct treatment with the normal aged in an institutional environment shows mixed results. O'Connell and O'Connell (1978) reported that overall change from direct treatment was slight. Thirty percent of their sample failed to profit from direct treatment, 50% were discharged before they reached maximum gains, and 20% made significant improvement. Hudson (1960), focusing on communication problems in the aged, reports positive results from treatment. Finlayson and Martin (1982) suggest that increased social stimulation and emotional support reduced depression in the elderly. And Hoyer, Kafer, Simpson, and Hoyer (1974) increased verbal performance in aged individuals by using operant procedures that involved administration of tokens.

Obler and Albert (1981) suggest teaching the normal elderly in an institution to use language strategies employed by the normal elderly who are not in an institution. The process, of course, requires training staff in what the strategies are and how to prompt their use by patients. A variety of techniques have been used in attempts to improve cognitive skills in the aged. The most successful are: modeling, watching use of cognitive strategies used by younger persons, and feedback of information about the correctness of a response. Direct instruction, noncognitive intervention, attempts to change response speed, attempts to motivate by giving money, and praise are not effective. Practice improves some skills, but not others.

Treatment for the normal aged in a communication-impairing environment has focused on the environment and the individual. Apparently, manipulation of both are necessary. And, as is true with most disorders, what should be done must flow from the patient—what the patient can tell us about his or her problem and what he or she can tell us about what should be done for it.

Language of Confusion

Because we expect confusional state to change, and because it usually does, few treatments have been developed for it. Probably, medical management that removes the cause of the confusion is the most appropriate treatment. Chedru and Geschwind's (1972) patients improved after the effects of alcoholic intoxication, barbituate intoxication, electroconvulsive therapy, and general anesthesia passed. In cases of trauma or surgical intervention, perhaps the time necessary for edema to subside is the appropriate treatment.

Reality orientation has been used with confused patients. Whether it is an efficacious treatment is debatable. It is employed during the confusional state and dropped when confusion is resolved. Whether reality orientation improves confusion or whether the patient becomes oriented because whatever caused the confusion has subsided in unknown. No controlled studies have been conducted.

I (1978) have suggested speech and language-specific treatment for the language of confusion. The principles involve finding appropriate stimulus and response modes that result in less confabulation and irrelevancy, using a hierarchy of tasks that permits more open-ended responses when the patient demonstrates that he or she is ready to roam verbally without confabulating, and confronting the patient with the veracity of the confabulation and the appropriateness of his or her irrelevance. Most of the confused patients I have seen improve when given this type of treatment. Whether they would have improved if I had left them alone, I do not know.

We offer the confused patient medical management if medicine has a treatment for what brings the patient to our hospital, in addition to reality orientation and speech and language specific therapy. Whether the latter two have any influence on the improvement we typically see, we do not know.

Schizophrenia

Because few schizophrenic patients are seen by speech pathologists, speech and language treatments are few. But others see these patients and they manage them. Finkel and Cohen (1982) relate that psychotherapy, behavioral modification, family psychotherapy, and pharmacotherapy are all useful approaches for managing the schizophrenic patient under the proper circumstances. Geschwind (1975) cautions that one must be certain the patient considered for these treatments is schizophrenic—and is only schizophrenic. He estimates that neurologic disorders account for 30% of all first admissions to mental hospitals, and some of these neurologic causes of psychiatric disorders respond to a neurologic treatment.

Speech and language deficits in a schizophrenic patient have been viewed in two contexts. By a few, they are considered symptoms requiring specific speech and language treatment. By most, they are considered symptoms that will indicate whether other treatment—drugs, psychotherapy—is working. Feldstein and Weingartner (1981) review the use of speech and language behavior to determine the efficacy of drug therapy with schizophrenic patients. Improvement in speech and language implies medication is working. Lack of improvement implies the need for a change in medicinal management.

Halpern (1980) is among those who advocate treating the schizophrenic patient's speech and language deficits. The techniques he suggests do not differ markedly from those used with other language disorders. He cautions that most schizophrenic patients are not concerned with their communication problems. Some need a highly structured treatment, and others require more informal approaches. Halpern advocates the use of reinforcements—food, coffee—to achieve change. He notes that progress is slow, but speech and language therapy is beneficial. Enlisting the aid of other staff, he believes, is essential to achieve carry-over outside the treatment session.

Some have used operant techniques to combat muteness in the schizophrenic patient. Isaacs, Thomas, and Goldiamond (1960) used operant techniques to reinstate verbal behavior in two patients. And, Sherman (1963) reports success in restoring speech in a mute schizophrenic patient. Operant conditioning in a 16-session treatment trial resulted in the patient's using his intact language, displayed in writing, orally.

We lack empirical evidence to demonstrate the efficacy of language therapy with the schizophrenic patient. Language deficit in schizophrenia may be like a patient's inability to run with a broken leg. Set the bone, immobilize it, wait, and, eventually, the patient will run. For schizophrenia, find the correct medicinal management and treat with psychotherapy, and the patient's language deficit may resolve. Whether this is the appropriate procedure for managing communicative deficit in schizophrenia, we do not know.

Right Hemisphere Involvement

The patient with right hemisphere involvement has been treated as interesting—and seldom treated. Myers (1981) suggests it is time for speech pathologists to relinquish this wallflower role in relation to the right hemisphere patient; it is time to dance the dance. She cautions that, prior to stepping onto the floor, we must remember what we are treating is not aphasia.

A variety of disciplines have intervened with the right hemisphere patient, and they have obtained mixed results. Taylor, Schaeffer, Blumenthal, and Grissel (1969) report no difference between treated and untreated right hemisphere patients following a program designed to improve perceptual and motor skills. LaPointe and Culton (1969) report success in remediating left neglect in a patient with a right hemisphere lesion. Diller and Weinberg (1977) were successful in training right hemisphere patients with hemi-inattention to compensate for their deficits.

Myers and West (1978) have listed the right hemisphere patient's specific deficits that may respond to rehabilitation. These include: lack of sensitivity, inappropriate behavior, denial of cognitive deficits, lack of motivation, lability, visual hallucinations, and dissociation between what is said and what is experienced. The few who have attempted to treat these problems differ in their rationale and their techniques.

Myers (1981) emphasizes that the problem of right hemisphere patients is not just perceptual, but perceptual in a broad sense. They need more than training designed to get them to look to the left or to match stimuli. Perceptual deficit impairs simultaneous discrimination and interpretation. Treatment tasks should emphasize context and its use to search for meaning. Myers advocates having right hemisphere patients use their good verbal ability to reverbalize what they experience. They will not use nonverbal cues to find meaning the way patients with a left hemisphere lesion do. Because of the right hemisphere patient's irrelevance and the inability to cope with open-ended tasks, Myers (1979) suggests maintaining rigid stimulus control in highly structured tasks and, gradually, permitting the patients more freedom on open-ended tasks when they demonstrate they are ready to deal with less structure.

Adamovich (1981) uses a more comprehensive approach in treating right hemisphere patients. She advocates treating perception, sequencing ability, auditory comprehension, verbal expression, reading, writing, organizational ability, problem solving, and auditory and visual memory. Her methodology employs developing task continua, from easy to difficult, according to cognitive and linguistic developmental hierachies.

Yorkston (1981) suggests using the right hemisphere patient's learning style to dictate how he or she is treated. Because the patient has poor generalization ability, she suggests using functional tasks; for example reading rather than canceling letters. And, because the patient can talk, she advocates having him or her provide verbal cues by talking his or her way through tasks. Because the patient tends to forget, she suggests massed practice to promote generalization. Next, because the right hemisphere patient is not very good at recognizing his or her errors and because the patient is impulsive, Yorkston uses sequential tasks that cannot continue unless errors are recognized and corrected. Finally, because the right hemisphere patient is not very good at reasoning and problem solving, she suggests breaking tasks down into numerous small steps, and if the patient fails to advance from one step to the next, adding additional steps. She asks her patients, constantly, "Have you finished this step?"

Many right hemisphere patients tend to ignore their left visual world, and because they do, they may have difficulty reading. Thus, some have focused on treating the right hemisphere patient's reading deficits. Collins (1976) has summarized the traditional techniques—encouraging oral reading and analyzing whether what is heard makes sense, using a brightly colored cardboard guide shaped like a carpenter's square to force attention to the left margin and focus on the line being read. Stanton, Yorkston, Kenyon, and Beukelman (1981) have developed a language-based reading program for right hemisphere patients with left neglect. They eschew the Diller, Ben-Yishay, Gerstman, Goodkin, and Gordon (1974) suggestion to use perceptual cues and employ Fordyce and Jones' (1966) observation that right hemisphere patients do better with verbal than with pantomime instructions. The Stanton et al. reading program requires overt verbalization—the patient cues himself or herself by talking aloud. When he fails to do so, the clinician intervenes and says, "Tell yourself." The program includes numerous small steps and employs intensive repetition. It is data based, in that the patient does not progress until he or she has reached criterion on each step. Stanton et al. provide data to demonstrate its efficacy with a sample of right hemisphere patients.

So, we are beginning to dance the dance with the right hemisphere patient. Presently, we are awkward, lack rhythm, step on toes, and know only a few steps. We are not ready to attend the cotillion, but we are looking in that direction.

Dementia

Miller (1977) has observed that dementia is usually diagnosed, but not treated. Except for those who have a treatable cause of dementia, behavioral therapy is employed in an attempt to slow dementia's progression. Mueller and Atlas (1972) report that the few gains resulting from behavioral treatment are lost when treatment stops. There have been a few efforts to find a drug or nutritional treatment for Alzheimer's patients. None has been successful. Thus, treatment for most demented patients is confined to reality orientation, or modification of demands made on the patient to permit him or her function as best he or she can.

Ratusnik, Lascoe, Herbon, and Wolfe (1979) used group sessions in an attempt to improve demented patients' awareness of themselves and others, awareness of time and place, word-finding and vocabulary usage, gestural communication, and to decrease verbal perseveration and inappropriate behaviors. The techniques included traditional stimulus-response activities and group discussion. Following approximately 2 months of treatment in 40-minute sessions 4 days a week, over half of their 16 patients improved in receptive and expressive language and in awareness of self and others. Less than half improved in memory and in orientation for time and place. Harris and Ivory (1976) used reality orientation in a 5-month treatment trial. They noted treated patients were significantly better than nontreated patients in six of nine verbal behaviors: spontaneous verbal interaction; using their own, the therapist's, and other patient's names correctly; compliance with simple requests; and correct verbalization of information pertaining to time. Schwartz et al. (1979) were unsuccessful in their attempt to teach demented patients to use their unimpaired syntax to cue semantic deficits.

General techniques for managing dementia have included attempting to keep the patient at home for as long as possible; providing proper nutrition and hydration; managing other medical problems immediately; and manipulating the environment to reduce emotional lability, promote cognition and memory, and regulate sleep and wake cycles. Bayles (1982b) has offered specific techniques for managing the demented patient. These include frequent family counselling; establishing and adhering to a fixed daily schedule; simplifying the environment but loading it with orientation materials—calendars, clocks, pictures; not arguing with the patient; using physical contact to provide support; and emphasizing health and diet. She suggests avoiding the use of verbal analogies, fragmented discourse, humor, sarcasm, indefinite referents, conversations with more than two persons, and open-ended questions. Finally, Bayles recommends periodic evaluations of the patient to detect and cope with changes in his behavior.

Thus, unless the cause of the dementia is treatable, what we have to offer is designed to slow deterioration of behavior or lessen demand as behavior deteriorates. Those of us who work with demented patients are aware of what we have to learn from the patient's family. They have lived with the disorder before it was brought to our attention. We need to set ourselves on "receive" rather than "send" when we talk with family members. We want to know what they have done that helps. We can assist them by arranging group sessions where families can gather to share.

Aphasia

Treatments for aphasia abound. A recent book (Chapey, 1981) contains at least 13 different types of aphasia therapy, and these barely scratch the literature's surface. Three chapters in this book discuss treatment of aphasic patients at various levels of severity. To avoid redundancy, I will summarize the general types of treatment used with aphasic patients and, then, consider treatment we may not call treatment, but which should be part of every aphasic patient's management.

How speech pathologists treat—and have treated—aphasic patients is influenced by their philosophy of aphasia therapy. There are probably as many philosophies of aphasia therapy as there are therapists. However, these can be organized into four broad groups. First, some treatment is "traditional." It incorporates proven methods of the past, most of which utilize a stimulus-response approach. Emphasis is placed on language content. Second, there has been a move to develop specific treatments for specific problems. Benson (1979b) suggested that speech pathologists look in this direction, and some have. These types of treatment are usually identified by easily remembered acronyms; Melodic Intonation Therapy (MIT) (Sparks, Helm, & Albert, 1974); Visual Action Therapy (VAT) (Helm & Benson, 1978); Voluntary Control of Involuntary Utterances (VCIU) (Helm & Barresi, 1980). Typically, they are applied with patients demonstrating a specific type of aphasia—MIT for the Broca's patient, VAT for the global patient. Third, some clinicians have extended the trend toward testing "functional" communication to administering "functional" treatment. The treatment developed by Davis and Wilcox (1981), Promoting Aphasics' Communicative Effectiveness (PACE), is an example of "functional" treatment. It emphasizes language context rather than language content. Fourth, larger caseloads have motivated busy clinicians to combine clients and conduct group therapy. Some (Aten, Kushner-Vogel, Haire, & Fitch-West, 1981; Bloom, 1962) believe that when three or more gather, more improvement occurs than when just two—patient and therapist—meet. Group treatments follow a variety of philosophies of aphasia therapy. Some are designed to create a social setting, and nothing more. Some are rigidly structured to lead group members, in unison, through what they might do if they were in individual treatment.

While an unassailable study on the efficacy of aphasia therapy has not been conducted, Darley's (1972) conclusion that it helps has received empirical support in recent clinical trails reports (Basso et al., 1979; Wertz et al., 1981) and numerous single-case studies. Of course, every clinician can tell tales of patients he has not helped, and some who were helped only a little. And, we continue to seek solutions to questions about when to treat, how much, where, and how. But, Benson's (1976b) conclusion that language therapy for the aphasic patient is, without a doubt, efficacious is an appropriate statement on the state of the art.

I believe there is a portion of the aphasic patient's management that we have ignored. We tend to treat language deficit, and when improvement in language slows or stops, we consider terminating treatment or moving the patient into a maintenance group. Perhaps we owe our patients more than just an attempt to improve their language skills. Perhaps we need to assist them in coping with the language deficit that remains after direct language therapy has done what it can. Figure 1-5 implies that two values may be emphasized in the management of aphasic patients. At one point, usually early postonset, we value the quality of language, and we seek its restoration through the treatment we administer. But, at some point, our value may change because improvement in the patient's language slows or stops. We change our value to the quality of the patient's life and emphasize coping with the language deficit that remains. We seek ways for the patient to live the best he or she can with his or her residual language deficits. We look for meaningful ways to help the patient fill his or her days, for family members to find freedom from constant care and attention. We do a lot of the first—attempts to restore language—but I am not certain we do much of the latter—assist in coping with disability. And, because aphasia goes on a long time, and language therapy fills only a small portion of that time, the most important thing we can do for our patients is what we probably do the least.

So the treatment of aphasia has blossomed in the last decade. It has been watered by numerous techniques and fed by alternatives to tradition. The clinician is no longer buffeted by storms that question whether treatment's soil is arable. Empirical evidence indicates it is. But, we continue to seek means for improving the product, and we need to consider treatment that may be necessary after the treatment we have demonstrated we do well has done what it can.

The State of the Art

Treatment implies we have something to do and that that something is, in fact, treatment—it improves whatever is being treated. There are

FIGURE 1-5
How the value emphasized in aphasia therapy may change over time (After Wertz, 1983b)

TREATMENT: A CURE-CARE CONUNDRUM

TIME

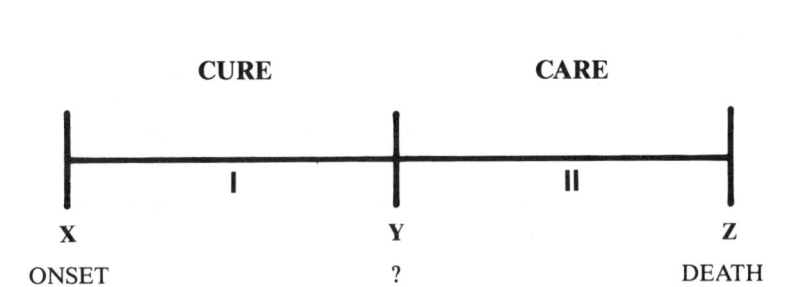

```
        CURE              CARE
    |----------|----------|----------|
    |    I     |    II    |
    X          Y          Z
  ONSET        ?        DEATH
```

           VALUES   EMPHASIS
I = QUALITY OF LANGUAGE   X - Y = RESTORATION OF
II = QUALITY OF LIFE   LANGUAGE
                            Y - Z = COPING WITH DISABILITY

---

many treatments for the aphasic patient, and the treatments administered appear to improve the patient's language. Such is not the case for the other language disorders being discussed here. For the normal aged in a communication-impairing environment, there appear to be several things we can do, both with the patient and with his or her environment. Whether what we can do will improve communication, we do not know. For the patient who suffers the language of confusion, there are fewer available techniques. While we could develop more, it is not clear that they are necessary. Confusion appears to clear in these patients. Whether treatment is the cause of this improvement or whether it speeds the course, we do not know. Language deficit in schizophrenia is seldom treated by the speech pathologist. Whether it should be, or could be, is not certain. We are beginning to see the patient with right hemisphere involvement for therapy. The patient's language, usually, is fairly intact. We are beginning to treat his or her failure to use this language to communicate. Fair enough! These patients have a problem, and it deserves remediation. Whether it is capable of being remediated awaits evidence. Finally, most demented patients are not expected to improve. The treatments we offer are designed to slow loss of communicative ability and to reduce demands to a level where the patient can use what he or she retains. This is treatment if it works. We seek evidence to support our belief that it does.

Some treatment techniques stand out by their resistance to classification. I have suggested a need for techniques that assist the patient to cope with residual deficits remaining after we have worked as much magic as we can. While this was discussed for aphasia, it is appropriate to consider it for the other language disorders. Our experience with assisting patients to cope is limited. Many of us are confined by our clinics and have little knowledge of need—let alone solutions—that exist beyond the setting in which we usually see patients. We need to learn from patients by seeing what they can do and cannot do in their natural habitats. Simply, we need to learn from patients. Linge (1980), a clinical psychologist who suffered head trauma in an automobile accident and made sufficient recovery to return to work, has told us about some things that hinder, and some that help. He suggests eliminating distractions (one thing at a time); developing a highly structured routine, imposing order and developing habit; creating a serene environment, removing emotional tension; keeping situations one-on-one (avoiding groups); if the patient is capable, encouraging excessive note taking; and using all possible sensory channels. Of course, what was best for Linge will not be best for all. But, many of our patients who have walked at least a portion of the road back may verify some of his suggestions, and they probably have others to offer. If we can compile a list, we can cull from it those things appropriate for today's patient.

Finally, we must remember that not all patients want, need, or can gain from treatment. Again, the presence of a problem does not indicate that there is a means for solving it. Too often, I believe, we put patients into treatment when they do not want to be nor should be there. Perhaps there is a message for us in the following AP wire bulletin.

> FT. WORTH, TEXAS (AP). The telephone rang as Mrs. F. A. Farnum was vacuuming her canary's cage. She wheeled to pick up the phone and—whoosh—up the vacuum cleaner nozzle went Joey Boy with one desperate "cheep!" Mrs. Farnum jerked the bag open, grabbed out her canary, and desperately shook off a little dust. Joey Boy was still unrecognizable, so she put him under the faucet. Then, to be sure the bird did not catch cold, she put him under her electric hair dryer. "He has not been singing since then," Mrs. Farnum said, "he just sits hunched over and stares a lot. But he is eating well."

How like many of our patients after they have been probed with PICAs, pelted with PACE, and massaged with MIT. Eating well. Not much singing, but a lot of staring. Sometimes, what follows a traumatic event transcends the trauma.

The State of The Clinical Art

What follows is repetitious, but that is what summaries tend to be. Pride will usually prevent a retreat even in some unimportant matter like doing the dishes before sitting down to dessert. Therefore, this is not a retreat but a reiteration.

The Disorders

I have listed and explored what I think we know about six language disorders that may be present in adults. Are there others? Perhaps. I continue to see patients I cannot classify. Are there too many? Some do not classify communicative deficit in schizophrenia as a language disorder. Some report the right hemisphere patient's language as not impaired; it is his failure to use his good language to communicate effectively that concerns us. Should the disorders listed be subdivided into subgroups? Some do this in aphasia. Some do not.

Little attention has been given to the possibility of coexisting disorders. I have argued against talking about the presence of one disorder *in* another. However, it is possible for a schizophrenic patient to suffer a left hemisphere CVA and demonstrate subsequent aphasia. Similarly, the demented patient who is undergoing gradual cortical atrophy may suffer a left hemisphere CVA and display, in addition to his generalized language deficit, signs of focal aphasia. Therefore, I have no reservations about one disorder coexisting *with* another.

I have not discussed the language of patients who suffer bilateral head trauma, or those who suffer a focal right hemisphere CVA and, later, a focal left hemisphere CVA. Many of these do not fit into the aphasic or demented bins. Where do we put what Eisenson (1947) has called an "inconsistent and unconventional lot?"

Six disorders have been discussed. The proof that aphasia and dementia should be on a list of language disorders has been demonstrated in the clinic and in the literature. Whether environmental influence on the communication of the normal aged, the language of confusion, schizophrenia, and right hemisphere involvement should reside on the list, awaits data and resolution of debate.

Appraisal

The purposes of appraisal, I believe, are to permit diagnosis, determine severity, state a prognosis, and, if appropriate, focus therapy. We do not have a single, economic measure that will accomplish these purposes for all of the language disorders discussed here. In fact, we do not have a battery of several, uneconomical measures that meets our purposes. We have measures for some of the disorders that will meet some of our purposes. Perhaps it is futile to seek the all-purpose appraisal measure. We may have to settle for developing one that tells us who is who, and once that question is answered, branch into appropriate batteries designed to meet the additional needs.

Our experience dictates that we should avoid using measures developed for one disorder to appraise another. Administer a test for aphasia and there is a high probability of observing aphasia in the normal aged, the confused patient, the schizophrenic patient, the patient with a right hemisphere lesion, the demented patient, and, sometimes, small appliances. There is a need to do what Bayles (1982b) has done: develop measures for the disorder being appraised.

Technology offers some hope. LaPointe (1983) has observed that neurology has undergone a technological revolution. PET and CT have contributed mightily to answer the riddle of "lesion, lesion, where is the lesion?" In fact, a new publication, *Journal of Cerebral Blood Flow and Metabolism*, has resulted from technological advance. The influence of technology on speech pathology, LaPointe observes, is nil. "We remain a Model A in a space shuttle world." When technology reaches us, and it will, we must remember it is the product, not the process, that will be productive.

So, we continue to seek the means to meet appraisal's purposes. In aphasia, we refine. In the other disorders, we develop. We attempt to change Mosher and Feinsilver's (1971) summary on schizophrenia: "Despite decades of effort, schizophrenia continues to defy adequate description and classification"—not only for schizophrenia, but also for other language disorders one sees in adults.

Diagnosis

Diagnosis should be more than a system for organizing our files. I have argued that what you call it makes a difference; a difference in prognosis, a difference in management. Aphasia, for example, has a different future and requires a different management than does dementia.

The labels we use and the arguments we have about them are more than exercises in semantics. What we call something is, increasingly, dictating whether there are funds available to pay for its treatment. Second-, third-, and, probably, 15th-party payers provide dollars to care for some disorders, but not others. The war continues to be waged to find funds to pay for aphasia therapy. Try finding support for treating communication deficit in the normal aged resulting from a communication-impairing environment. A physician friend has told me of a dilemma he experienced during World War II, and his solution for it. Regulations restricted the use of penicillin to treat venereal disease in fighter pilots. This "keep them in the air" philosophy shunned many who needed the drug. His solution was a simple, but effective one. His medical unit experienced an epidemic of "gonorrhetic pneumonia." There may be a need, therefore, to relax rigidity and accept "Alzheimer's aphasia" or "environmental aphasia."

It is necessary for us to argue our diagnostic differences to agreement. We need a list of labels that are applied correctly and uniformly. The implications in the diagnosis of one clinician should not require inferences by another.

Treatment

I continue to stress, here and elsewhere (Wertz, 1983a), the need to determine whether our treatment is treatment; that we have something to do for language disorders in adults and that that something works. Some—usually speech and language clinicians—tell me what we do is efficacious. Others—usually physicians and biostatisticians—tell me there is no unassailable evidence that treatment works. I can agree with both, specifically, for the treatment of aphasia. Those I cannot agree with are the ones who suggest we should stop asking the question. The test of repair is whether the broken gets fixed. We ask this of our mechanics, and our patients ask it of us. And, we have some answers for the treatment of aphasia. But, we have little data to back the need for our deeds with other language disorders in adults.

Changes in the treatment of language disorders have come in Toffleresque profusion and have led, in some cases, to Kafkaesque confusion. We seem eager to change our treatments, but we have lost the art of preservation. Rosenbek (1979) has listed some of our cherished treatments that may be abandoned for the new. He suggests looking both ways, to the past and to the future, in the search for methods to mend broken language. The true have not, necessarily, been tried. Neither have the new. Rosenbek advises clinicians to plant their feet in the stream of clinical change and not emerge until they find a few facts about what does, and what does not, work in the management of language-impaired adults.

Along with my suggestion to avoid appraising one disorder with a measure designed for another, I believe we should be wary about administering treatment methods demonstrated to be effective for one disorder to rehabilitate another. We need to refine and to define, to determine what works for whom. Reality orientation cannot be a panacea for all language deficits. The meager literature implies it is. Some have failed to tell us who got oriented, except that they were old. Helm (1978) developed and tested careful selection criteria for patients who profit from MIT. Similar efforts are necessary for the methods we develop and administer to combat the other langauge disorders suffered by adults. In addition, we want to know more than just what works for whom. There is a need to know when, where, and for how long. Should we intervene early postonset or later? Is treatment for a specific disorder done best in the individual treatment session or in a group session, or, perhaps, in the patient's home? How long should treatment go on? Often, it is easier to get a patient into treatment than to get him or her out of it. Often patients have only so many dollars to spend on treatment. Should these be spent early postonset or later; in an intensive, short treatment trial or spaced less intensively over a longer period? I do not think we know.

Finally, there is a need to assist patients beyond treatment's duration. We have focused our efforts on mending language and have done little to assist patients in living with the deficits that cannot be mended. Only recently have we focused our therapy on function. I suggest we extend this to function after therapy has ended. Our source for developing this assistance is a simple one, the patient. The human brain is designed to enable us to accept someone else's experience, celebrate that acceptance, and be someone else for at least an hour. Much of what I know about successful treatment of language disorders in adults I learned by accepting the experience of patients, celebrating that acceptance, and *being* a patient for as long as it took to plan appropriate treatment. Suffering a language disorder, for some, is the straw that breaks. For others, it is the tie that binds. Many we see in treatment leave it to fill their days as best they can, but fill them they do. We can learn from them to save others from emptiness.

The State of This State of the Clinical Art

Most state-of-the-art statements end with "Perhaps in the next 10 years. . . ." Many of the questions and several of the needs posed here are answered and met in the other chapters in this book. Rosenbek (1983) has written an appropriate ending. He acknowledges that we are developing a data base, but we need not fear that all of the questions will soon be answered. As we learn more and more, we learn we need to learn more and more. We have been active. The sparks spread in this chapter have not been stolen from the ashes of inertia. This has represented my view of the state of the art—what it is and what I hope it will become. You, with different biases and more knowledge, will have a different view. That is as it should be, and that is good.

References

Adamovich, B.L. Language versus cognition: The speech-language pathologist's role. In R. H. Brookshire (Ed.), *Clinical Aphasiology: Proceedings of the Conference*. Minneapolis: BRK Publishers, 1981, 277-281.

Adamovich, B. L., & Brooks, R. L. A diagnostic protocol to assess the communication deficits of patients with right hemisphere damage. In R. H. Brookshire (Ed.), *Clinical Aphasiology: Proceedings of the Conference*. Minneapolis: BRK Publishers, 1981, 244-253.

Adelson, R., Nasti, A., Sprafkin, J. N., Marinelli, R., Primavera, L. H., & Gorman, B. S. Behavioral ratings of health professional's interactions with the geriatric patient. *The Gerontologist*, 1982, *22*, 277-281.

Alajouanine, T., Castaigne, P., Lhermitte, F., Escourolle, R., & Ribancourt, B. Etude de 43 cas d'aphasie post traumatique. *Encephale*, 1957, *46*, 1-45.

Alexander, M. P. & Lo Verme, S. R. Aphasia after left hemispheric intracerebral hemorrhage. *Neurology, 30*, 1980, 1193-1202.

Anderson, T., Bourestom, N., & Greenberg, R. Rehabilitation predictors in completed stroke. Final Report. *American Rehabilitation Foundation,* Minneapolis, 1970.

Appell, J., Kertesz A., & Fishman, M. Language in Alzheimer patients. Paper presented to the Academy of Aphasia, London, Ontario, 1981.

Archibald, Y. M., & Wepman, J. M. Language disturbance and nonverbal cognitive performance in eight patients following injury to the right hemisphere. *Brain*, 1968, *91*, 117-127.

Aten, J., Kushner-Vogel, D., Haire, A., & Fitch-West, J. Group treatment for aphasia: A panel discussion. In R. H. Brookshire (Ed.), *Clinical Aphasiology: Proceedings of the Conference*. Minneapolis: BRK Publishers, 1981, 141-154.

Baker, H., & Leland, B. *Detroit Test of Learning Aptitude.* Indianapolis: Bobbs-Merrill, 1967.

Basso, A., Capitani, E., & Vignolo, L. Influence of rehabilitation on language skills in aphasic patients. A controlled study. *Archives of Neurology*, 1979, *36*, 190-196.

Bayles, K. A. Language function in senile dementia. *Brain and Language*, 1982, *16*, 265-280. (a)

Bayles, K. A. Language and dementia producing diseases. *Communicative Disorders: A Journal for Continuing Education*, 1982, *7*,131-146. (b)

Bayles, K. A., & Boone, D. R. The potential of language tasks for identifying senile dementia. *Journal of Speech and Hearing Research*, 1982, *47*, 210-217.

Beasley, D. S., & Davis, G. A. *Aging: Communication processes and disorders*. New York: Grune & Stratton, 1981.

Benson, D. F. Psychiatric aspects of aphasia. *British Journal of Psychiatry*, 1973, *123*, 555-556.
Benson, D. F. Disorders of verbal expression. In D. F. Benson & D. Blumer (Eds.), *Psychiatric aspects of neurologic disease.* New York: Grune & Stratton, 1975, 121-137.
Benson, D. F. *Aphasia, alexia, and agraphia.* New York: Churchill Livingstone, 1979. (a)
Benson, D. F. Aphasia rehabilitation. *Archives of Neurology*, 1979, *36*, 187-189. (b)
Benton, A. L., Van Allen, M. W., & Fogel, M. L. Temporal orientation in cerebral disease. *Journal of Nervous and Mental Disorders*, 1964, *139*, 110-119.
Blazer, D., & Williams, C. D. Epidemiology of dysphoria and depression in an elderly population. *American Journal of Psychiatry*, 1980, *137*, 439-444.
Bloom, L. M. A rationale for group treatment of aphasic patients. *Journal of Speech and Hearing Disorders*, 1962, *27*, 11-16.
Bollinger, R. L. Communication disorders of "chronic brain injured" patients. Unpublished doctoral dissertation, University of Washington, 1970.
Borkowski, J. G., Benton, A. L., & Spreen, O. Word fluency and brain damage. *Neuropsychologia*, 1967, *5*, 135-140.
Branch, C., Milner, B., & Rasmussen, T. Intercarotid sodium amytal for the lateralization of cerebral dominance. *Journal of Neurosurgery*, 1964, *21*, 399-405.
Brandt, S. D., Rose, P., & Lucas, R. Speech-language consultation as part of a multidisciplinary team in long-care facilities. *Communicative Disorders: A Journal for Continuing Education*, in press.
Brosin, H. Acute and chronic brain syndromes. In A. Friedman & H. Kaplan (Eds.), *Comprehensive textbook of psychiatry.* Baltimore: Williams & Wilkins, 1967, 708-711.
Brown, R. Schizophrenia, language, and reality. *American Psychologist*, 1972, *28*, 395-403.
Buschke, H. Method for evaluating language competence in neurological patients. *Transactions of the American Neurological Association*, 1975, *100*, 169-171.
Caton, C. L. M. Effect of length of inpatient treatment for chronic schizophrenia. *American Journal of Psychiatry*, 1982, *139*, 856-861.
Chaika, E. A linguist looks at schizophrenic language. *Brain and Language*, 1974, *1*, 257-276.
Chapey, R. (Ed.). *Language intervention strategies in adult aphasia.* Baltimore: Williams & Wilkins, 1981.
Chapman, J. The early symptoms of schizophrenia. *British Journal of Psychiatry*, 1966, *112*, 225-251.
Chedru, F. & Geschwind, N. Disorders of higher cortical functions in acute confusional states. *Cortex*, 1972, *8*, 395-411.
Citrin, R. & Dixon, D. Reality orientation: A milieu therapy used in an institution for the aged. *The Gerontologist*, 1977, *17*, 39-43.
Collins, M. J. The minor hemisphere (A discussion session). In R. H. Brookshire (Ed.), *Clinical Aphasiology: Proceedings of the Conference.* Minneapolis: BRK Publishers, 1976, 339-352.
Critchley, M. Speech and speech-loss in relation to the duality of the brain. In V. B. Mountcastle (Ed.), *Interhemispheric relations and cerebral dominance.* Baltimore: The Johns Hopkins Press, 1962. 208-213.
Crosson. B., & Warren, R. L. Use of the Luria-Nebraska Neuropsychological Battery in aphasia: A conceptual critique. *Journal of Consulting and Clinical Psychology*, 1982, *50*, 22-31.
Damasio, A. The nature of aphasia: Signs and syndromes. In M. T. Sarno (Ed.), *Acquired aphasia.* New York: Academic Press, 1981, 51-65.
Darby, J. K. (Ed.). *Speech evaluation in psychiatry.* New York: Grune & Stratton, 1981.
Darley, F. L. *Aphasia.* Philadelphia: W. B. Saunders, 1982.

Darley, F. L. (Ed.). *Evaluation of appraisal techniques in speech and language pathology.* Reading, Massachusetts: Addison-Wesley, 1979. (a)

Darley, F. L. The differential diagnosis of aphasia. In R. H. Brookshire (Ed.), *Clinical Aphasiology: Proceedings of the Conference.* Minneapolis: BRK Publishers, 1979, 23-29. (b)

Darley, F. L. The efficacy of language rehabilitation in aphasia. *Journal of Speech and Hearing Disorders*, 1972, *37*, 3-21.

Darley, F. L. Aphasia: Input and output disturbances in speech and language processing. Paper presented to the American Speech and Hearing Association, Chicago, 1969.

Darley, F. L. *Diagnosis and appraisal of communication disorders.* Englewood Cliffs, NJ: Prentice-Hall, 1964.

Davis, G. A., & Wilcox, J. M. Incorporating parameters of natural conversation in aphasia treatment. In R. Chapey (Ed.), *Language intervention strategies in adult aphasia.* Baltimore: Williams & Wilkins, 1981. 169-194.

Deal, J. L., & Deal, L. A. Efficacy of aphasia rehabilitation: Preliminary results. In R. H. Brookshire (Ed.), *Clinical Aphasiology: Proceedings of the Conference.* Minneapolis: BRK Publishers, 1978, 66-77.

Deal, J. L., Deal, L. A., Wertz, R. T., Kitselman, K., & Dwyer, C. Right hemisphere PICA percentiles: Some speculations about aphasia. In R. H. Brookshire (Ed.), *Clinical Aphasiology: Proceedings of the Conference.* Minneapolis: BRK Publishers, 1979, 30-37.

Deal, L. A., Deal, J. L., Wertz, R. T., Kitselman, K., & Dwyer, C. Statistical prediction of change in aphasia: Clinical application of multiple regression analysis. In R. H. Brookshire (Ed.), *Clinical Aphasiology: Proceedings of the Conference.* Minneapolis: BRK Publishers, 1979, 95-100.

Deal, J. L., Wertz, R. T., & Spring, C. Differentiating aphasia and the language of generalized intellectual impairment. In R. H. Brookshire (Ed.), *Clinical Aphasiology: Proceedings of the Conference*, Minneapolis: BRK Publishers, 1981. 166-173.

Delis, D. C., & Kaplan, E. The assessment of aphasia with the Luria-Nebraska Neuropsychological Battery: A case critique. *Journal of Consulting and Clinical Psychology*, 1982, *50*, 32-39.

Denny-Brown, D., Meyer, J. S., & Horenstein, S. The significance of perceptual rivalry resulting from a parietal lesion. *Brain*, 1952, *75*, 433-471.

DeRenzi, E. & Vignolo, L. A. The Token Test: A sensitive test to detect receptive disturbances in aphasia. *Brain*, 1962, *85*, 665-678.

Diller, L., Ben-Yishay, Y., Gerstman, L., Goodkin, R., Gordon, W., & Weinberg, J. Studies in cognition and rehabilitation in hemiplegia. *Rehabilitation Monograph*, 1974, *50*.

Diller, L., & Weinberg, J. Hemi-inattention in rehabilitation: The evolution of a rational remediation program. In E. A. Weinstein & R. P. Friedland (Eds.), *Advances in Neurology, volume 18, Hemi-inattention and hemisphere specialization.* New York: Raven Press, 1977, 63-82.

Di Simoni, F. G., Darley, F. L., & Aronson, A. E. Patterns of dysfunction in schizophrenic patients on an aphasia test battery. *Journal of Speech and Hearing Disorders*, 1977, *42*, 498-513.

Dresser, A. C., Meirowsky, A. M., Weiss, G. H., Mc Neel., M. L., Simon, G. A., & Caveness, W. F. Gainful employment following head injury: Prognostic factors. *Archives of Neurology*, 1973, *29*, 111-116.

Duffy, J. R. What is aphasia? (A discussion session). In R. H. Brookshire (Ed.), *Clinical Aphasiology: Proceedings of the Conference.* Minneapolis: BRK Publishers, 1981, 327-329.

Duffy, J. R. & Keith, R. Performance of non brain-injured adults on the PICA: Descriptive data and comparison to patients with aphasia. *Aphasia Apraxia Agnosia*, 1980, *2*, 1-30.

Eisenson, J. Aphasics: Observations and tentative conclusions. *Journal of Speech and Hearing Disorders*, 1947, *12*, 290-292.
Eisenson, J. Prognostic factors relating to language rehabilitation in aphasic patients. *Journal of Speech and Hearing Disorders*, 1949, *14*, 262-264.
Eisenson, J. *Examining for Aphasia.* New York: The Psychological Corp., 1954.
Eisenson, J. Language and intellectual modifications associated with right cerebral damage. *Language and Speech*, 1962, *5*, 49-53.
Eisenson, J. Aphasia: A point of view as to the nature of the disorder and factors that determine prognosis for recovery. *International Journal of Neurology*, 1964, *4*, 287-295.
Elmore, C. M., & Gorham, D. R. Measuring the impairment of the abstracting function with the proverbs test. *Journal of Clinical Psychology*, 1957, *13*, 263-266.
Emerick, L. *Appraisal of language disturbance.* Marquette, MI: Northern Michigan University Press, 1971.
Ernst, B., Dalby, M. A., & Dalby, A. Aphasic disturbances in presenile dementia. *Acta Neurologica Scandinavia*, 1970, *46*, 99-100.
Fairbanks, H. Studies in language behavior. II. The quantitative differentiation of samples of spoken language. *Psychological Monographs*, 1944, *56*, 19-38.
Farber, R., & Reichstein, M. B. Language dysfunction in schizophrenia. *British Journal of Psychiatry*, 1981, *139*, 519-522.
Feldstein, S., & Jaffee, J. Vocabulary diversity of schizophrenics and normals. *Journal of Speech and Hearing Research*, 1962, *5*, 76-78.
Feldstein, S., & Weingartner, H. Speech and psychopharmacology. In J. K. Darby (Ed.), *Speech evaluation in psychiatry.* New York: Grune & Stratton, 1981, 369-396.
Finkel, S. I., & Cohen, G. Guest editorial: The mental health of the aging. *The Gerontologist*, 1982, *22*, 227-228.
Finlayson, R. E., & Martin, L. M. Recognition and management of depression in the elderly. *Mayo Clinic Proceedings*, 1982, *57*, 115-120.
Foley, J.M. Differential diagnosis of the organic mental disorders in elderly patients. In C.M. Gaitz (Ed.), *Aging and the brain.* New York: Plenum Press, 1972, 153-161.
Folsom, J. Reality orientation for the elderly mental patient. *Journal of Geriatric Psychiatry*, 1968, *1*, 291-307.
Fordyce, W., & Jones, R. The efficacy of oral and pantomine instructions for hemiplegic patients. *Archives of Physical Medicine and Rehabilitation*, 1966, *61*, 359-365.
Forer, S., & Miller, L. Rehabilitation outcome: Comparative analysis of different patient types. *Archives of Physical Medicine and Rehabilitation*, 1980, *61*, 359-365.
Freeman, F. R., & Rudd, S. M. Clinical features that predict potentially reverseable progressive intellectual deterioration. *Journal of the American Geriatrics Society*, 1982, *30*, 449-451.
Friedland, R. Cerebral metabolic indices of dementia pathophysiology. Paper presented to the Veterans Administration Audiology and Speech Pathology Educational Conference, Martinez, CA, October, 1982.
Fromkin, V.A., A linguist looks at "A linguist looks at 'schizophrenic language'." *Brain and Language*, 1975, *2*, 498-503.
Gardner, H. *The shattered mind.* New York: Knopf, 1975.
Gerson, S. N., Benson, D. F., & Frazier, S. H. Diagnosis: Schizophrenia versus posterior aphasia. *American Journal of Psychiatry*, 1977, *134*, 966-969.
Geschwind, N. Writing disturbances in acute confusional states. In N. Geschwind (Ed.), *Selected papers on language and the brain.* Dordrecht, Holland: D. Reidel Publishing Co., 1974. 482-497. (a)
Geschwind, N. *Selected papers on language and the brain.* Dordrecht, Holland: D. Reidel Publishing Co., 1974. (b)

Geschwind, N. The borderland of neurology and psychiatry: Some common misconceptions. In D. F. Benson & D. Blumer (Eds.), *Psychiatric aspects of neurologic disease.* New York: Grune & Stratton, 1975, 1-9.

Golden, C. J., Hammeke, T. A., & Purisch, A. D. *The Luria-Nebraska Neuropsychological Battery: Manual.* Los Angeles: Western Psychological Services, 1980.

Golper, L. A. A study of verbal behavior in recovery of aphasic and nonaphasic persons. In R. H. Brookshire (Ed.), *Clinical Aphasiology: Proceedings of the Conference.* Minneapolis: BRK Publishers, 1980, 28-38.

Goodglass, H, & Kaplan, E. *The assessment of aphasia and related disorders.* Philadelphia: Lea & Febiger, 1972.

Gordon, E., Drenth, V., Jarvis, L., Johnson, J., & Wright, V. Neuropsychologic syndromes in stroke as predictors of outcome. *Archives of Physical Medicine and Rehabilitation*, 1978, *59*, 339-403.

Halpern H. The differential diagnosis of speech and language impairment in the adult neuropsychiatric patient. *Communicative Disorders: An Audio Journal for Continuing Education*, 1980, *5*.

Halpern, H., Darley, F. L., & Brown, J. Differential language and neurological characteristics in cerebral involvement. *Journal of Speech and Hearing Disorders*, 1973, *38*, 162-173.

Halstead, W. C., Wepman, J. M., Reitan, R. M., & Heimburger, R. F. *Halstead Aphasia Test, Form M.* Chicago: University of Chicago Industrial Relations Center, 1949.

Harris, C. & Ivory, P. An outcome evaluation of reality orientation therapy with geriatric patients in a state mental hospital. *The Gerontologist*, 1976, *16*, 496-503.

Harrison, R. J., & Holmes, R. L. (Eds.), *Progress in anatomy* (Vol. 1). London: Cambridge University Press, 1981.

Hartman, J. Measurement of early spontaneous recovery from aphasia with stroke. *Annals of Neurology*, 1981, *9*, 89-91.

Hecaen, H., & Albert M. L. *Human neuropsychology.* New York: John Wiley & Sons, 1978.

Hecaen, H., MaGurs, G., Remier, A., et al. Aphasic croisée chez un sujet droitier bilingue. *Revue Neurologique*, 1971, *124*, 319-323.

Hecaen, H. and Marcie, P. Disorders of written language following right hemisphere lesions: Spatial dysgraphia. In S. Diamond & L. Beaumont (Eds.), *Hemisphere function in the human brain.* London: Paul Elek, 1974, 345-366.

Helm, N. Criteria for selecting aphasia patients for melodic intonation therapy. Paper presented to the American Academy for the Advancement of Science, Washington, DC, 1978.

Helm, N, & Barresi, B. Voluntary control of involuntary utterances: A treatment approach for severe aphasia. In R. H. Brookshire (Ed.), *Clinical Aphasiology: Proceedings of the Conference.* Minneapolis: BRK Publishers, 1980, 308-315.

Helm, N., & Benson, D. G. Visual action therapy for global aphasia. Paper presented to the Academy of Aphasia, Chicago, IL, 1978.

Holland, A. L. Factors affecting functional communication skills of aphasic and nonaphasic individuals. Paper presented to the American Speech and Hearing Association, San Francisco, 1978.

Holland, A. L. *Communicative Abilities in Daily Living.* Baltimore: University Park Press, 1980.

Holland, A. L. Aphasia in head injury. Paper presented to the Clinical Aphasiology Conference, Oshkosh, Wisconsin, 1982. (a)

Holland, A. L. A criticism of the language of the Luria—Nebraska Battery. A paper presented to the Veterans Administration Regional Medical Education Conference on Neuropsychology, Northport, NY, 1982. (b)

Holland, A.L. Observing functional communication of aphasia adults. *Journal of Speech and Hearing Disorders*, 1982, *47*, 50-56. (c)

Holland, A. L. Language intervention in adults: What is it? In J. Miller, D. Yoder, & R. Schiefelbusch (Eds.), *Contemporary Issusses In Language Intervention*, *ASHA Reports 12*. Rockville, MD: The American Speech-Language-Hearing Association, 1983, 3-14.

Hooper, E. *The Hooper Visual Organization Test*. Los Angeles: Western Psychological Services, 1958.

Horner, J., & Heyman, A. Aphasia associated with Alzheimer's dementia. Paper presented to the International Neuropsychological Society, Pittsburgh, 1982.

Horsfall, G. H. An investigation of selected language performance in adult schizophrenic subjects. Unpublished doctoral dissertation, University of Florida, 1972.

Hoyer, W. J., Kafer, R. A., Simpson, S. C., & Hoyer, F. W. Reinstatement of verbal behavior in elderly mental patients using operant procedures. *The Gerontologist*, 1974, *14*, 149-152.

Hudson, A. Communication problems of the geriatric patient. *Journal of Speech and Hearing Disorders*, 1960, *25*, 238-248.

Hughes, C. P., Berg, L., Danziger, W. L., Coben, L. A., & Martin, R. L. A new clinical scale for the staging of dementia. *The British Journal of Psychiatry*, 1982, *140*, 566-572.

Issacs, W., Thomas, J., & Goldiamond, I. Application of operant conditioning to reinstate verbal behavior in psychotics. *Journal of Speech and Hearing Disorders*, 1960, *25*, 8-12.

Jaffe, J. The psychiatrist's approach to managing the aphasic patient. In R. T. Wertz (Ed.), Aphasia: Interdisciplinary approach, *Seminars, Speech, Language, Hearing*, 1981, *2*, 249-258.

Jellinek, H. M., & Harvey, R. F. Vocational/educational services in a medical rehabilitation facility: Outcomes in spinal cord and brain injured patients. *Archives of Physical Medicine and Rehabilitation*, 1982, *63*, 87-88.

Joynt, R.J., & Goldstein, M. N. The minor cerebral hemisphere. In W. J. Friedlander (Ed.), *Advances in neurology, volume 7: Current reviews of higher nervous system dysfunction*. New York: Raven Press, 1975, 147-183.

Kahn, R., Goldfarb, A., Pollack, M., & Peck, A. Brief objective measures for the determination of mental status in the aged. *American Journal of Psychiatry*, 1960, *117*, 326-328.

Kaplan, E., Goodglass, H., & Weintraub, S. *Boston Naming Test*. Experimental edition, 1976.

Keenan, J. S. Communicative disorders and institutionalized geriatric patients. *Communicative Disorders: An Audio Journal for Continuing Education*, 1979, *4*.

Keenan, J. S., & Brassell, E. G. A study of factors related to prognosis for individual aphasic patients. *Journal of Speech and Hearing Disorders*, 1974, *39*, 257-269.

Keenan, J. S., & Brassell, E. G. *Aphasia Language Performance Scales*. Murfeesborough, TN: Pinnacle Press, 1975.

Kertesz, A. *Aphasia and associated disorders: Taxonomy, localization , and recovery*. New York: Grune & Stratton, 1979.

Kertesz, A. *Western Aphasia Battery*. New York: Grune & Stratton, 1982.

Kertesz, A., & McCabe, P. Recovery patterns and prognosis in aphasia. *Brain*, 1977, *100*, 1-18.

Kitselman, K. Language impairment in aphasia, delirium, dementia, and schizophrenia. In J. K. Darby (Ed.), *Speech evaluation in medicine*. New York: Grune & Stratton, 1981, 199-214.

Kleist, K. Schizophrenic symptoms and cerebral pathology. *Journal of Mental Science*, 1960, *106*, 246-255.

Klonoff, H., Fibiger, C. H., & Hutton, G. H. Neuropsychological patterns in chronic schizophrenia. *Journal of Nervous and Mental Disease*, 1970, *150*, 291-300.

Labouvice-Vief, G., Hoyer, W. J., Baltes, M. M., & Baltes, P. B. Operant analysis of intellectual behavior in old age. *Human Development*, 1974, *17*, 259-272.

LaPointe, L. L. Aphasia intervention with adults: Historical, present, and future approaches. In J. Miller, D. Yoder, & R. Schiefelbusch (Eds.), *Contemporary Issues In Language Intervention, ASHA Reports 12.* Rockville, MD: The American Speech-Language-Hearing Association, 1983, 127-136.

LaPointe, L. L., & Culton, G. L. Visual-spatial neglect subsequent to brain injury. *Journal of Speech and Hearing Disorders*, 1969, *34*, 82-86.

LaPointe, L. L. & Horner, J. *Reading Comprehension Battery for Aphasia.* Tigard, OR: C. C. Publications, 1979.

Linge, F. R. What does it feel like to be brain damaged? *Canadian Mental Health*, 1980, 4-7.

Lomas, J., & Kertesz, A. Patterns of spontaneous recovery in aphasic groups: A study of adult stroke patients. *Brain and Language*, 1978, *5*, 388-401.

Lorenze, E., & Canero, P. Dysfunction in visual perception with hemiplegia: Its relation to activities of daily living. *Archives of Physical Medicine and Rehabilitation* , 1962, *43*, 514-517.

Lubinski, R. Speech language and audiology programs in home health care agencies and nursing homes. In D. S. Beasley & G. A. Davis (Eds.), *Aging: Communication processes and disorders.* New York: Grune & Stratton, 1981, 339-356.

Lubinski, R., Morrison, E. B., & Rigrodsky, S. Perception of spoken communication by elderly chronically ill patients in an institutional setting. *Journal of Speech and Hearing Disorders*, 1981, *46*, 405-412.

Ludlow, C. L. Identification and assessment of aphasic patients for language intervention. In J. Miller, D. Yoder, & R. Schiefelbusch (Eds.), *Contemporary Issues In Language Intervention, ASHA Reports 12.* Rockville MD: The American Speech-Language-Hearing Association, 1983, 75-91.

Luria, A. R. *Restoration of function after brain injury.* New York: Macmillan, 1963.

Luria, A. R. *Traumatic aphasia.* The Hague: Mouton, 1970.

MacDonald, M. L. Environmental programming for the socially isolated aging. Paper presented to the 2nd Annual Convention of the Midwestern Association of Behavior Analysis, Chicago, IL, 1976.

McNeil, M. R., & Prescott, T. E. *Revised Token Test.* Baltimore: University Park Press, 1978.

Mayo Clinic, *Clinical examinations in neurology* (4th Ed.). Philadelphia: W. B. Saunders, 1976.

Meehl, P. E. Seer over sign: The first good example. *Journal of Experimental Research In Personality*, 1965, *1*, 27-32.

Metzler, N. G., & Jelinek, J. E. Writing disturbances in patients with right cerebral hemisphere lesions. In R. H. Brookshire (Ed.), *Clinical Aphasiology: Proceedings of the Conference.* Minneapolis: BRK Publishers, 1977, 214-225.

Miller, E. The management of dementia: A review of some possibilities. *British Journal of Social and Clinical Psychology*, 1977, *16*, 77-83.

Mills, R. H. & Drummond, S. S. Analysis of impaired naming in language of confusion. Paper presented to the American Speech-Language-Hearing Association, Detroit, 1980.

Mosher, L. R., & Feinsilver, D. *Special report on schizophrenia.* Publication (HSM) 72-9042. Bethesda, MD: U.S. Department of Health, Education and Welfare, National Institute of Mental Health, 1971.

Moss, C. S. *Recovery With aphasia: The aftermath of my stroke.* Urbana: University of Illinois Press, 1972.

Mueller, D., & Atlas, L. Resocialization of regressed elderly residents: A behavioral management approach. *Journal of Gerontology*, 1972, *27*, 361-363.

Mueller, P. B. Communicative disorders in a geriatric population. Paper presented to the American Speech and Hearing Association, San Francisco, 1978.

Mueller, P. B., & Peters, T. J. Needs and services in geriatric speech-language pathology and audiology. *Asha*, 1981, *23*, 627-632.

Myers, P. S. Analysis of right hemisphere communication deficits: Implications for speech pathology. In R. H. Brookshire (Ed.), *Clinical Aphasiology: Proceedings of the Conference*. Minneapolis: BRK Publishers, 1978, 49-57.

Myers, P. S. Profiles of communication deficits in patients with right cerebral hemisphere damage. In R. H. Brookshire (Ed.), *Clinical Aphasiology: Proceedings of the Conference*. Minneapolis: BRK Publishers, 1979, 38-46.

Myers, P. S. Treatment of right hemisphere damaged patients: A panel presentation and discussion. In R. H. Brookshire (Ed.), *Clinical Aphasiology: Proceedings of the Conference*. Minneapolis: BRK Publishers, 1981, 272-276.

Myers, P. S., & Linebaugh, C. W. Comprehension of ideomatic expressions by right-hemisphere-damaged adults. In R. H. Brookshire (Ed.), *Clinical Aphasiology: Proceedings of the Conference*. Minneapolis: BRK Publishers, 1981, 254-261.

Myers, P. S. & West, J. F. The speech pathologist's role with right hemisphere damaged patients. In R. H. Brookshire (Ed.), *Clinical Aphasiology: Proceedings of the Conference*. Minneapolis: BRK Publishers, 1978, 364-365.

Nelson, H. E., & O'Connell, A. Dementia: The estimation of premorbid intelligence levels using the New Adult Reading Test. *Cortex*, 1978, *14*, 234-244.

Obler, L. K, & Albert, M. L. Language and aging: A neurobehavioral analysis. In D. S. Beasley & G. A. Davis (Eds.), *Aging: Communication processes and disorders*. New York: Grune & Stratton, 1981, 107-122.

O'Connell, P., & O'Connell, E. Speech-language pathology services in a skilled nursing facility. Paper presented to the American Speech and Hearing Association, San Francisco, 1978.

Ojemann, G. A. Subcortical language mechanisms. In H. Whitaker & H. A. Whitaker (Eds.), *Studies in neurolinguistics, volume 2*. New York: Academic Press, 1975, 103-138.

Orzeck, A. Z. *Orzeck Aphasia Evaluation*. Los Angeles: Western Psychological Services, 1964.

Osler, W. The Gulstonian Lectures on malignant endocarditis. *British Medical Journal*, 1885, *1*, 467-470, 522-526, 577-579.

Ostwald, P. F. *Soundmaking: The acoustic communication of emotion*. Springfield, IL: Charles C. Thomas, 1963.

Parsons, O. Current perspectives in neuropsychology. Paper presented to the Veterans Administration Conference on Multidisciplinary Approaches to the Brain Impaired Patient, Topeka, KN, 1982.

Pollack, M., Levenstein, D. S. W., & Klein, D. F. A three-year posthospital follow up of adolescent and adult schizophrenics. *American Journal of Orthopsychiatry*, 1968, *38*, 94-110.

Porch, B. E. *Porch Index of Communicative Ability*. Palo Alto, CA: Consulting Psychologists Press, 1973.

Porch, B. E., Collins, M. J., Wertz, R. T., & Friden, T. Statistical prediction of change in aphasia. *Journal of Speech and Hearing Research*, 1980, *23*, 312-322.

Porch, B. E., Friden, T., & Porec, J. Objective differentiation of aphasic versus nonorganic patients. Paper presented to the International Neuropsychological Society, Santa Fe, NM, 1976.

Porch, B. E., Wertz, R. T., & Collins, M. J. Recovery of communicative ability: Patterns and prediction. Paper presented to the Academy of Aphasia, Albuquerque, NM, 1973.

Porch, B. E., Wertz, R. T., & Collins, M. J. A statistical procedure for predicting recovery from aphasia. In B. E. Porch (Ed.), *Clinical Aphasiology: Proceedings of the Conference*. Albuquerque, NM: Veterans Administration, 1974, 27-37.

Prins, R., Snow, C., & Wagenaar, E. Recovery from aphasia: Spontaneous speech versus language comprehension. *Brain and Language*, 1978, *6*, 192-211.
Rathbone-McCuan, E. Geriatric day care: A family perspective. *The Gerontologist*, 1976, *16*, 517-521.
Ratusnik, D., Lascoe, D., Herbon, M., & Wolfe, V. Group language stimulation for patients with senile dementia, a pilot project. *Aphasia Apraxia Agnosia*, 1979, *1*, 14-29.
Rausch, M. A., Prescott, T. E., & De Wolfe, A. S. Schizophrenic and aphasic language: Discriminable or not? *Journal of Consulting and Clinical Psychology*, 1980, *48*, 63-70.
Raven, J. C. *Coloured Progressive Matrices*. London: H. K. Lewis & Co., 1962.
Rebok, G. W., & Hoyer, W. J. The functional context of elderly behavior. *The Gerontologist*, 1977, *17*, 27-34.
Rioch, M. J., & Lubin, A. Prognosis of social adjustment for mental hospital patients under psychotherapy. *Journal of Consulting Psychology*, 1959, *23*, 313-318.
Rochester, S. R., Martin, J. R., & Thurston, S. Thought process disorder in schizophrenia: The listener's task. *Brain and Language*, 1977, *4*, 95-114.
Rochford, G. A study of naming errors in dysphasic and in demented patients. *Neuropsychologia*, 1971, *9*, 437-443.
Rosenbek, J. C. Wrinkled feet. In R. H. Brookshire (Ed.), *Clinical Aphasiology: Proceedings of the Conference*. Minneapolis: BRK Publishers, 1979, 163-176.
Rosenbek, J. C. Some challenges for clinical aphasiologists. In J. Miller, D. Yoder, & R. Schiefelbusch (Eds.), *Contemporary Issues In Language Intervention, ASHA Reports 12*. Rockville, MD: The American Speech-Language-Hearing Association, 1983, 317-325.
Rubens, A. B. Aphasia with infarction in the territory of the anterior cerebral artery. *Cortex*, 1975, *11*, 239-250.
Sarno, M. T. *Functional Communication Profile*. New York: Institute of Rehabilitation Medicine, New York University Medical Center, 1969.
Sarno, M. T., & Levita, E. Recovery in aphasia during the first year post stroke. *Stroke*, 1979, *10*, 663-670.
Schuell, H. A short examination for aphasia. *Neurology*, 1957, *7*, 625-634.
Schuell, H. *The Minnesota Test for Differential Diagnosis of Aphasia*. Minneapolis: University of Minnesota Press, 1965. (a)
Schuell, H. *Differential diagnosis of aphasia with the Minnesota Test*. Minneapolis: University of Minnesota Press, 1965. (b)
Schuell, H., Jenkins, J. J., & Carroll J. B. A factor analysis of the Minnesota Test for Differential Diagnosis of Aphasia. *Journal of Speech and Hearing Research*, 1962, *5*, 349-369.
Schuell, H., Jenkins, J. J., & Jimenez-Pabon, E. *Aphasia in adults: Diagnosis, prognosis, and treatment*. New York: Hoeber Medical Division, Harper, 1964.
Schwartz, M. F., Marin, O. S. M., & Saffran, E. M. Disassociation of language function in dementia: A case study. *Brain and Language*, 1979, *7*, 277-306.
Sherman, J. A. Reinstatement of verbal behavior in a psychotic by reinforcement methods. *Journal of Speech and Hearing Disorders*, 1963, *28*, 398-401.
Sklar, M. *Sklar Aphasia Scale*. Los Angeles: Western Psychological Services, 1966.
Snyder, L. H., Pyrek, J., & Smith, K. C. Vision and mental function of the elderly. *The Gerontologist*, 1976, *16*, 491-495.
Solomon, K. Social antecedents of learned helplessness in the health care setting. *The Gerontologist*, 1982, *22*, 282-287.
Sparks, R., Helm, N., & Albert, M. Aphasia rehabilitation resulting from melodic intonation therapy. *Cortex*, 1974, *10*, 303-316.

Spiers, P. A. Have they come to praise Luria or bury him?: The Luria-Nebraska Battery controversy. *Journal of Consulting and Clinical Psychology*, 1981, *49*, 331-341.

Spreen, O., & Benton, A. L. *Neurosensory Center Comprehensive Examination for Aphasia.* Victoria B.C.: University of Victoria Neuropsychology Laboratory, 1969.

Stanton, K. M., Yorkston, K. M., Kenyon, V. T., & Beukelman, D. R. Language utilization in teaching reading to left neglect patients. In R. H. Brookshire (Ed.), *Clinical Aphasiology: Proceedings of the Conference*. Minneapolis: BRK Publishers, 1981, 262-271.

Steinhauer, M. B. Geriatric foster care: A prototype design and implementation issues. *The Gerontologist*, 1982, *22*, 293-300.

Strohner, H., Cohen, R., Kelter, S., & Woll, G. "Semantic" and "acoustic" errors of aphasic and schizophrenic patients in a sound-picture matching task. *Cortex*, 1978, *14*, 391-403.

Swisher, L. P., & Sarno, M. T. Token test scores of three matched patient groups: Left brain-damaged with aphasia, right brain-damaged without aphasia, nonbrain damaged. *Cortex*, 1969, *5*, 264-273.

Taylor, M. A., Greenspan, B., & Abrams, R. Lateralized neuropsychological dysfunction in affective disorder and schizophrenia. *American Journal of Psychiatry*, 1979, *136*, 1031-1034.

Taylor, M. M., Schaeffer, J. N., Blumenthal, F. S., & Grissel, J. L. Controlled evaluation of perceptual and motor training therapy after stroke resulting in left hemiplegia. Final Report, Social and Rehabilitation Service, RD 2215-M. Department of Health, Education and Welfare, Washington, DC, 1969.

Todt, E. H., & Howell, R. J. Vocal cues as indices of schizophrenia. *Journal of Speech and Hearing Research*, 1980, *23*, 517-526.

Vignolo, L. A. Evolution of aphasia and language rehabilitation: A retrospective study. *Cortex*, 1964, *1*, 344-367.

Watson, R. T., & Heilman, K. M. The differential diagnosis of dementia. *Geriatrics*, 1974, *29*, 145-154.

Watson, J. M. & Records, L. E. The effectiveness of the Porch Index of Communicative Ability as a diagnostic tool in assessing specific behaviors of senile dementia. In R. H. Brookshire (Ed.), *Clinical Aphasiology: Proceedings of the Conference*. Minneapolis: BRK Publishers, 1978, 93-105.

Weinstein, E. A. Affections of speech with lesions of the non-dominant hemisphere. *Research Publication Association for Research of Nervous and Mental Disorders*, 1964, *42*, 220-225.

Weisbroth, S., Esibill, N., & Zuger, R. R. Factors in the vocational success of hemiplegic patients. *Archives of Physical Medicine and Rehabilitation*, 1971, *52*, 441-446, 486.

Wells, C. E. Refinements in the diagnosis of dementia. *American Journal of Psychiatry*, 1982, *139*, 621-622.

Wepman, J. M, & Jones, L. V. *The Language Modalities Test for Aphasia*. Chicago: Education-Industry Service, 1961.

Wertz, R. T. Neuropathologies of speech and language: An introduction to patient management. In D. F. Johns (Ed.), *Clinical management of neurogenic communicative disorders*. Boston: Little, Brown & Company, 1978, 1-101.

Wertz, R. T. Language deficit in aphasia and dementia: The same as, different from, or both. Paper presented to the Clinical Aphasiology Conference, Oshkosh, WI, 1982.

Wertz, R. T. Language intervention context and setting for the aphasic adult: When? In J. Miller, D. Yoder, & R. Schiefelbusch (Eds.), *Contemporary Issues In Language Intervention, ASHA Reports 12*. Rockville, MD: The American Speech-Language-Hearing Association, 1983, 196-220. (a)

Wertz, R. T. A philosophy of aphasia therapy: Some things patients have not said but you can see if you listen. *Communication Disorders: A Journal for Continuing Education*, 1983, *8*, 1-17. (b)

Wertz, R. T., Collins, M. J., Weiss, D., Kurtzke, J. F., Friden, T., Brookshire, R. H., Pierce, J., et al. Veterans Administration cooperative study on aphasia: A comparison of individual and group treatment. *Journal of Speech and Hearing Research*, 1981, *24*, 580-594.

Wertz, R. T., Kitselman, K. P., & Deal, L. A. Classifying the aphasias: Contributions to patient management. Paper presented to the Academy of Aphasia, London, Ontario, 1981.

Wertz, R. T., & Rosenbek, J. C. Appraising apraxia of speech. *Journal of the Colorado Speech and Hearing Association*, 1971, *5*, 18-36.

Yarnell, P., Monroe, P., & Sobel, L. Aphasia outcome in stroke: A clinical neuroradiological correlation. *Stroke*, 1976, 514-522.

Yorkston, K. M. Treatment of right hemisphere damaged patients: A panel presentation and discussion. In R. H. Brookshire (Ed.), *Clinical Aphasiology: Proceedings of the Conference*. Minneapolis: BRK Publishers, 1981, 281-283.

Yorkston, K. M., & Beukelman, D. R. A system for quantifying verbal output of high-level aphasic patients. In R. H. Brookshire (Ed.), *Clinical Aphasiology: Proceedings of the Conference*. Minneapolis: BRK Publishers, 1977, 175-180.

G. Albyn Davis

Effects of Aging on Normal Language

Aphasia usually arises in persons who already have been undergoing gradual and hardly perceptible changes in their cognitive systems. These changes continue relentlessly throughout the rest of an aphasic individual's life. The changes of aging, a combination of development and decline, reflect the genetically programmed predisposition of the human species to have a limited life span of around 100 years. Diseases, accidents, bad habits, and pollution contribute to a longevity or life expectancy in the United States of around 74 years. Aging of the language function is of particular interest to the speech-language pathologist because of its potential contribution to language behaviors in aphasic clients. It poses a special problem of differential diagnosis within a patient, namely, between the deficits of aphasia and the normal "deficits" which arise from simply being old. Unfortunately, we have little information with which to make this differentiation. As Cohen (1979) observed recently, "Geriatric psycholinguistics is virtually an unexplored territory" (p. 412).

Few investigators have set out intentionally to study the effect of aging on the language behaviors involved in diagnosis and assessment of aphasia. However, several have explored the relationship between aging and language functions indirectly, while answering questions about verbal learning, memory, or problem solving skill. Because language processing is a cognitive function, constrained by short-term memory and involving long-term memory, the study of cognitive changes has some relevance for

©College-Hill Press, Inc. All rights, including that of translation, reserved. No part of this publication may be reproduced without the written permission of the publisher.

the study of language changes. Language research with middle-aged and elderly adults is at a level that is similar to psycholinguistic research of the early 1960s; issues about sentence processing are raised more often with respect to memory than with respect to comprehension. This chapter shows that a few indications are available concerning the effect of aging on the language behaviors impaired in aphasia, such as digit memory span, sentence comprehension, picture naming, and word fluency.

What is Meant By Aging?

There is a fuzzy distinction between normal aging and the pathologies of aging. The physiological changes of each are similar. Certain changes underlying Alzheimer's dementia, for example, simply are exaggerations of the changes associated with normal aging. Also, the heightened prevalence of disease processes in old age makes it difficult to separate the effects of disease from the effects of species-specific programmed decline and simple wear-and-tear on the neurophysiological systems supporting cognitive function. To some extent, we may have to accept susceptibility to disease as part of the normal dynamics of aging. One way of making a distinction between normal and pathological aging is to consider whether cognitive changes are either not significant enough to prohibit independent functioning or, on the other hand, are serious enough to impair independent living sometimes to an extent that requires institutionalization. Still, there is overlap with this criterion, as "the ability to live independently in the community does not by itself rule out the early stages of dementia" (Jacoby, Levy, & Dawson, 1980, p. 249). Some changes of language function in normal aging may be considered to represent a *decline* of function, while pathological changes such as in dementia may be thought of as *deficits* of function.

Many factors contributing to variations of cognitive function are independent of chronological age per se but, nevertheless, often accumulate with increasing age. Living environment, depression, and medications can contribute to the appearance of decline or deficit in cognitive function. In an instructive lesson on medication in the elderly, Salzman (1982) noted that 22% of drug prescriptions in the United States are received by persons of age 65 and older. Almost two-thirds of these involve five to 12 medications every day. Chronological age is not a good predictor of a person's cognitive status, because cognitive status is influenced by so many other factors. One consistent result in research on aging is an increase in variability of performance with increasing age. It is difficult to describe a typical 70-year-old, an age at which one could be a physically fit president of the United States or a legally incompetent resident of a nursing home. The most trustworthy depiction of aging cognition may require (1) identifying functions that develop, remain stable, or decline throughout the life span, (2) comparing the relative rates of development or decline among some functions, and (3) not counting on being able to identify the changes with chronological age per se.

Because of the number of factors that contribute to changes associated with aging, subjects for studying cognitive change should be carefully selected. The typical design for investigating cognitive functions is called a *cross-sectional design*, in which groups of different ages are compared. Different subjects are selected for each group, and so all ages are tested during the same time period. Sometimes only two groups are compared: a young adult group of college age and an elderly group of subjects at least 60 or 65 years of age. Frequently, three groups are used, identified as young, middle-aged, and old. A middle-aged group usually averages around 45 to 50 years of age. As Schaie (1980) noted, it is difficult to obtain data on normal aging beyond the late 60s, because it is more difficult to find old subjects with a health status that is reasonably comparable to young and middle-aged adults.

The principal confounding factor in a cross-sectional design is the *cohort effect* in which certain inherent differences between age-defined populations are present because they were born at different times. A factor such as education level can contribute to differences on cognitive tasks shown by different age groups. The population born between 1915 and 1925 has received less formal education than the population born between 1955 and 1965. Education has been a difficult variable to control, and some investigators have had to settle for reporting educational as well as age differences in describing their subjects. In Borod, Goodglass, and Kaplan's (1980a) norms for the *Boston Diagnostic Aphasia Examination* (Goodglass & Kaplan, 1972), variability of performance was shown to be influenced by age and education. Sometimes different age groups are equated on one measure before being compared with another measure (Feier & Gerstman, 1980). The education variable may be factored out in the statistical analysis of cross-sectional data (Botwinick, West, & Storandt, 1975), or groups are made comparable by creating two young and two old groups of high- and low-education levels (Cohen, 1979).

A basic question in this chapter is how much of an aphasic patient's deficit, if any, can be attributed to aging? A comparison between aphasic subjects and an age-matched normal control group may answer this question in part, but the language function in question may be one that maintains at a constant level across the life span, or one that declines. Therefore, the question cannot be answered confidently until the language function is measured across the life span. Furthermore, generalizations about the intrusion of a naturally declining language function on a deficit of aphasia should be considered with respect to the average age of a peacetime aphasic population. The average aphasic patient is around 55 years of age (Davis & Holland, 1981) and some age-related cognitive changes do not seem to occur until after 60 years. Therefore, aphasia is likely to occur before any significant interaction with aging is possible.

The Classic Aging Pattern

A broad range of cognitive functions is measured with intelligence tests such as the *Wechsler Adult Intelligence Scale* (WAIS). These tests often are divided into verbal and nonverbal (performance) skills, and the effects of aging on these general categories have been studied frequently (for an excellent review, see Schaie, 1980). The classic aging pattern is for verbal measures to maintain a constant level or even increase, and for nonverbal measures to decline gradually, especially in speed of performance. Verbal skills sometimes are referred to as "hold" functions while nonverbal skills are functions that "don't hold." When young adults and old adults are matched in overall score on the WAIS, elderly subjects are better than the young on verbal scores, while young subjects are better than the elderly on nonverbal scores. In longitudinal studies, in which a single group is tested repeatedly over many years, overall IQ is maintained until the decade of the 70s.

Further suggestion of decline in nonverbal functions comes from the norms for Raven's *Coloured Progressive Matrices*. This measure of visuospatial thinking is often given to aphasic adults (see Kertesz & McCabe, 1975). Peak performance of normal adults is reached in the early 20s; and then a decline begins at about age 30, and continues gradually to 85 years (Raven, Court, & Raven, 1976). Johnson, Cole, Bowers, et al. (1979) found age-related decline in music recognition. Because visuospatial and musical abilities are managed primarily by the right cerebral hemisphere, Johnson et al. concluded that the aging process includes a decline of right hemisphere function. In dichotic listening, older subjects were shown to be poorer than younger subjects in recalling digits presented to the left ear, presumably to the right hemisphere (Clark & Knowles, 1973). Kocel (1980) proposed that aging is accompanied by an increased reliance on the left hemisphere as reflected in maintained or improving verbal abilities.

One verbal behavior commonly cited as being maintained, or even increasing, is vocabulary tested by having the examinee define several words.

Suspecting that qualitative scoring of such tests might better capture changes than simple quantitative scoring, Botwinick et al. (1974, 1975) developed a scoring system that was more descriptive of nuances in definitional responses. Their qualitative scoring included attention to the "superior synonym" as the best response, with explanations and descriptions receiving lower scores. First, they compared a younger group ($\overline{X} = 18.4$, 17–20 years) and an older group ($\overline{X} = 70.6$, 62–83 years) matched for quantitative level of vocabulary performance. The elderly group gave significantly fewer superior synonyms. Later, Botwinick et al. (1975) investigated qualitative responses over the life span with groups representing each decade from the 20s throught the 70s. A gradual decline in use of superior synonyms did not appear; instead, quantitative and qualitative scores were maintained at the same level until the 70s, when a sharp decline did occur. These studies demonstrate the value of obtaining data across the life span rather than only from young and old groups. We cannot assume that all changes between young and old age are characterized by gradual decline. Expressing nuances of word meaning appears to hold until rather late in life.

As indicated by nonverbal performance scores across the life span, the most consistent behavioral change seen with advanced age is a decline in success with fast-paced tasks and a "generalized slowness of behavior" (Birren, 1964; Crook, 1979). Regarding intellectual and problem-solving abilities, Schaie (1980) concluded:

> When all is said and done, we conclude . . . [that there is] little change until midlife, except for the need to take somewhat more time to achieve equal levels of accuracy. Slowing sensory and perceptual processes may make it likely that older people, particularly those beyond the early seventies, will tend to make mistakes by simplifying their conceptual frameworks even when this is maladaptive and by failing to spend as much time as their central nervous sytem requires to obtain adequate solutions because of real or perceived pressures "to get on with it." (p. 279)

The Possibility Of An Aging Language Function

If cognitive processes simply slow down in late adulthood, the prospect for an interesting discussion of aging and language function appears to be somewhat restrained. The processes of language comprehension and production may simply be caught up in the generalized slow down.

However, it would be of interest to determine the regions of linguistic performance in which central slowing has an impact on linguistic accuracy and style. Furthermore, we should not rely on the extensive results from intelligence testing as the final word on aging and language function. Such verbal tests are often confounded by demands on general knowledge and problem solving, and they are not aimed at subtle linguistic dimensions of syntax and semantics. Cohen (1979) argued that the verbal subtests of IQ batteries, especially the vocabulary subtest "yield very little insight into the vastly more complex process involved in ordinary language functions such as the comprehension of discourse and written texts" (p. 412). However, the well-established findings on the aging of sensory systems, the central nervous system, and memory are suggestive of the possibility that language function changes with advancing age.

Sensory Functions

Reductions of auditory and visual sensitivity are a common feature of aging. Hearing loss due to aging is called *presbycusis*, and visual acuity decline, similarly, is called *presbyopia*. Elderly people often benefit from hearing aids, lipreading, and special auditory training. They also may require more lighting in a room, and large-print or magnifiers for reading. A gradual decline of color perception begins between ages 30 and 40 with loss of blue-green discrimination and, then, red-green deterioration, beginning around age 55-60 (Voke, 1982).

Much has been written on hearing loss as a function of aging (Beasley & Davis, 1981; Bergman, 1980; Henoch, 1979; Maurer & Rupp, 1979). Such changes certainly affect ability to comprehend. Obler and Albert (1981) relied on hearing loss in the elderly in order to conclude that "language comprehension appears both to deteriorate and to change with aging" (p. 110). However, change in language comprehension was not demonstrated in normally hearing older subjects in Obler and Albert's review. Adequate hearing sensitivity and speech perception are prerequisites for auditory language comprehension, but are not the processes of auditory language comprehension. In order to analyze the linguistic mechanisms of comprehension, processses common to auditory comprehension and reading should be considered.

The Central Nervous System

Slowing of cognitive processes in aging may be attributed to changes in the central nervous system. Valenstein (1981) described certain gross morphological changes. Brain weight increases rapidly until three years, and then increases slowly until 18 years; it remains stable for three decades and "then slowly declines, so that the average brain weight in persons over 86 is 11% less than the mean brain weight of younger adults" (p. 88). Ventricular size is larger in elderly adults, and the cerebral cortex atrophies. Atrophy begins to reach statistically significant proportions around age 50 (Yamaura, Ito, Kubota, & Matsuzana, 1980). The appearance of these changes on CT scans (computed tomography) is important because of the continuing need for age-related normative CT data (Jacoby, Levy, & Dawson, 1980). Certain microscopic changes have also been recorded (Adams, 1980; Valenstein, 1981). Schulz and Hunziker (1980) found atrophy of neurons in the precentral gyrus for subjects aged 85 to 94, but not in subjects aged 65 to 74. Gross morphological atrophy may be attributed, in part, to neuronal dropout or loss of neurons. However, dropout occurs only in certain areas including prefrontal cortex and the hippocampus. The temporal lobe has not been shown to lose neurons in the normally aging brain. In addition, lipofuscin, a yellow-brown pigment, accumulates in nerve and glial cells; neurofibrillary tangles appear in the hippocampus of the normally aging brain; and neuritic or "senile" plaques are seen in the amygdala of the corpus striatum deep within the brain.

Adams (1980) advised: "Aging affects all parts of the body and, in view of the interdependency of organs, there is a certain artificiality in discussing the changes in the nervous system in isolation. Aging in the pituitary and endocrine glands, the liver, heart, and lungs are all capable of altering function and structure of the brain" (p. 149).

Physiological changes have been measured from the aging brain (Michalewski, Thompson, & Saul, 1980; Valenstein, 1981). In the healthy old person, little relationship has been demonstrated between intellect and EEG. Alpha activity decreases over the life span; and in 30% to 70% of the normal elderly, episodic abnormalities of EEG occur over the temporal region. Other changes in EEG are associated with dementia. Several changes in evoked potentials have been observed. The clearest changes are in passive response to visual stimuli; amplitude of early components of the cortical measure increase, and later components decrease. Response latencies are longer. During active processing of stimuli, more latency than amplitude changes are seen. Valenstein (1981) noted that changes in cerebral blood flow occur primarily in adults with dementia.

Memory

The literature on aging contains many vague and sometimes erroneous statements about changes in memory. The normal aging of memory carries important implications for the possibility of aging language function, because this function is supported by the different components of the memory system. An accurate portrayal of aging memory involves attention to its different components. However, memory has been portrayed in two slightly different ways. Thorough reviews of aging memory include one based on a *multistore* memory model (Smith & Fullerton, 1981) and another based on *depth of processing* in primary and secondary memory (Craik, 1977). The multistore model divides memory into sensory memory, short-term memory, and long-term memory. The attention mechanism selects information from sensory memory to be processed in the limited capacity short-term memory. The active processes of language comprehension and expression are carried out within the constraints of short-term memory. The depth of processing orientation, on the other hand, states that variations of capacity and time in memory are related to the extent to which material is processed. Memory is seen to be more of a continuum than a segmentation of qualitatively distinct components.

Attention

Only a portion of information in sensory memory is selected for the depth of processing occurring in short-term memory. Investigators have been interested in the level of processing applied to relatively unattended stimuli. One research paradigm is the dichotic presentation of word lists or messages (see Craik, 1977). Subjects are instructed to recall the stimulus to one ear first, and the other ear second. Stimuli to the second ear are not attended to as well as those to the first ear. The elderly are equal to young adults in recall from the first ear, but show a decline of recall from the second ear. Craik emphasized that the elderly have immediate recall problems under conditions of divided attention. Parkinson, Lindholm, and Urell (1980) found that when the young and old are equated in digit span, the age difference in dichotic listening is eliminated. They concluded that immediate recall of digits, and dichotic memory, are mediated by a common storage mechanism which may decline somewhat with age.

Short-Term Memory

In multistore models, short-term memory (STM) is considered to represent active or working memory which has a limited capacity and in which traces are retained no longer than 30 seconds (Norman, 1976). In the depth of processing orientation, time of storage is seen as continuum; primary memory, which is similar to STM, is considered to represent information that is "in mind," still being rehearsed, and the focus of attention (Craik, 1977).

The possibility of STM deficit has been seized upon as a basis for predicting declines of auditory language comprehension (Cohen, 1979; Feier & Gerstman, 1980). In an article on comprehension, Nash and Wepman (1973) stated: "One aspect of auditory functioning which has been well documented is auditory memory. Short-term memory declines with age" (p. 244). Cohen (1979) cited a common notion that STM in the elderly is more vulnerable to interference than in younger subjects, but Craik (1977) stressed that there is no empirical evidence for this view.

Capacity traditionally has been measured with a test of immediate memory span for digits. Digit span does not change much with age. Craik (1977) cited Botwinick and Storandt's (1974) findings regarding digit spans across several decades: 6.7 (20s), 6.2 (30s), 6.5 (40s), 6.5 (50s), 5.5 (60s), and 5.4 (70s). These findings are fairly consistent. More recently, college students averaged 6.4 digits, and elderly subjects averaged 5.8 digits, a difference which lacked statistical significance (Parkinson, Lindholm, & Urell, 1980). Also, in immediate recall of supraspan word lists, the recency effect, which indicates recall from STM or primary memory, remains unchanged by normal aging (Smith & Fullerton, 1981). Digit span backwards, on the other hand, does decline with advanced age. A consistent conclusion is that significant changes in STM capacity occur only in conditions of divided attention or when reorganization of the material is required.

Scanning of sequences in STM is one process of working memory which may be involved in sentence comprehension. In studies of this process, the subject is presented a set of subspan digits and then must decide whether a particular digit was contained in the set. Scanning is assumed to be the process by which the subject mentally compares the test digit with each item in the remembered set. Response time is taken as a measure of rate of scanning and also to determine whether each set is scanned exhaustively, or only partially. Aging has been shown to decrease the rate of scanning (Anders, Fozard, & Lillyquist, 1972; Madden & Nebes, 1980). A significant decrease is evident by middle-age (Anders et al., 1972). Search time in the elderly is double that of college-age adults. The mode of process, however, does not change with increasing age. Scanning has been studied with aphasic adults, also (Swinney & Taylor, 1971; Warren, Hubbard, & Knox, 1977). Aphasic subjects scan items in STM at a slower rate than age-matched normal controls. Scanning speed in aphasia, therefore, may be a result of focal brain injury and the aging process.

Long-Term Memory

Aging with respect to long-term memory (also, secondary memory) involves several issues. Proponents of multistore and depth-of-processing models agree that we should consider acquisition of information (learning), storage, and retrieval from storage. Smith and Fullerton (1981) made an additional distinction between episodic and semantic memory. Episodic memory pertains to remembering specific events, and is observed in the laboratory with verbal learning tasks of word list recall and paired-associate recall. Semantic memory refers to our general knowledge of the world, and investigators are most interested in how concepts are organized in relatively permanent storage. Semantic memory is studied with respect to recognition and recall of sentence and word meanings.

In general, experimental paradigms require either *recognition* (identification of to-be-remembered material from some choices) or *recall* (production of to-be-remembered material). Recognition has been considered to reflect acquisition, while recall requires acquisition, search for the item in LTM, and retrieval. Recognition usually produces more accurate memory scores. For some time, aging was believed to affect recall but not recognition, because recall is a more demanding function requiring search and retrieval processes. However, in a thorough and forceful critique of research on aging of long-term memory, Burke and Light (1981) cited evidence that recognition memory also declines during adulthood, but to a lesser degree than recall. These reviewers argued that recognition is more complex than it may seem, because it also involves search and retrieval during the initial encoding of information.

Aging appears to affect *acquisition* of new information for long-term storage. Acquisition is facilitated by the application of encoding[1] strategies to stimuli. We may memorize lists with the help of mnemonic devices, such as visual imagery; and when experimental subjects are asked to learn word lists, they recall the most words when they can use visual imagery or their semantic knowledge to organize the words during the acquisition process. It has been suggested that organization and mnemonics are not utilized as spontaneously by the elderly as they are by younger adults (Craik, 1977). That is, the elderly are able to use encoding strategies, but they must often be instructed to do so. Smith and Fullerton (1981) suggested that reduced encoding occurs primarily in acquisition for episodic memory.

While the decline of spontaneous encoding for LTM acquisition has been proposed frequently as a specific characteristic of aging, Burke and Light's (1981) examination of the relevant research produced a different conclusion. The elderly still do not recall as well as the young when instructed to encode word lists. Therefore, aging may reduce the ability to organize new information, even when this ability is not applied spontaneously. Burke and Light suggested that this reduced ability can be thought of as a retrieval problem, namely, in the retrieval of organizational cues from semantic memory that are used to encode information during acquisition.

Aphasic adults fail to use organizational cues from word lists to facilitate recall (Tillman & Gerstman, 1977). Aging acquisition strategies may contribute to the aphasic impairment, but language-disordered patients still are much more impoverished in this mental ability than age-matched controls. Many of Tillman and Gerstman's aphasic subjects ($\overline{X} = 56.6$, 32–82 years) were younger than the elderly groups in many studies of normal aging. Aphasia may eliminate encoding for memory acquisition at any age, while aging simply reduces its efficiency or frequency of use. Also, aphasic subjects failed to benefit from training in the use of organizational cues, while elderly normal adults sometimes did better with such training, but still not as well as younger adults.

Storage of episodic memories has been studied with respect to the susceptibility of memory traces to interference in LTM. As with STM, there is no evidence to support the idea that aging increases vulnerability to interference. Regarding semantic memory, Smith and Fullerton (1981) suggested that amount of information stored probably increases with advancing age. Vocabulary size probably increases, for example (Riegel, 1968). However, organization of sematic memory has not been studied directly with adults of different age groups.

Although the free word association paradigm may be an indicator of semantic organization, the nature of associates given by different subjects is also likely to reflect a preference for using certain aspects of semantic organization. Age differences have been observed with respect to tendencies in providing paradigmatic (in-class) and syntagmatic (other class) responses (Riegel, 1968). The age-related changes include an increase in variability of word associates given by older individuals. Young adults tend to give fairly standard paradigmatic responses, but with advancing age there is a shift to idiosyncratic and more syntagmatic responses. The elderly still use more paradigmatic than syntagmatic responses; the change occurs in the proportion of use of syntagmatic responses. The elderly tend to provide more verbs in response to concrete nouns and to provide more concrete nouns in response to adjectives. They also give more subjective responses, including personal statements and expressions of feelings, attitudes, and stereotypes. Such changes have been interpreted as a response to changing needs and environmental demands as a person proceeds through adulthood. Paradigmatic responses come more readily from young adults who are still influenced by formal education's organization of information according to within-class hierarchical category relationships. The elderly may be more oriented to adapting to real-life situations and, therefore, tend to prefer concrete functional relationships. Smith and

Fullerton (1981) suggested that slight changes in semantic organization may occur, partly due to increases in vocabulary size.

Acquisition and retention of semantic information from complex sentences was studied by Walsh and Baldwin (1977). One sentence was *The rock which rolled down the mountain crushed the tiny hut at the edge of the woods.* An elderly group ($\overline{X} = 67.3$ years) performed as well as young adults ($\overline{X} = 18.7$ years) in acquisition and retention of the semantic content in such sentences, in spite of the older group's inferior performance on the primacy portion of a free recall task. The investigators felt that tests of semantic memory are more valid than tests of episodic memory as measures of memory in one's everyday environment. Therefore, memory may function better for the elderly in real life than in the laboratory, with respect to word lists.

Retrieval from episodic memory involves recall of specific events from the past, and the elderly often appear to recall from the remote past more readily than from the recent past. As Craik (1977) explained, such anecdotal evidence is suspect, because remote events may have been rehearsed more; and so, retrieval comes from the most recent rehearsal. Craik reviewed a few studies in which subjects of various ages were asked to recall either names of high school teachers or news events. Older subjects recalled fewer episodes than younger subjects; and, in the study of news events, recall declined with increasing remoteness of the event dating from one month to two years prior to testing. Smith and Fullerton (1981) suggested that a decline in retrieval reflects the decline of encoding during acquisition of information. Craik (1977) concluded that aging does involve a decline of retrieval from episodic memory.

Retrieval from general knowledge (semantic memory) was studied by Lachman, Lachman, and Thronesbery (1979) who asked subjects to answer 190 questions about history, geography, the Bible, literature, sports, mythology, famous people, news events, and general information. There was no difference in accuracy of recall among young, middle-aged, and elderly adults. This type of investigation leads us into investigations of language function as it is commonly assessed with aphasic patients. Studies of picture naming have been considered to represent retrieval from semantic memory (Burke & Light, 1981; Smith & Fullerton, 1981). These investigations will be reviewed later in this chapter.

Conceptual Style

As was suggested in regard to free word association, experimental behaviors based on the static organization of semantic memory may also be indicative of how one chooses to use semantic memory. Organization of concepts may be structured according to their paradigmatic and syntagmatic relationships to each other, and yet a subject's use of these relationships may be based on other considerations such as their pragmatic value. In addition, investigation of an aphasic's semantic memory is limited because of the language disorder; it is difficult for an experimenter to present words to represent concepts, when the aphasic subject may have trouble comprehending the words. This, in turn, prohibits the investigator's inferences about semantic memory in aphasia. Therefore, studies of semantic organization in aphasia have included pictures to represent concepts, instead of words. Pictures also have been used to study semantic organization styles in young and old normal adults.

Young adults (males, 21.8 years; females, 20.3 years) were compared with old adults (males, 71.3 years; females, 71.6 years) by Kogan (1974) who administered an object-sorting task. Fifty cards with black-and-white line drawings of common objects were used. Subjects were asked to group the pictures however they wished, and results were analyzed with reference to three possible conceptual styles. The elderly subjects formed fewer groups, which Kogan interpreted as indicative of low concept differentiation. The higher differentiations by adults were considered to be suggestive of literalness and weaker imagination. Young adults had a strong inclination toward using one style, namely, *categorical-inferential*, in which each group member is an example of a concept, such as grouping pots and knives as kitchen utensils. The relationship among the members of such groups is often referred to as a class relationship. Around 13% of the young adults' groupings were *relational-thematic*, in which group membership was defined according to functional relationship, such as a match goes with a pipe. Even fewer groupings were *analytic-descriptive*, in which members were defined according to an attribute, such as shape. Like the young adults, the elderly subjects had a strong preference for categorical-inferential groups, but there was a significant shift in the use of relational-thematic strategy to around 25% by the elderly subjects. Kogan's interpretation was similar to interpretation regarding shifts in free word association. The categorical-inferential style was similar to paradigmatic word association, and the relational-thematic style was similar to syntagmatic word pairs. Kogan suggested that the elderly had become more adventuresome in organizing concepts.

Cicirelli (1976) repeated the object-sorting task and compared children (5-7 years), young adults (19-21 years), and three groups of elderly adults (60-69, 70-79, 80-89 years). His results indicated that the shift to more thematic conceptualization is not a gradual one, but occurs during the period of old age. The 60-year-old subjects maintained the same level of thematic organization as the young adults. The increase in thematic classification (and reciprocal decrease in categorical classification) occurred between the 60s and 80s. Also, the elderly left more objects ungrouped; and this characteristic, as well as their style preference, were similar to the children's groupings. Cicirelli suggested that, perhaps, the elderly's strategy represents a decline during old age to an early stage of cognitive development rather than a preference because of needs and demands typical of old age.

Whichever is the case, normal aging does seem to result in a change of conceptual organization style. This consideration might be applied to interpretating aphasic performance in tasks involving the classification and pairing of objects. There has been interest in whether the word retrieval deficit of, at least, certain types of aphasia is related to disorganization of semantic memory (Goodglass & Baker, 1976). Grober, Perceman, Kellar, and Brown (1980) compared anterior and posterior aphasias by asking subjects to decide whether a pictured object belongs to a particular category presented by the experimenter. Aphasic subjects took longer to decide than two normal controls; however, age-related shifts in conceptual style were not considered in design and interpretation. Age of the subjects was not reported. Categorical-inferential and relational-thematic classifications were addressed by Semenza, Denes, Lucchese, and Bisiacchi (1980) with Broca's and Wernicke's aphasics and age-matched controls. Again, ages of the subjects were not reported. A picture-matching task was employed in which one of two choices was matched with a target picture. The relationship of objects within the picture triads was based on either class membership (categorical-inferential) or theme membership (relational-thematic). Broca's aphasics had more difficulty with thematic relationships; Wernicke's aphasics had difficulty with both, but much more so with class relationships. Therefore, a pronounced double dissociation occurred with respect to conceptual style. One is left to wonder whether the normal elderly's tendency to use thematic style has anything to do with these results. The problem may be worth considering, especially because Broca's aphasics tend to be at least a decade younger than Wernicke's aphasics (Harasymiw, Halper, & Sutherland, 1981; Holland, 1980; Kertesz & Sheppard, 1981; Obler, Albert, Goodglass, & Benson 1978).

Studies Of Language Function

Investigations of memory and aging present different prospects as to whether language functions change through adulthood. The effect of aging on language may vary, depending on which language function is being considered, and on the complexity of that function. Certainly with adequate compensation for hearing loss, the elderly should have enough STM capacity to process language, although slowed scanning speed may affect comprehension at some level and in certain situations. Increased vocabulary size and subtle reshaping of semantic organization may enhance flexibility of language use as we become older. Retrieval from semantic memory, as observed in verbal responses, may change primarily with respect to the kind of information a person is retrieving. Changes in language behavior may be due to declining perceptual-motor processes, instead of declining comprehension and retrieval processes. Finally, changes may be due to changing real-life demands as an individual retires, adjusts goals, and moves to a different living environment.

Aphasia Test Norms

A few comprehensive aphasia tests are accompanied by information regarding the performance of age-matched normal adults in order to permit comparison with aphasic performance. For example, Schuell's diagnostic battery was administered to 50 normal adults, and their scores are contained in the test manual (Schuell, 1973). Age was depicted in terms of percentages, with 50% age 60 or older, and 38% below and 62% above age 50 (Schuell, Jenkins & Jimenez-Pabon, 1964). Many tests were performed without error, but tendencies to make mistakes occurred primarily on subtests which are related to formal education, including paragraph reading, oral and written spelling, and writing sentences. Aphasia test norms tell us only about the basic language abilities of a general population of adults representing a wide age range. In order to make them comparable in age to the aphasic population, ages of the normal subjects are skewed in the direction of older adulthood with an average age around the late 50s. As they are generally presented, these data tell us little about whether the language skills on these tests change with increasing age.

On the *Porch Index of Communicative Ability* (Porch, 1967), normal adults with an average age of 56.8 achieve an overall score of 14.46 and a small standard deviation of .33 (Duffy, Keith, Shane, & Podraza, 1976). This score represents performance on a scale from 1 to 16 (15 is the best typical performance) averaged from 18 subtests which cover auditory comprehension, reading, speaking, and writing. Relative to the traditional subtest categories, average performance on gestual subtests is 14.66 (SD = .31); verbal subtests, 14.55 (SD = .33); and graphic subtests, 14.12 (SD = .71). The lowest subtest score is for writing sentences, a 12.57 (SD = 1.78); the only other scores below 14.00 are on verbal description of object function (13.72, SD = 1.01) and demonstrating object function (13.68, SD = 1.31). Therefore, adults generally appear to hold at a high level of performance with the language skills measured by the PICA. The lowest score could be based on varying education levels, as was indicated with Schuell's norms. Because the scoring system is rather rigid, verbal description variation is likely to result from variations of style.

Nevertheless, Duffy et al. (1976) found significant negative correlations between age and PICA scores. The correlations were small, however, with a −.34 for the overall score being typical. The interaction between age and education probably was strong, because education also was correlated significantly with the overall score and was relatively strong for the writing category (r = .53).

Normal adult performance on the *Boston Diagnostic Aphasia Examination* (BDAE) was reported by Borod, Goodglass, and Kaplan (1980a). Age and education contributed to scores on several subtests, and age alone was related only to repeating low probability sentences, word fluency measured by animal naming, narrative writing, and most of the primarily visuospatial parietal lobe tests. The result with parietal tests is consistent with the "don't hold" status of nonverbal intelligence tests. In an unpublished report, these norms were presented according to five age groups: 25-39 years, 40-49 years, 50-59 years, 60-69 years, and 70-85 years (Borod, Goodglass, & Kaplan, 1980b).

If a few basic language functions change as a person ages, then we might want our clinical assessment manuals to include normal adult performance differentiated according to age. Perhaps, scores for young, middle, and late adulthood would be sufficient. Whether this is warranted depends on the susceptibility of language functions to change with aging.

Comprehension

Except for the barriers created by auditory and visual sensory declines, comprehension of words and basic sentences appears to be unaffected by the aging process. Comprehension of sentences by adults is indicated in the norms for the *Auditory Comprehension Test for Sentences* (Shewan, 1979). Over a broad age range of 21 to 76 years (median = 61) adults scored 20.07 of 21 points with little variability (SD = 1.17). In Borod and associates' (1980b) BDAE norms, there was no significant change from the 30s through the 70s in the auditory comprehension subtests. A slight drop can be seen in the 70s for "complex ideational material," which includes yes/no questions about short paragraphs, but this change was not statistically significant. Age and education had a significant impact on the subtest for reading sentences and paragraphs; the age effect occurred again as a drop in the 70s, as opposed to a gradual decline over the life span. This is the same pattern across the decades shown with superior synonym definitions.

Studies of Memory

It is tempting to infer an aging effect on comprehension from certain studies of semantic memory. Equal accuracy among young, middle-aged, and elderly adults in answering questions indicates that there is no change in understanding them (Lachman et al., 1979). Camp (1981) studied ability to answer visually presented "direct-access" questions such as *What man's wife was turned into a pillar of salt?* (answer: Lot) and "inferential" questions such as *What U.S. President was the first to see an airplane fly?* (answer: T. Roosevelt). Access to semantic memory was tested in two recognition paradigms. Subjects included members of MENSA and emeritus professors. Elderly and young adult groups did not differ in accuracy of response for both types of questions, but the elderly group was slower in responding when yes/no answers were required. Camp interpreted slower responses as slower processing of the problem in addition to slower perceptual-motor speed. In such a task, comprehension is not observed as purely as the psycholinguist would like; the subject's task involves dealing with one's fund of knowledge, known to be highly variable among individuals.

Ability to encode inferences from sentences was examined in a study of sentence list recall (Till & Walsh, 1980). Young ($\overline{X} = 20.4$ years) and old ($\overline{X} = 68.4$ years) subjects were compared in free and cued recall of 16 sentences, such as (1) *The pupil carefully positioned the thumbtack on the chair* and (2) *The chauffeur drove on the left side*. In the condition of cued recall, the subject was given a cue to the sentence to be produced. Cues were based on information that could be inferred from the sentence, such as *prank* from (1) and *England* from (2). Young adults recalled more sentences in the cued condition than in the free recall condition, indicating that they encoded inferences from the sentences. However, the old adults recalled fewer sentences in the cued condition than in the free recall condition, indicating some difficulty in detecting inferences from sentences.

It is not clear whether Till and Walsh's finding can be generalized to drawing inferences during sentence comprehension. In a subsequent experiment, these investigators had their subjects engage in a "comprehension" task during sentence list acquisition (Till & Walsh, 1980). Subjects were asked to produce written responses that might reflect sentence meanings. Then, in cued recall of these sentences, the previous age difference was eliminated as the old adults equalled recall by the young adults. Comprehension abilities during list presentations were not compared; however, we might infer that aging does not affect comprehension of inferences as much as it affects the use of encoding in the learning and recall process.

Sentence Comprehension

We begin to get a look at comprehension directly in an investigation of recoding with a verbal-pictorial verification task. Nebes (1976) was concerned about the elderly's tendency not to use imagery or elaborative encoding strategies in acquisition of information for episodic memory. Would the elderly exhibit a similar decline in simply recoding a verbal stimulus into a pictorial code during a verification task? Models of the mental processes underlying sentence verification have included two stages: (1) encoding the stimuli into mental representations, and (2) comparing the mental codes of the two stimuli. Response times have been assumed to include time to carry out each of these stages. In Nebes's study, elderly adults ($\overline{X}=69$ years) took longer than young adults ($\overline{X}=19$ years) in determining a match between a phrase *(square outside circle)* and a picture, and in matching two pictures. The verbal-picture condition took longer than the picture-picture condition, and this additional time was assumed to consist of the formulation of a mental pictorial image from the phrase. This time difference between conditions was the same for the young and old adults, indicating that aging does not affect encoding in this task. Nebes's analysis indicated that the mental process of comparing the two pictorial cues was the locus of slower processing by the elderly.

Sentence verification has been of some interest in the study of comprehension in aphasia (Brookshire & Nicholas, 1980; Just, Davis, & Carpenter, 1977), and effect of aging on this function might be worth exploring further. We might anticipate that aging will affect latency but not accuracy, while aphasia affects latency and accuracy.

Walsh and Baldwin's (1977) previously cited study involved recalling meaning derived from some fairly complex sentences such as *The warm breeze blowing from the sea stirred the heavy evening air.* In a measure of comprehension accuracy, no differences were found between old adults ($\overline{X}=68$ years) and young adults ($\overline{X}=19$ years). A similarly complex comprehension level was tested by Feier and Gerstman (1980). Adult subjects heard sentences with center-embedded and right branching relative clauses about animals doing a variety of unusual things. Each type of clause was either subject relative or object relative:

1. The giraffe that bumped into the cow kicked the hippo.
2. The lion that the elephant pushed jumped over the horse.

3. *The giraffe kicked the hippo that bumped into the cow.*
4. *The lion jumped over the horse that the elephant pushed.*

Young adults (18–25 years) and older adults (52–58) years, 63–69 years, 74–80 years) indicated comprehension by manipulating small animal or human figures. Comprehension accuracy held between the young adult period and the 50s; it dropped in the 60s, and dropped further in the 70s. There was no interaction between sentence type and age. Feier and Gerstman's study was the first indication of an effect of aging on comprehension accuracy. Lack of pragmatic reality in these sentences may combine with their complexity to produce this aging effect.

One might predict that a similar effect would occur with the Token Test (DeRenzi & Vignolo, 1962), especially with the complex instructions of Part V. This test of auditory comprehension also possesses little pragmatic reality in instructions to manipulate tokens of different color, size, and shape. When this test was given to nonbrain-injured adults, age was found not to be a factor in test performance (DeRenzi, 1979; Orgass & Poeck, 1966; Swisher & Sarno, 1969). Instead, DeRenzi (1979) found that years of schooling had a greater effect. Noll and Randolph (1978) gave the test to 25 normal adults ($\overline{X} = 54$, 29–76 years), and these subjects averaged only 2.2 errors on Part V. They averaged 59.7 of 62 points on the whole test with a standard deviation of 2.2 (range 52–62). There is little evidence of age-related decline in Token Test performance. We could be suspicious of the decline in color discrimination cited earlier as possibly influencing Token Tests scores after age 60.

An age effect on reading comprehension occurred with lengthy sentences describing an event and containing one date and one country name. Such sentences were used in a study of recall, but a test of comprehension was included (Gordon, 1975). Four multiple choice questions were asked about each of five sentences, such as *In the year 1958 a crisis in Denmark occurred when rural lobbyists tried to persuade the parliament to increase duties on man-made textiles.* Elderly adults ($\overline{X} = 71$ years) were less accurate than young adults ($\overline{X} = 21$ years).

Cohen (1979) asked subjects to detect semantic anomalies in sentences such as *Mary had lost weight—her dress was too small.* Subjects were grouped according to age and education level: old and highly educated ($\overline{X} = 68$, 65–79 years), old with low education ($\overline{X} = 79$, 70–95 years), young and highly educated ($\overline{X} = 24$, 20–29 years), and young with low education ($\overline{X} = 24$, 18–29 years). Both elderly groups made significantly more errors than their respective young adult groups, with the difference being greater between the less-educated age groups. Cohen added that the most striking aspect of the less-educated elderly's performance was "the large number of value judgements which were based on irrelevant moral grounds rather than on semantic or logical considerations . . . it seems as if personal values are more salient than semantic coherence for this group" (p. 423). Whether the moral grounds were irrelevant may be a judgment by the experimenter. Nevertheless, there are some similarities here with the findings with free word association, namely, the tendency to give idiosyncratic and evaluative responses.

Paragraph Comprehension

A few investigators have found aging effects at the discourse level of comprehension. As in some aphasia tests, this level is tested by having subjects listen to, or read, a short paragraph, and then answer questions about the content in the paragraph. A few specific issues were addressed in the studies: (1) Does aging have a differential effect on comprehension of explicit and implicit meaning in a text (Belmore, 1981; Cohen, 1979)? The previously cited difficulty in detecting inferences for cued recall indicates that aging may impinge upon comprehension of implicit information more than explicit information. (2) Aging may affect task performance, especially when a paragraph is read to subjects, because of a decline in recall of the paragraph, rather than because of a decline in comprehension (Belmore, 1981; Taub, 1979). (3) As indicated by Cohen's study on detecting semantic anomalies in sentences, aging may be a factor, depending on the education level or basic lifelong language ability of the subject (Taub, 1979). (4) Does aging affect the ability to comprehend jokes (Schaier & Cicirelli, 1976)?

In studies of inferencing, subjects are asked two types of questions about a paragraph. One type asks about facts or information explicitly stated in the paragraph. The other type asks about inferences or information implied by a paragraph. Explicit and implicit questions are used in the *Reading Comprehension Battery for Aphasia* (LaPointe & Horner, 1979). Cohen's (1979) normal subjects were divided according to education level, described in the previous section. He found an age-related reduction in accuracy for implicit questions but not for explicit questions in high- and low-educated groups.

While Cohen's study involved listening to paragraphs, Belmore (1981) examined inferencing with a reading task in which subjects verified true and false statements about a paragraph. Here is one example (p. 318):

STIMULUS PARAGRAPH: Everyone sat down for dinner.
There was a crystal vase on the long

	table. The guests all admired the lovely roses.
TRUE PARAPHRASE:	There was a vase on the table.
TRUE INFERENCE:	There were roses in the vase.

Belmore measured accuracy and response latency for an old ($\overline{X} = 67$ years) and young ($\overline{X} = 18$ years) group. With respect to accuracy, the dependent variable in Cohen's study, there was no age effect when statements were verified immediately after reading the paragraph. However, when only the statements were presented again, requiring a much greater demand on paragraph retention, the old group was less accurate than the young group. Unexpectedly, the age-related reduction occured more for explicit information (the paraphrase) than for implicit information (inference). The older subjects took significantly longer than the younger subjects to verify both types of statements. Belmore concluded that the general decline in speed was not specific to explicit or implicit meaning. In the condition of immediate comprehension testing, whether there is an age effect on inferencing is equivocal. This effect may depend on how paragraph comprehension is tested. "clearly, such an impairment is not an inevitable result of the aging process" (Belmore, 1981 p. 321).

Belmore's study points to the conclusion that age effects in paragraph comprehension are related more to recall demands than to comprehension per se. An investigator may look for changes in comprehension as evidence that the age effect in a recall task occurs at the acquisition (encoding) stage. Taub (1979) studied paragraph comprehension in three conditions: (1) questions were presented with the paragraph, and unlimited time was given to read and answer; (2) unlimited time for paragraph reading was provided, but questions were presented after the paragraph was removed, and (3) after the first condition, the same questions were presented, placing an even greater demand on paragraph retention. Without demands on retention, called the "comprehension" condition, there was greater accuracy than with (2) and (3). Old subjects ($\overline{X} = 70$ years) were less accurate than young subjects ($\overline{X} = 27$ years) in comprehension and in the recall conditions (2) and (3). Also, the elderly were less reliable in their answers. That is, they tended to change their answers in condition (3), which involved the same questions as condition (1). Taub concluded that the age effect in discourse comprehension requiring recall can be attributed to inadequate acquisition of the paragraph when presented.

Furthermore, Taub (1979) found that the age-related reduction in paragraph comprehension occurred with subjects classified as low and middle in giving definitions on the WAIS vocabulary test. The subjects classified as high in vocabulary did not show an age effect. This is similar to Cohen's finding that recognition of anomalous sentences produced an age effect for the less educated subjects. Therefore, aging may influence language comprehension only in individuals with lower verbal abilities throughout adulthood. However, this is not necessarily so, because Belmore's (1981) subjects were relatively well educated.

A person may have to do some inferencing in order to get the point of a joke. Schaier and Cicirelli (1976) compared three older groups in their 50s, 60s, and 70s as to their ability to comprehend paragraph-length jokes. Twelve jokes were based on Piagetian concepts of conservation of mass, weight, or volume; and these were compared with 12 "noncognitive" jokes. Here are two of the conservation jokes:

> MASS: Mr. Jones went in to a pizza parlor and ordered a whole pizza for his dinner. When the waiter asked if he wanted it cut into 6 or 8 pieces, Mr. Jones said: "Oh, you'd better make it 6! I could never eat 8 pieces."
>
> WEIGHT: George and Bob had a raft they made out of old logs. One day they took the raft out into the middle of the lake for a picnic lunch. As soon as they finished their lunch the raft began to sink. George said, "Oh, no! We've eaten too much" (p. 579).

Schaier and Cicirelli measured appreciation of the jokes with a rating scale for funniness. Comprehension was determined by asking subjects to explain what was funny about each joke.

What was funny about the results was that with less comprehension of humor, there was more appreciation. In comparing the two types of jokes, conservation jokes were comprehended better, but appreciated less. The following age effects were found: (1) the group aged 50-59 appreciated the jokes less than the older groups, (2) there was an age-related decline in comprehension, and (3) gender interacted with the comprehension results, as the reduction in females occurred between the 60s and 70s, while the reduction in males occurred sooner, between the 50s and 60s. Schaier and Cicirelli concluded that decline in humor comprehension accompanies a decline in cognitive ability, while appreciation increases until the cognitive demands of the joke are too great and the joke is not understood at all.

Summary

Compared with the voluminous research on adult psycholinguistics with college students as subjects, very little has been done to study aging and comprehension of language. It appears that comprehension accuracy for sentences holds throughout the life span, except for semantically unusual and syntactically complex sentences. With these special sentences, decline may begin in the 60s. Depth of comprehension, especially for discourse, may be reduced with old age in the derivation of inferences from statements and paragraphs. In tasks of discourse comprehension, when new information must be acquired for answering questions, retention may be more of a factor than comprehension per se. However, there is some evidence that comprehension at this level declines, a conclusion sometimes phrased in terms of encoding at the acquisition stage of a recall task.

The term "decline" should be used carefully, especially to depict results from the usual comparison of only a young and an old group. This comparison does not tell us whether the change is gradual from early adulthood, begins at middle age, or begins even later in adulthood. Many of the studies already done need to be replicated with groups between youth and old age, and with elderly groups divided into decades, as in the study of joke comprehension. Changes did not occur until the 60s or 70s for object sorting, giving definitions, and sentence comprehension. Also, education and/or intelligence may interact with aging of the language function, another variable leading to qualification of any age effect.

Word Retrieval

The response form in previously mentioned studies of semantic memory has been word retrieval. The paradigms included free word association and question answering. Aging is accompanied by a shift to more syntagmatic and idiosyncratic word associations than in young adulthood. Retrieving answers about stored knowledge does not appear to change, but accuracy when inferencing is involved appears to drop beginning in the 60s. There is some slowing of response time. Aging of word retrieval per se has been investigated with respect to picture naming and word fluency, usually in order to examine retrieval from semantic memory.

Convergent Retrieval

Word retrieval is often assessed by having subjects converge on one lexical item. The most common clinical paradigm is object naming, called *confrontation naming*. There was no effect of age on the BDAE subtests of responsive naming (answering questions) and body part naming (Borod et al., 1980a, 1980b). Age-related norms were determined for the *Boston Naming Test* (Kaplan, Goodglass, & Weintraub (1976) consisting of 85 line drawings for words of varied frequency of use. In terms of number correct, the following average scores were obtained: 72.8 (under 40 years),

76.5 (40-49), 75.6 (50-59), 70.8 (60-69), and 63.2 (over 70). Again we see a decline beginning in the 60s. However, the authors warned that education could have been a factor, because the oldest groups had fewer years of schooling. Education was a significant factor: 57.0 (0 -8 years), 71.3 (9-12 years), and 75.9 (13-16 years). Furthermore, only six subjects were in the group over age 70, while 30 subjects were in the 60-69 age group. Nevertheless, Borod, et al. (1980a) suggested that the cut-off score for diagnosing aphasia be lowered for adults age 60 and older.

Thomas, Fozard, and Waugh (1977) analyzed the few errors made by their subjects on a picture-naming task. Five age groups were studied: 25-35, 36-45, 46-55, 56-65, and over 65. In the four groups from age 25 to 65, 76% of the errors were semantic confusions, errors in the same semantic category as the correct word. Only 12% of the errors were perceptual, a name of an object that was perceptually similar to the pictured object. In the oldest group, over age 65, there was an increase in perceptual errors to 35%. Therefore, in this age group, confrontation naming may be influenced by the visual decline common in the elderly.

Distinguishing between perceptual-motor processing and the central process of interest has been an important consideration in aging research. Anatomical and physiological aging definitely produce changes in perceptual-motor processing, and the status of a central psycholinguistic process must be extracted from tasks that include perceptual-motor functions. Thomas et al. (1977) attempted this distinction in measuring picture-naming latency. They had found that naming latency increases with age. Picture-naming latency was assumed to consist of perceptual-motor time (picture recognition + word formulation) and lexical search and retrieval time. Presenting the word with the picture to be named was assumed to generate perceptual-motor time only. This assumption was reinforced by the finding that word frequency did not affect naming latency in this condition, but did affect latency in naming the picture only. The age effect on confrontation naming latency was greater for picture naming than for picture + word naming. Thomas et al. concluded that while an age-related decline of perceptual-motor speed is a component of decreased speed in picture naming, aging also affects speed of lexical search and retrieval. In addition, practice in naming the same pictures reduced the diferences among age groups.

Eysenck (1975) analyzed word retrieval time by comparing naming of a category and letter, such as "fruit-A," with recognition of correct category-instance pairs, such as "fruit-apple." The recognition condition was assumed to represent a "decision" component of the retrieval process, namely, deciding whether the lexical search process was successful. Older subjects (55-65 years) took longer than the younger subjects (18-30 years) in the recognition task but not in the retrieval task. Eysenck concluded that the decision process is affected by aging, but not the search process. However, if we are to assume that decision is included in the process of naming to category + letters, then decrease in decision time should be reflected in this condition, also. Therefore, either the recognition condition did not truly assess a decision process, or a decision process is not a component of word retrieval in the category + letter-naming task.

Familiarity of objects contributes to the speed in naming them. Poon and Fozard (1978) looked into whether familiarity interacts with age to produce variation in object naming latency. They compared young (18–22 years), middle-aged (45–54 years), and older (60–70 years) adults in their naming of contemporary and dated objects. Pictures of dated objects were selected from 1910 commercial catalogues. Dated unique objects (churn, wringer) were compared with contemporary unique objects (calculator, hair dryer). Objects common to each period, in old and new versions, also were presented (razor, shoes). Young adults named contemporary unique objects faster than did the older adults, while the older adults named dated unique objects faster. Age did not affect the speed of naming common contemporary objects. Therefore, object familiarity is another variable that determines whether there will be an age effect in ease of lexical retrieval.

Divergent Retrieval

Divergent behavior involves a quantity and variety of responses instead of a convergence on one response (Chapey, Rigrodsky, & Morrison, 1977). Word fluency is a common measure of divergent word retrieval. In tests of word fluency, the subject is asked to produce as many words as possible which begin with a particular letter or belong to a particular concept category. Usually there is a brief time limit. Kamin (1957) found that elderly persons had lower word fluency scores than high schoolers when given an initial letter. Institutionalized elderly had lower scores than the elderly living in the community. Borod et al. (1980a, 1980b) found a gradual decline across the life span in animal naming, a word fluency activity which is affected by even nonspecific sites of brain damage. Adults under age 40 average 26.6 animal names in 60 seconds, while adults in their 50s produce 21.4, and adults in their 70s produce 18.6. An aging component, therefore, is likely to exist in an aphasic patient's performance on this task. This component probably is small, because aphasic persons produce an average of only 6.3 names with a standard deviation of 6.0 (Goodglass & Kaplan, 1972).

Stones (1978) used word fluency with categories and letters to study aging and semantic memory. In a unique effort to control for cohort effects, each older subject ($\overline{X} = 49$ years) was the parent of at least one subject in the younger group ($\overline{X} = 17$ years). The middle-aged group was significantly more diversified in its responses than the younger group. It is not clear from the article as to exactly what this meant with respect to the nature of word fluency responses. Nevertheless, Stones suggested that there are two sources of explanation. One is that the processes of semantic memory change. The second is that environmental influences change from the formal education period to the individual differences of experience by middle age.

Battig and Montague (1969) presented norms for the production of words from 56 categories. These norms were obtained from university undergraduate students. Howard (1980) investigated whether these norms would be applicable to middle-aged and old adults. The *dominance* of a response was of particular interest, namely, the order of frequency with which different words are produced in each category. Howard presented 21 of the 56 categories to young (20-39 years), middle-aged (40-59 years), and elderly (60-79 years) adults. The groups were comparable in education level. Many of Battig and Montague's categories were omitted partly in order to eliminate any obvious cohort effects that might occur with categories such as "A type of dance." Subjects were given 30 seconds to write their words for each category. Howard found a significant decrease in the average number of responses per category with increasing age: young, 7.05; middle-age, 7.12; and old, 6.06. This decrease was indicative of slower performance with age. However, the dominance of category members was similar among the age groups. Also, unlike free word association, variability of word fluency between subjects did not increase with age. Howard concluded that the Battig and Montague norms would be valid for research with any adult age group.

Summary

There may be some decline of accuracy in confrontation naming after age 60, especially when tested with a wide range of word frequency. Word retrieval speed certainly decreases, perhaps due to a combination of effects on peripheral and central (cognitive) processes. The decrease in speed explains the reduction in number of responses on word fluency tasks which are administered with a time limit of 60 seconds. Variables that influence performance by the elderly on tasks of word retrieval include: (1) the perceptual-motor changes of aging, (2) educational differences, and (3) familiarity with objects that are uniquely contemporary.

Sentence Production

Age did not affect the speed or gramaticality of sentence production when subjects were asked to incorporate word pairs in creating their sentences (Nebes and Andrews-Kulis, 1976). However, elderly subjects performed less well than young adults when discourse was investigated in a story-retelling task (Cohen, 1979). Again, responses depended in part on retention of experimental stimuli. The elderly provided fewer correct propositions, fewer modifiers, and fewer summary propositions representing the gist of the story. These differences were seen in Cohen's high- and low-educated groups. Also, the elderly, especially in the low-educated group, made many more "errors of anaphoric reference" such as the use of pronouns for which the referent was unclear. Buckingham (1979), by the way, had found that "indefinite anaphora" is a common occurrence in the fluent language of anomic aphasia. We should consider, nevertheless, that the reduction of encoding for episodic memory may contribute to the changes of verbal expression observed by Cohen.

With a picture-description task in a study of aphasia, Yorkston and Beukelman (1980) presented some pertinent data concerning amount of information conveyed in connected discourse and efficiency of communication. Younger normal adults ($\overline{X}=31$ years) were compared with older normal adults ($\overline{X}=73$ years) as control groups. These groups did not differ in amount of information expressed nor in number of syllables per minute. However, regarding message efficiency, the older group produced significantly fewer content units (basic ideas) per minute than the younger group.

Functional Communication

So far, aging has been considered with respect to linguistic function measured in experimental paradigms which minimize natural communicative context. With Holland's (1980) norms for *Communicative Abilities in Daily Living* (CADL), we can begin to consider whether aging affects ability to understand and convey messages by any means, including language. The CADL consists of a series of communication problems based on real-life situations in which extralinguistic context can be used to comprehend, and any communicative mode can be used to get a message across. The norms include 130 normal adults classified according to age and according to living environment (institutionalized versus noninstitutionalized). Holland found that both factors contribute to performance on the CADL. The group over 65 scored significantly below three younger age groups (below 46, 46-55, 56-65). Also, in the two oldest age groups, noninstitutionalized subjects tended to score higher than the institutionalized subjects. We might assume that institutionalized subjects are more affected by the aging process. In sum, however, it appears that aging has some influence on communicative abilities that are more general than language function per se.

Concluding Remarks

If aging has a significant impact on language function, there would be at least three conspicuous clinical implications: (1) If test scores are to be used to identify language deficit (as opposed to decline), norms and cutoff scores should be differentiated according to age. This has been done with the CADL (Holland, 1980) and has been suggested for the BDAE (Borod et al., 1980a). (2) Once aphasia has been identified in a patient, the clinician may need to identify the degrees to which aging and aphasia contribute to performances with different language functions. This review indicates that paragraph comprehension, naming, and word fluency might be targets of concern, especially for patients over 60 years old. (3) The degree to which aging is a factor may influence prognosis and decisions about emphasis in treatment.

Though there are some definite signals from the research that aging influences language functions, we should be careful about searching for aging language in our patients until more data are obtained. We are on firmer ground when we consider perceptual and motor factors in language performances. A life-span psycholinguistics has not blossomed into a data-rich field of study. Our theories of adult language processing have been built almost exclusively from data produced by college-age subjects. In the study of aging, more effort has gone into investigations of learning and memory, instead of the immediate comprehension and production that occurs in a conversation. However, sometimes purely linguistic behaviors have been the means by which investigators have examined issues in learning and memory, and so the relevant psycholinguistic questions have to be applied to this research on a post hoc basis. Currently keywords for finding research on word retrieval, for example, include "semantic memory" or "recall."

A life-span psycholinguistics would focus increased attention on the possibility of hearing loss and presbyopia in elderly subjects. Just as attempts are made to equate age groups on education, these groups might also be equated on auditory and visual perception. Several issues can be addressed in this research. One is whether changes occur as a gradual decline over the life span or as a decline beginning in old age. A gradual decline would impact on aphasic patients of both middle and old age, while a later decline would impact primarily on elderly patients. We need to learn more about when the slowing of processing speed begins to be accompanied by reductions in accuracy. One specific question pertains to the slowing of STM scanning rate. This decline may only affect comprehension of complex sentences, such as those investigated by Feier and Gerstman. As has been found with studies of problem solving, the elderly may retain all necessary cognitive abilities to perform as younger subjects if input is slowed down and more time is available for response.

If aging does contribute meaningfully to certain clinical behaviors such as tasks involving paragraph retention and word fluency, it may be of greatest concern for mild aphasias occurring in the age span from 60 to 70. The percentage of impact is likely to be greatest in mild aphasia, and some changes appear to occur only in old age. Given the areas of research reported in this chapter, investigators of aphasia might at least begin to report age of their aphasic subjects more often. We also might heighten our desire to include age-matched normal controls in aphasia research. However, increasing variability of performance, reflecting wide individual variation in rate of normal aging, indicates that chronological age-matching may not mean a great deal. It may be more accurate, but less realistic, to match brain-injured subjects with normal subjects possessing an equivalent physiological age of the central nervous system. After all, a stroke may arise from a CNS that is "older" than the CNS of a healthy age-matched control. We should, at least, be careful about interpreting differences between aphasic subjects and a small number of age-matched normal subjects.

Age has been of greatest concern in clinical aphasiology as one indicator of prognosis. Based on CNS and cognitive changes, our intuition that increasing age has a detrimental effect on recovery seems relatively secure. Aging probably does provide a magnet which draws recovery backward to some extent. It is disconcerting that most attempts to examine the relationship between chronological age and recovery have failed to produce a significant correlation (Davis & Holland, 1981). However, it is aging and not age that makes a difference.

Note

[1]The term *encoding*, as used in cognitive psychology, can be confusing to speech-language pathologists who were weaned on a different conception of the term. In communication models, encoding has referred to production as opposed to the "decoding" of input. However, in the study

of memory and cognition, encoding refers to the mental representation of stimuli, that is, the process of developing an internal code which is a kind of "mental response" to stimuli. The term decoding is not used; and, in fact, psychologists' use of encoding is similar to the communicologist's use of decoding.

References

Adams, R. D. The morphological aspects of aging in the human nervous system. In J. E. Birren and R. B. Sloane (Eds.), *Handbook of mental health and aging.* Englewood Cliffs, NJ: Prentice-Hall, 1980.

Anders, T. R., Fozard, J. L., & Lillyquist, T. D. Effects of age upon retrieval from short-term memory. *Developmental Psychology,* 1972, *6,* 214-217.

Battig, W. F., & Montague, W. E. Category names for verbal items in 56 categories. *Journal of Experimental Psychology Monographs*, *80,* 1969.

Beasley, D. S., & Davis, G. A. (Eds.). *Aging: Communication processes and disorders.* New York: Grune & Stratton, 1981.

Belmore, S. M. Age-related changes in processing explicit and implicit language. *Journal of Gerontology*, 1981, *36,* 316-322.

Bergman, M. (Ed.). *Aging and the perception of speech.* Baltimore, MD: University Park Press, 1980.

Birren, J. E. *The psychology of aging.* Englewood Cliffs, NJ: Prentice-Hall, 1964.

Borod, J. C., Goodglass, H., & Kaplan, E. Normative data on the Boston Diagnostic Aphasia Examination, Parietal Lobe Battery, and the Boston Naming Test. *Journal of Clinical Neuropsychology*, 1980, *2,* 209-215. (a)

Borod, J. C., Goodglass, H., & Kaplan, E. Normative data on neuropsychological tests. Boston V. A. Medical Center: Unpublished manuscript 1980. (b)

Botwinick, J., & Storandt, M. Vocabulary ability in later life. *Journal of Genetic Psychology*, 1974, *125,* 303-308.

Botwinick, J., West, R., & Storandt, M. Qualitative vocabulary test responses and age. *Journal of Gerontology*, 1975, *30,* 574-577.

Brookshire, R. H., & Nicholas, L. E. Verification of active and passive sentences by aphasic and nonaphasic subjects. *Journal of Speech and Hearing Research*, 1980, *23,* 878-893.

Buckingham, H. W. Linguistic aspects of lexical retrieval disturbances in the posterior fluent aphasias. In H. Whitaker & H. A. Whitaker (Eds.), *Studies in neurolinguistics* (Vol. 4). New York: Academic Press, 1979.

Burke, D. M., & Light, L. L. Memory and aging: The role of retrieval processes. *Psychological Bulletin*, 1981, *90,* 513-546.

Camp, C. J. The use of fact retrieval vs. inference in young and elderly adults. *Journal of Gerontology*, 1981, *36,* 715-721.

Chapey, R., Rigrodsky, S., & Morrison, E. B. Aphasia: A divergent semantic interpretation. *Journal of Speech and Hearing Disorders*, 1977, *42,* 287-295.

Cicirelli, V. G. Categorization behavior in aging subjects. *Journal of Gerontology*, 1976, *31,* 676-680.

Clark, L., & Knowles J., Age differences in dichotic listening performance. *Journal of Gerontology*, 1973, *28,* 173-178.

Cohen, G. Language comprehension in old age. *Cognitive Psychology*, 1979, *11,* 412-429.

Craik, F. I. M. Age differences in human memory. In J. E. Birren & K. W. Schaie (Eds.), *Handbook of the psychology of aging*. New York: Van Nostrand Reinhold, 1977.

Crook, T. H. Psychometric assessment in the elderly. In A. Raskin & L. F. Jarvik (Eds.), *Psychiatric symptoms and cognitive loss in the elderly*. Washington: Hemisphere, 1979.

Davis, G. A., & Holland, A. L. Age in understanding and treating aphasia. In D. S. Beasley & G. A. Davis (Eds.), *Aging: Communication processes and disorders*. New York: Grune & Stratton, 1981.

DeRenzi, E. A shortened version of the Token Test. In F. Boller & M. Dennis (Eds.), *Auditory comprehension : Clinical and experimental studies with the Token Test*. New York: Academic Press, 1979.

DeRenzi, E. & Vignolo, L. A. The Token Test: A sensitive test to detect receptive disturbances in aphasics. *Brain*, 1962, *85*, 665-678.

Duffy, J. R., Keith, R. L., Shane, H., & Podraza, B. L. Performance of normal (non-brain-injured) adults on the Porch Index of Communicative Ability. In R. H. Brookshire (Ed.), *Clinical Aphasiology Conference Proceedings*. Minneapolis: BRK, 1976.

Eysenck, M. W. Retrieval from semantic memory as a function of age. *Journal of Gerontology*, 1975, *30*, 174-180.

Feier, C. & Gerstman, L. Sentence comprehension abilities throughout the adult life span. *Journal of Gerontology*, 1980, *35*, 722-728.

Goodglass, H., & Baker, E. Semantic field, naming, and auditory comprehension in aphasia. *Brain and Language*, 1976, *3*, 359-374.

Goodglass, H., & Kaplan, E. *The assessment of aphasia and related disorders*. Philadelphia: Lea & Febiger, 1972.

Gordon, S. K. Organization and recall of related sentences by elderly and young adults. *Experimental Aging Research*, 1975, *1*, 71-80.

Grober, E., Perceman, E., Kellar, L., & Brown, J. Lexical knowledge in anterior and posterior aphasics. *Brain and Language*, 1980, *10*, 318-330.

Harasymiw, S. J., Halper, A., & Sutherland, B. Sex, age, and aphasia type. *Brain and Language*, 1981, *12*, 190-198.

Henoch, M. A. (Ed.). *Aural rehabilitation for the elderly*. New York: Grune & Stratton, 1979.

Holland, A. L. *Communicative abilities in daily living*. Baltimore: University Park Press, 1980.

Howard, D. V. Category norms: A comparison of the Battig and Montague (1969) norms with the responses of adults between the ages of 20 and 80. *Journal of Gerontology*, 1980, *35*, 225-231.

Jacoby, R. J., Levy, R. & Dawson, J. M. Computed tomography in the elderly: I. The normal population. *American Journal of Psychiatry*, 1980, *136*, 249-255.

Johnson, R. C., Cole, R. E., Bowers, J. K., Foiles, S. V., Nikaido, A. M., Patrick, J. W., & Woliver, R. E. Hemispheric efficiency in middle and later adulthood. *Cortex*, 1979, *15*, 109-119.

Just, M. A., Davis, G. A., & Carpenter, P. A. A comparison of aphasic and normal adults in a sentence-verification task. *Cortex*, 1977,*13*, 402-423.

Kamin, L. J. Differential changes in mental abilities in old age. *Journal of Gerontology*, 1957, *12*, 66-70.

Kaplan, E., Goodglass, H., & Weintraub, S. *Boston Naming Test* (experimental edition). Boston: Veterans Administration Medical Center, 1976.

Kertesz, A., & McCabe, P. Intelligence and aphasia: Performance of aphasics on *Raven's Coloured Progressive Matrices* (RCPM). *Brain and Language*, 1975, *2*, 387-395.

Kertesz, A., & Sheppard, A. The epidemiology of aphasic and cognitive impairment in stroke: Age, sex, aphasia type and laterality differences. *Brain*, 1981, *104*, 117-128.

Kocel, K. M. Age-related changes in cognitive abilities and hemispheric specialization. In J. Herron (Ed.), *Neuropschology of left-handedness*. New York: Academic Press, 1980.

Kogan, N. Categorizing and conceptualizing styles in younger and older adults. *Human Development*, 1974, *17*, 218-230.

Lachman, J. L., Lachman, R., & Thronesbery, C. Metamemory through the adult life span. *Developmental Psychology*, 1979, *15*, 543-551.

LaPointe, L. L., & Horner, J. *Reading Comprehension Battery for Aphasia*. Tigard, OR: C. C. Publications, 1979.

Madden, D. J., & Nebes, R. D. Aging and the development of automaticity in visual search. *Developmental Psychology*, 1980, *16*, 377-384.

Maurer, J. F., & Rupp, R. R. *Hearing and aging: A guide to rehabilitation*. New York: Grune & Stratton, 1979.

Michalewski, H. J., Thompson, L. W., & Saul, R. E. Use of the EEG and evoked potentials in the investigation of age-related clinical disorders. In J. E. Birren & R. B. Sloane (Eds.) *Handbook of mental health and aging*. Englewood Cliffs, NJ: Prentice-Hall, 1980.

Nash, M., & Wepman, J. M. Auditory comprehension and age. *The Gerontologist*, 1973, Summer, 243-247.

Nebes, R. D. Verbal-pictorial recoding in the elderly. *Journal of Gerontology*, 1976, *31*, 421-427.

Nebes, R. D., & Andrews-Kulis, M. S. The effect of age on the speed of sentence formation and incidental learning. *Experimental Aging Research*, 1976, *2*, 315-331.

Noll, J. D., & Randolph, S. R. Auditory semantic, syntactic, and retention errors made by aphasic subjects on the Token Test. *Journal of Communication Disorders*, 1978, *11*, 543-553.

Norman, D. A. *Memory and attention: An introduction to human information processing* (2nd Ed.). New York: John Wiley & Sons, 1976.

Obler, L. K., & Albert, M. L. Language and aging: A neurobehavioral analysis. In D. S. Beasley & G. A. Davis (Eds.), *Aging: Communication processes and disorders*. New York: Grune & Stratton, 1981.

Obler, L. K., Albert, M. L., Goodglass, H., & Benson, D. F. Aging and aphasia type. *Brain and Language*, 1978, *6*, 318-322.

Orgass, B., & Poeck, K. Clinical validation of a new test for aphasia: An experimental study of the Token Test. *Cortex*, 1966, *2*, 222-243.

Parkinson, S. R., Lindholm, J. M., & Urell, T. Aging, dichotic memory and digit span. *Journal of Gerontology*, 1980, *35*, 87-95.

Poon, L. W., & Fozard, J. L. Speed of retrieval from long-term memory in relation to age, familiarity, and datedness of information. *Journal of Gerontology*, 1978, *33*, 711-717.

Porch, B. E. *Porch Index of Communicative Ability, Volume I: Theory and development*. Palo Alto, CA: Consulting Psychologists Press, 1967.

Raven, J. C., Court, J. H., & Raven, J. *Manual for Raven's Progressive Matrices and Vocabulary Scales, Section 1: General overview*. London: H. K. Lewis, 1976.

Riegel, K. F. Changes in psycholinguistic performances with age. In G. A. Talland (Ed.), *Human aging and behavior*. New York: Academic Press, 1968.

Salzman, C. A primer on geriatric psychopharmacology. *American Journal of Psychiatry*, 1982, *139*, 67-74.

Schaie, K. W. Intelligence and problem solving. In J. E. Birren & R. B. Sloane (Eds.), *Handbook of Mental Health and Aging*. Englewood Cliffs, NJ: Prentice-Hall, 1980.

Schaier, A. H., & Cicirelli, V. G. Age differences in humor comprehension and appreciation in old age. *Journal of Gerontology*, 1976, *31*, 577-582.

Schuell, H. M. *Differential diagnosis of aphasia with the Minnesota Test* (2nd Ed., rev. by J. W. Sefer). Minneapolis: University of Minnesota Press, 1973.

Schuell, H. M., Jenkins, J. J., & Jiménez-Pabón, E. *Aphasia in adults*. New York: Harper & Row, 1964.

Schulz, U., & Hunziker, O. Comparative studies of neuronal perikaryon size and shape in the aging cerebral cortex. *Journal of Gerontology*, 1980, *35*, 483-491.

Semenza, C., Denes, G., Lucchese, D., & Bisiacchi, P. Selective deficit of conceptual structures in aphasia: Class versus thematic relations. *Brain and Language*, 1980, *10*, 243-248.

Shewan, C. M. *Auditory Comprehension Test for Sentences*. Chicago: Biolinguistics Clinical Institutes, 1979.

Smith, A., & Fullerton, A. M. Age differences in episodic and semantic memory: Implications for language and cognition. In D. S. Beasley & G. A. Davis (Eds.), *Aging: Communication processes and disorders*. New York: Grune & Stratton, 1981.

Stones, M. J. Aging and semantic memory: Structural age differences. *Experimental Aging Research*, 1978, *4*, 125-132.

Swinney, D. A., & Taylor, O. L. Short-term memory recognition search in aphasics. *Journal of Speech and Hearing Research*, 1971, *14*, 578-588.

Swisher, L. P., & Sarno, M. T. Token Test scores of three matched patient groups: Left brain-damaged with aphasia; right brain-damaged without aphasia; non-brain damaged. *Cortex*, 1969, *5*, 264-273.

Taub, H. Comprehension and memory of prose material by young and old adults. *Experimental Aging Research*, 1979, *5*, 3-13.

Thomas, J. C. Fozard, J. L., & Waugh, N. C. Age-related differences in naming latency. *American Journal of Psychology*, 1977, *90*, 499-509.

Till, R. E. & Walsh, D. A. Encoding and retrieval factors in adult memory for implicational sentences. *Journal of Verbal Learning and Verbal Behavior*, 1980, *19*, 1-16.

Tillman, D., & Gerstman, L. J. Clustering by aphasics in free recall. *Brain and Language*, 1977, *4*, 355-364.

Valenstein, E. Age-related changes in the human central nervous system. In D. S. Beasley & G. A. Davis (Eds.), *Aging: Communication processes and disorders*. New York: Grune & Stratton, 1981.

Voke, J. A brief review of age changes in colour discrimination. *The Optician*, 1982, January 18.

Walsh, D. A., & Baldwin, M. Age differences in integrated semantic memory. *Developmental Psychology*, 1977, *13*, 509-514.

Warren, R. L., Hubbard, D. J., & Knox, A. W. Short-term memory scan in normal individuals and individuals with aphasia. *Journal of Speech and Hearing Research*, 1977, *20*, 497-509.

Yamaura, H., Ito, M., Kubota, K., & Matsuzana, T. Brain atrophy during aging: A quantitative study with computed tomography. *Journal of Gerontology*, 1980, *35*, 494-498.

Yorkston, K. M., & Beukelman, D. R. An analysis of connected speech samples of aphasic and normal speakers. *Journal of Speech and Hearing Disorders*, 1980, *45*, 27-36.

Craig W. Linebaugh

Mild Aphasia

An Opening Dilemma

As one begins reading a chapter on *mild* aphasia, he or she ought to ask—and legitimately so—What is *mild* aphasia? Who among my patients is *mildly* aphasic? Is it those whose PICA (Porch, 1967) overall performance is above the 90th percentile? Or should it be the 80th percentile? Is it the patient who responds in the negative when asked if a hammer is good for cutting wood, but fails to recognize why the bugler had trouble finding friends (from the *Boston Diagnostic Aphasia Examination*, Goodglass & Kaplan, 1972)? Is it a 62-year-old, noninstitutionalized male with a *CADL* (Holland, 1980) score above 112 but below 124? Is it those my standard aphasia battery proclaims to be "within normal limits," but my communicative experience with them tells me otherwise?

Please excuse the hyperbole, for it is born of the desire to emphasize a dilemma we share as clinicians and researchers. The dilemma is this: The "mildness" of the mildly aphasic person's aphasia depends not on his or her score on some standardized test. Rather, it depends on the degree to which the aphasia impairs his or her ability to communicate at the level demanded by personal, social, vocational, educational, and recreational needs. The degree to which we can quantify a patient's aphasia in absolute terms, using some standardized measure, is reduced to a person-by-person relativism in the realm of functional communication. Language performance which is "unimpaired" for a person with few verbal needs may

©College-Hill Press, Inc. All rights, including that of translation, reserved. No part of this publication may be reproduced without the written permission of the publisher.

be a "mild" impairment for one with somewhat greater needs. What is a "mild" impairment for that one may be a "moderate," even disabling, impairment for the lawyer, teacher, or politician.

This was the conclusion of the participants in a round-table discussion at the 1978 Clinical Aphasiology Conference (Wertz, 1978) when confronted with the same question: What is mild aphasia? It was valid then, and it is valid as you read this chapter. Indeed, its validity is eternal.

A second conclusion reached by the participants in that round-table discussion was that we had far to go in our understanding, assessment, and treatment of mildly aphasic persons. This chapter represents a tour of the ground that has been covered in the four years which have since elapsed. The section on Phenomenology is intended to draw clinical implications from the recent data regarding the performance of mildly aphasic patients. The Assessment and Treatment sections are intended to familiarize the reader with recently developed procedures. All three sections are intended to provide sufficient information to allow the reader to decide whether or not a study or procedure has applications to his or her own clinical and research endeavors.

Phenomenology

Auditory Comprehension

Recent studies of auditory comprehension in mildly aphasic patients have dealt with two areas. The first has been that of context. In a 1978 study, Wilcox, Davis, and Leonard investigated aphasic subjects' comprehension of indirect requests presented via a videotape depicting a natural communicative situation. The indirect requests used were of the type "Can you move the table?" or "Will you close the door?" The context in which the requests were made was such that the conveyed intention was indeed a request for some action, rather than the literally interpreted request for information. In addition, the investigators assessed the influence of affirmative versus negative surface forms of the request.

This study included 10 aphasic subjects described as having a high level of auditory comprehension. This designation was based on their having scored 60% or above "on a battery of standard comprehension tests requiring literal interpretation" (Wilcox et al., 1978, p. 366). Results showed significantly better performance by the high level aphasic subjects than the low level subjects. This difference was attributed to the low level group's generally depressed comprehension abilities. In a second experiment in which the effects of positive versus negative intent of the requests was studied, the results were similar. Here, too, the high level subjects performed significantly better than the low level subjects. These results essentially mirror the differences between high and low level aphasic patients on standard tests and, as such, are less than startling. What is of particular significance, however, is the degree to which context appeared to facilitate comprehension. On the standard tests, the high level group performed at a mean accuracy level of approximately 76%. In comprehending contextually supported requests, the mean accuracy level was nearly 95%. For the record, the low level group showed an even more impressive gain when contextual support was available. What may be inferred from these findings is that aphasic persons can successfully employ the extralinguistic cues available in natural communicative situations to enhance their auditory comprehension. Particular to this discussion, even mildly aphasic persons appear to benefit significantly from contextual information.

A second series of experiments concerning the role of context in the auditory comprehension of mildly impaired aphasic patients was conducted by Waller and Darley (1978a, 1978b, 1979). These investigators assessed the effects of pictorial, verbal, and combined pictorial and verbal prestimulation on sentence and paragraph comprehension. The prestimulation served to establish a context appropriate to the stimulus which followed. Results of this study indicated that verbal prestimulation significantly enhanced paragraph comprehension by aphasic individuals. No facilitative effects were observed for sentence comprehension. Also of note is the deleterious effect of pictorial prestimulation as compared to a control condition (no prestimulation). The authors speculate that this seemingly incongruous finding may have resulted from difficulty encountered by the aphasic subjects in attempting to recode the pictures verbally, using their disrupted language systems. Normal controls performed equally well in the picture and control conditions. That interference was exerted by pictorial prestimulation is at odds with recent findings of Elmore-Nicholas and Brookshire (1981). These investigators reported a facilitating effect for the presence of a sentence-relevant picture on a sentence verification task. The differences in these two studies may be related to the greater complexity of the pictures used by Waller and Darley, and to their having removed the picture prior to presentation of the stimulus. Under Waller and Darley's conditions, the need for verbal recoding of the picture would have been substantially greater than in the conditions employed by Elmore-Nicholas and Brookshire.

The second area of recent activity has been studies of the effects of extraneous factors on the auditory comprehension of the mildly aphasic. In particular, the effects of a distractor task and those of competing auditory signals have been investigated. The former were assessed in a study by DeRenzi, Faglioni, and Previdi (1978). These researchers investigated the ability of mildly aphasic subjects to carry out commands under three conditions: no delay, with a 20-second unfilled delay, and with a 20-second delay during which the subject was counting backwards by ones, twos, or threes. No significant differences were found among normal control, brain-damaged nonaphasic, and aphasic subjects' ability to carry out the commands in the no-delay and unfilled-delay conditions. All subjects, however, experienced significant performance decrements in the filled-delay condition. Here, the normal and brain-damaged nonaphasic subjects experienced mean decrements of 24% and 27%, respectively. Aphasic subjects showed a mean decrement of 48%, indicating their greater susceptibility to a distractor task.

In a study of the effects of competing auditory signals on Token Test performance, Basili, Diggs, and Rao (1980) assessed the relative effects of white noise and speech babble. Normal controls, right cerebral hemisphere-damaged, and left hemisphere-damaged aphasic subjects were administered the Token Test in quiet, in the presence of white noise, and in the presence of speech babble. As expected, the aphasic subjects performed at a lower level than either of the other two groups in all conditions. Regarding the three conditions, the aphasic subjects performed at comparable levels in quiet and in the presence of white noise, but experienced a decrease in performance in the presence of speech babble. The authors suggest that the differential effects exerted by white noise and speech babble may be related to difficulty in separating the acoustically more complex babble from the primary speech stimulus, or to difficulty in ignoring the linguistic nature of the babble.

Verbal Expression

Among the most frequently observed deviations in the verbal output of mildly aphasic individuals are residual word retrieval difficulties and disruptions of the flow of speech. Most clinicians who work with aphasic patients have at one time or another suspected that the two were somehow related, but until recently this relationship had not been examined empirically. A 1981 study by Brown and Cullinan begins to fill this void. Brown and Cullinan examined the performance of 24 anomic aphasic patients, 21 of whom were described as having mild or minimal speech deficits, on three tasks. The tasks were (1) naming 38 objects, 15 actions, and 9 colors, (2) describing pictures, and (3) engaging in a conversation, usually with one of the experimenters. The latter two tasks were employed to obtain samples of connected speech which were subsequently analyzed for the presence of various types of dysfluency. Two categories of dysfluency were analyzed, the first consisting of dysfluencies likely to be considered as "stuttering" (e.g., vocal-segregate repetitions, part-word repetitions, prolongations), and the second consisting of types likely to be considered "normal dysfluencies" (e.g., revisions, word and phrase repetitions, parenthetic remarks). Hesitations were considered separately.

The subjects' performances on the naming task were examined for both accuracy and latency of response. These variables were then correlated with various measures of the frequency of occurrence of the dysfluency types. These analyses revealed a significant relationship between word retrieval difficulty and dysfluency. That is, as the number of correct naming responses decreased and latency increased, the number of dysfluencies increased. In addition, the proportion of stuttering-like dysfluencies increased as both word-retrieval difficulty and the total number of dysfluencies increased. These findings led the authors to suggest that the aphasic individual is reacting to both word-retrieval difficulty and the incidence of dysfluencies, thereby casting himself into a whirlpool of increasing disruption of speech flow.

A second area of investigation has dealt with the ability of mildly aphasic persons to produce connected discourse. Ulatowska and her colleagues (1980, 1981) have reported an elaborate study investigating the ability of 10 aphasic subjects to produce narrative and procedural discourse. Narratives were elicited by asking the subjects to recount a memorable experience, tell a story concerning a sequence of pictures, and to retell a story following an examiner's reading of it. Procedural descriptions concerned routine, frequently performed tasks, such as brushing teeth or combing hair, and procedures learned by special instruction and possibly never performed (bowling, changing a tire).

Variables related to the complexity of the language produced, and to discourse length and structure, were analyzed for both narratives and descriptions. The primary findings of this study may be summarized as follows: The subjects produced well-formed narrative and procedural discourse, including all the elements essential to discourse superstructure. Discourse errors produced by the aphasic subjects differed from those of normal controls in number, but not in kind. The aphasic subjects produced language that was both less copious and less complex than was the language of normal controls. Reduced complexity was made particularly evident by less embedding. The reduction in quantity of language appeared to be, at least in part, selectively distributed. This is particularly apparent for the narratives, where the reduction in language was primarily displayed on nonessential, elaborative portions of the narrative. In procedural descriptions, however, language reduction resulted in the omission of essential, as well as ancillary, steps. For a full elaboration of the findings of this study, the reader is referred to Ulatowska, North and Macaluso-Haynes (1981).

In a separate study of 11 mildly aphasic subjects, Ulatowska, Hildebrand, and Haynes (1978) compared spoken and written language in both isolated sentences and connected discourse. The results of this study are consistent with the study just discussed. Here, too, aphasic subjects were observed to produce less complex language than normal controls, especially in writing. The aphasic subjects in this study were also observed to produce more preposition and semantic errors than the controls, the greater difference again being in written language. Overall, the aphasic subjects produced fewer errorless word sequences of the type being analyzed in writing than they did in spoken language. (The unit of linguistic analysis in this and the preceding study was the T-unit. A T-unit is defined as one independent clause and its dependent modifiers.) Nevertheless, on ratings of communicative adequacy, which focused on the intelligibility and specificity of the message apart from any disruptions of form, a majority of aphasic individuals were rated better or equal in written, as compared to spoken, language. Moreover, the aphasic subjects' communicative adequacy for both written and spoken language was substantially higher than their overall level of linguistic function as measured on the *Boston Diagnostic Aphasia Examination* (BDAE) (Goodglass & Kaplan, 1972). What is critical to note, however, is that the high level of communicative adequacy achieved by the mildly aphasic subjects was done so only at the expense of considerable time. In one example cited by the investigators, two samples of written discourse, rated equally for communicative adequacy, required of their normal and aphasic authors 3 and 30 minutes, respectively.

Studies of discourse thus provide us with several bits of important information regarding mild aphasia. First, both the spoken and written discourse of mildly aphasic persons is reduced in amount and complexity of language. In addition, substantial percentages of word sequences (T-units) produced contain some form of linguistic error. In spite of these disruptions of language, however, mildly aphasic subjects tend to preserve the discourse superstructure necessary to provide information in a coherent manner. Indeed, they are able to achieve a high degree of communicative adequacy. To do so, however, they must be allowed substantially longer amounts of time to accomplish communicative tasks than is required by their nonaphasic counterparts.

Coverbal Behavior

Katz, LaPointe, and Markel (1978) have reported a study in which they assessed the integrity of the coverbal behavior of aphasic patients. Coverbal behaviors are those such as head nodding, shaking, or tilting, and eyebrow raising, which are produced in association with speech. Katz et al. made video-tape recordings of aphasic and control subjects as they alternately told what they thought about 20 common words (e.g., "What do you think about laughing/black/friend?"). Several of the 10 aphasic subjects studied had relatively mild language deficits. Coverbal behaviors selected for study included eye contact, eyebrow raising, smiling, head nodding, head shaking, and head tilting. No significant differences in frequency of occurrence of these behaviors separated the aphasic and control subjects. The aphasic subjects, however, did tend to engage in a given coverbal behavior for a longer time period than did the controls.

Regarding mildly aphasic patients, the data on eye contact is particularly interesting. Those aphasic subjects who had milder verbal expressive deficits maintained eye contact for shorter durations than did those subjects with greater degrees of verbal involvement. The authors suggest that this may indicate that the subjects with milder impairments were less dependent on eye contact to maintain their speaking turn than were those with more severe deficits. For aphasic persons, in general, it was suggested that the preservation of coverbal behavior contributes to their being better communicators than language users.

Communicative Burden

It is generally recognized that successful communication by an aphasic speaker is to some extent dependent on his listeners' assuming a greater share of the burden of communication than might have been necessary prior to the onset of aphasia. In a recent study, Linebaugh, Kryzer, Oden, and Myers (1982) sought to objectively assess this reapportionment of communicative burden. As a measure of communicative burden, these investigators used the percentage of communicative exchanges initiated by the aphasic speaker as compared to his nonaphasic listener. A communicative exchange was operationally defined as an "utterance (in any modality or combination of modalities) produced by one participant in a communicative interaction, and the other's response to it." Percentages of exchanges initiated by the aphasic speakers were obtained from communicative interactions that were essentially narrative in form. Five different topics were discussed by the aphasic speakers. Several of the 12 subjects could be described as mildly aphasic.

The percentage of communicative exchanges initiated by the aphasic speakers ranged from 42 to 91%. These percentages were correlated to a significant degree with the subjects' scores on the *CADL* (Holland, 1980). This indicated that the amount of communicative burden which the aphasic individual was able to assume was directly related to his functional communicative abilities, as measured by the *CADL*. Specific to this discussion, the mildly aphasic subjects were able to carry the bulk of the communicative burden in the type of interaction assessed. Nevertheless, the listener occasionally had to probe for essential bits of information, indicating his need to assume at least a slightly greater amount of the communicative burden.

Implications

The following implications can be drawn from the recent reasearch on mild aphasia:

1. Mildly aphasic individuals benefit from the context provided in natural communicative situations and through verbal prestimulation. The effectiveness with which a patient can utilize contextual information should be assessed. The patient can be taught strategies by which he or she can derive maximum benefit from contextual information. Those with whom the patient routinely communicates can be trained to provide additional contextual information when appropriate.

2. Mildly aphasic individuals are highly susceptible to distractor tasks and competing signals. The effects of these deterrents to optimal performance should be assessed for the individual patient. He or she should be prepared to deal with them as they are encountered in natural communicative situations.

3. The dysfluency experienced by some mildly aphasic patients may be related both to word retrieval difficulty and to the occurrence of dysfluencies. To minimize dysfluency, patients should learn to deal productively with instances of anomia. For example, one can use a delay to search for the desired, or synonymous, word or to formulate a circumlocution. The patient should also try to control any negative emotional reactions to his dysfluencies which may exacerbate the disruption of his flow of speech.

4. Mildly aphasic patients preserve the essential elements of discourse, in spite of using language that is reduced in amount and complexity. This contributes to their ability to communicate more effectively than might be inferred from their linguistic performance alone.

5. Mildly aphasic patients, as a group, appear able to communicate with a high degree of adequacy, but they require substantially more time to do so than do their normal counterparts. Patients with mild aphasia must, therefore, be trained to indicate their need for more time, and those with whom they communicate should be encouraged to provide it.

6. That aphasic patients' communicative skills exceed their language skills may be attributable in part to the preservation of coverbal behaviors.

Clinicians should seek to develop their patients' purposeful use of these behaviors to enhance communication.

7. While able to carry the bulk of the burden of communication in some interactions, mildly aphasic speakers must nevertheless rely on their communication partners to assume an additional share of the burden in other interactions. This depends on several factors, including the type of interaction, the subject matter, and the familiarity of the partner with both the aphasic speaker and the topic. The aphasic speaker should be trained in recognizing the need to shift some portion of the burden, and in acceptable ways of doing so.

Assessment

Assessment of the language and communication skills of mildly aphasic patients has long been a major problem for clinicians. Traditionally, we have relied on measures such as the Token Test (DeRenzi & Vignolo, 1962) or the Word Fluency Measure (Borkowski, Benton, & Spreen, 1967), or "home-made" measures, such as answering questions about a reading passage or retelling a story. The former are limited by the wide range of normal performance on such measures and their questionable relevance to functional communication. The latter are suspect because of their obvious lack of standardization. In this section, we shall consider several recent attempts to provide more sensitive measures of mild aphasia, as well as the applicability of some recently published tests to this population.

Auditory Comprehension

The Token Test was designed to be, and has long been, a standard measure of mild auditory comprehension deficits. Perhaps no other test of aphasia has undergone closer scrutiny or more revisions. Two recent efforts to enhance the Token Test bear particular mention.

The first was undertaken by Brookshire (1978). He developed a "Token Test Battery," which consisted of six versions of the standard Token Test (DeRenzi & Vignolo, 1962). These included three basic test conditions using two response modes. The three test conditions were (1) the standard version of the Token Test, (2) a configurational condition in which the subject pointed to the one of four groupings of the tokens shown on a card which best fit a command, and (3) a visual condition in which the subject matched a configuration of tokens representing a command to one of four choices. The two response modes were immediate and delayed, in which the tokens were covered during presentation of the command, and for 10 seconds thereafter.

Brookshire administered this battery to 25 aphasic, 10 right hemisphere-damaged, and 10 normal subjects. The normal subjects responded accurately and promptly on essentially all test items. The aphasic subjects performed worst in the standard condition, followed by the configurational and, then, the visual conditions. The right hemisphere-damaged group reversed this order of difficulty. Both groups of brain-damaged subjects had greater difficulty in the delayed response mode. Brookshire developed "order-of-difficulty matrices" which permit an individual patient's performance on the six subtests to be compared with that of the group. He suggested that marked deviations from the group pattern are indicative of the presence of associated problems. For example, if an aphasic patient showed greater-than-expected difficulty in all the delayed response conditions, one might suspect a more general memory deficit. To date, no additional studies using this Token Test Battery have been reported, and one can only speculate on its true clinical utility.

A second attempt to enhance the power and usefulness of the Token Test has received much wider attention and study. Recognizing the psychometric shortcomings of the original Token Test, McNeil and Prescott (1978) undertook development of the *Revised Token Test* (RTT). Among the RTT's improvements are standardized administration procedures, a multidimensional scoring system, percentile scores based on large samples of normal, left brain-damaged, and right brain-damaged subjects, and guidelines for test interpretation. If not familiar with the RTT, the reader is encouraged to study the test manual carefully, and determine the usefulness of the RTT in his or her clinical practice.

A second recently published test which this clinician has found useful with mildly aphasic patients is the *Auditory Comprehension Test for Sentences* (ACTS) (Shewan, 1980). This test is based on the work of Shewan and Canter (1971), who examined the relative influence of length, vocabulary, and syntax on the auditory comprehension of aphasic subjects. Two aspects of the ACTS, in particular, provide useful information regarding mildly aphasic persons. First, the most difficult sentences for each of the three factors represent a rather severe test of the aphasic patient's auditory comprehension in the absence of contextual support. Regrettably, the test includes only three items at the most complex level of each factor (length, vocabulary, and syntax), and there are no stimulus sentences by which the cumulative effects of increased difficulty in two or three factors can be assessed. While the author is to be commended for the economy of her test, one cannot help but wish for more items of greater difficulty so that different patterns of auditory processing deficits at the most complex levels could be identified.

The second aspect of the ACTS, which is particularly revealing, is not a part of the test per se. For each test item, a picture accurately depicting the content of the stimulus is presented along with three foils. Each foil differs from the correct response by a single element. This configuration allows the examiner to determine which stimulus element the subject apparently failed to comprehend. In many instances, the difference between the correct picture and a foil is rather obscure in the context of the whole picture. (Indeed, these minor differences may limit the applicability to certain, particularly visually impaired, patients.) As a result, the patient must carefully scan each response alternative, paying close attention to detail. Whether serendipitously or by design, Shewan has given us a convenient vehicle to observe patients' ability to organize their analysis of a group of alternative responses, while they maintain a high degree of attention to detail over a series of stimuli of varying complexity.

Another instrument which may be employed to assess the auditory comprehension of mildly aphasic patients in the Advanced Auditory Battery (AAB) proposed by Berry (1976). Designed as a supplement to the *Porch Index of Communicative Ability* (PICA) (Porch, 1967), the AAB includes 10 tasks, each comprising items, which sample a subject's comprehension of auditory stimuli of various levels of complexity. The battery uses the objects from the PICA, and a scoring system based on the PICA's 16-point multidimensional scale, but tailored to each of the 10 subtests. Berry (1976) provides a description of the test items and the scoring system in sufficient detail to allow accurate replication.

Recently Tompkins, Rau, Marshall, Lambrecht, Golper, and Phillips, (1980) investigated a number of considerations regarding the AAB. These investigators compared the performances of 24 aphasic subjects with mild auditory comprehension deficits with those of three nonbrain-damaged controls. They found that the two groups differed significantly on four of the subtests. These included subtests involving (1) three nouns, a verb, a locative preposition, and a temporal preposition denoting sequence; (2) three nouns to be responded to in sequence; (3) two nouns, two verbs, and a temporal preposition denoting sequence; and (4) two nouns and a locative preposition. Five subtests yielded scores different from those obtained on PICA subtests VI (pointing by function) and X (pointing by name). These included the four subtests listed above, plus one involving two nouns and a temporal adverb. These five subtests, therefore, were found to provide information not available from the PICA. Tompkins et al. concluded that, with appropriate revisions, the AAB could be a useful clinical tool for assessing mild auditory comprehension deficits. Specifically they called for further research on an abbreviated form of the battery using the most discriminating subtests, and also suggested refinement of the scoring system.

Verbal Expression

Two potentially useful tools for the assessment of the verbal expression of mildly aphasic patients have appeared recently. One is the Reporter's Test developed by DeRenzi and Ferrari (1978). At its most basic level, the Reporter's Test can be described as the Token Test in reverse. The subject's task is to describe what the examiner has done with a configuration of tokens in sufficient detail so that a person who could not see the tokens would be able to replicate the maneuver. There are five parts to the Reporter's Test. The first four parallel the first four parts of the standard Token Test. Part V required substantial revision of Part V of the Token Test because the commands did not lend themselves to the reporter format. Seven standard Token Test items were retained and three new items added. Scoring is done on a pass/fail basis for the entire response and in Parts I-IV a weighted score is also derived based on the patient's response to each critical element in the stimulus (e.g. color, size, shape).

DeRenzi and Ferrari reported data from the administration of the Reporter's Test to 70 nonbrain-damaged hospital patients, 60 left brain-damaged adults with mild to moderate expressive deficits, 20 nonaphasic, left brain-damaged adults, and 20 right brain-damaged adults. The scores of all subjects were corrected for the influence of educational background. Comparison of the Reporter's Test with various other measures of verbal expression, including visual confrontation, naming, and word fluency, revealed it to be a powerful discriminator between aphasic and nonaphasic subjects.

The second measure to be developed recently, of use in assessing mild expressive impairments, has perhaps greater functional relevance than does the Reporter's Test. Yorkston and Beukelman (1977, 1980) have developed a means for quantifying subjects' descriptions of the "Cookie Theft" picture from the BDAE. Using transcripts of Cookie Theft descriptions from 78 normal speakers, these investigators compiled a list of 57 content units expressed by at least one of the normal speakers. A content unit was defined as a "grouping of information that was always expressed as a unit by normal speakers."

Three measures were generated from the descriptions. These were (1) number of content units that indicated the amount of information conveyed, (2) syllables per minute, and (3) content units per minute that served as a measure of rate of information transfer. These measures were calculated for five groups of subjects: (1) 48 normal adult speakers ranging in age from 19 to 49 years, (2) 30 normal geriatric speakers ranging in age from 58 to 93 years, (3) 17 mildly aphasic speakers with PICA verbal percentiles ranging from the 81st to 99th percentile, (4) 16 high-moderate aphasic speakers with PICA verbal percentiles ranging from the 66th to 80th percentile, and (5) 17 low-moderate aphasic speakers with PICA verbal percentiles ranging from the 50th to 65th percentile. The mildly aphasic group did not differ from the two normal groups in terms of the number of content units produced. The mildly aphasic subjects did, however, produce significantly fewer syllables and content units per minute than either of the normal groups. These findings indicate that while the mildly aphasic subjects conveyed as much information as did the normals, they did so much less efficiently. Again we see, as we did earlier in the work of Ulatowska and her colleagues (1980, 1981), that the mildly aphasic individual communicates at an essentially normal level of adequacy, but needs substantially more time than do normal speakers.

I employ an additional count of syllables per content unit. Approximate means of 4.8, 5.7, and 6.3 syllables per content unit for the normal, geriatric, and mildly aphasic groups, respectively, can be derived from Yorkston and Beukelman's data. This measure has proven especially useful for documenting increasing communicative efficiency over time for patients who used excessive amounts of verbalization. For such patients, the goal of treatment was to move their inflated number of syllables per content unit in the direction of the mean of the age-appropriate normal group. These values can likewise serve as goals for nonfluent patients whose mean length of utterance needs expansion.

In addition to their content-based analysis, Yorkston and Beukelman (1978) have developed a system for assessing the grammaticality of connected speech samples. This analysis was based on the mean length of uninterrupted grammatical strings. A *string* was defined as a "series of words which have a grammatical relationship to each other." An elaborate set of rules for determining mean string length is provided by the authors.

Analyzing the Cookie Theft descriptions from their previous study, Yorkston and Beukelman found that mildly aphasic subjects fell below normals for mean length of grammatical string. Review of the transcripts, however, suggested that in several instances, strings were broken by errors which were not necessarily due to a failure to apply grammatical rules. As a result, the mean length of grammatical string was reduced by factors other than faulty syntax. The normal and mildly aphasic subjects were then compared on a second measure, "mean of the three longest strings." On this measure there was no significant difference between the mildly aphasic and normal subjects. These findings suggest that while mildly aphasic patients are similar to normals in their ability to produce long grammatical strings, their overall performance is reduced in efficiency. Whether this is because of a loss of syntactic knowledge, faulty application of this knowledge, or other nongrammatical problems remains unclear.

In a 1980 study, Golper, Thorpe, Tompkins, Marshall, and Rau also sought to extend the types of information that could be extracted from descriptions of the Cookie Theft picture. In addition to the content and grammaticality analyses of Yorkston and Beukelman, these investigators used five measures intended to assess the flow of verbal propositions. Golper et al. used the performance deviations employed by Loban (1967) for describing language development for this analysis. The measures included word and phrase interruptions or revisions, sequence interrupters in words and phrases (noncontentive utterances such as "uh" or "I mean"), and morpho/syntactic deviations. They also included a category of "phonetic error" which encompassed phonemic substitutions, omissions, and any unintelligible phonemes.

Transcripts of Cookie Theft picture descriptions obtained from 10 mildly aphasic subjects (PICA overall percentiles between 79th and 95th percentile), five of whom were fluent and five nonfluent, 10 right hemisphere-damaged subjects, and 10 normal geriatric subjects were analyzed. These analyses revealed that the aphasic subjects produced significantly more of each type of deviation than did either of the other two groups. Fluent and nonfluent aphasic subjects differed only in their incidence of word and phrase interrupters, with the nonfluent aphasic subjects producing more. The authors suggested that these additional measures may be useful for assessing mildly aphasic patients and for documenting their improvement over time.

Communicative Efficiency

In the preceding discussion it has been stated that mildly aphasic speakers generally are able to convey amounts of information comparable to those conveyed by normal speakers, but that they do so with reduced efficiency. Yorkston, Beukelman, and Flowers sought to address the matter of communicative efficiency more directly in a 1980 study. These investigators video tape-recorded aphasic speakers answering specific questions asked by a listener who was not able to see a series of stimulus pictures. After the listener had asked the designated question, he and the aphasic individual were free to use any means they chose to achieve the transfer of information. When the listener thought he had the desired information, or when a time limit had expired, he wrote his answer on a response sheet.

The listener's written answer was scored for accuracy, and the duration of the interaction was timed separately for each picture in the series. The investigators developed a method for comparing the relative efficiency of two communication samples based on a rank ordering procedure. This readily replicated method is described by Yorkston et al. (1980). The authors also provide case illustrations by which they demonstrate the usefulness of their method in assessing differences in a given patient's communicative efficiency over time and with different communication partners. This procedure appears to have considerable potential for both documenting improvement and identifying successful communication strategies.

Treatment

The literature of recent years contains little in the way of treatment procedures targeted on the mildly aphasic patient. One source rich in treatment approaches for the mildly aphasic was a panel discussion held at the 1980 Clinical Aphasiology Conference (Darley, Helm, Holland, & Linebaugh, 1980). Among the suggestions offered were (1) having the aphasic patient "teach" the clinician about his area of expertise, (2) retelling and summarizing stories of increasing length, (3) writing letters and keeping a diary, (4) forming sentences using designated words, (5) performing multiple-step verbal cognitive tasks such as giving directions, (6) writing captions for cartoons, (7) interpreting metaphors and idioms, (8) various divergent semantic tasks (Chapey, 1977), and (9) working on specific job-related tasks. In addition to these suggestions, three more elaborate descriptions of specific treatment approaches have also appeared recently.

The first of these is a program designed to improve word retrieval called SORRT (Logue & Dixon, 1979). SORRT is an acronym for semantic, oppositional, and rhyming retrieval training. As part of their program, Logue and Dixon provide a set of probes consisting of four single-word response tasks and one conversational analysis procedure. From these probes, the clinician is able to determine the primary types of response and retrieval strategies used by the patient, as well as those that are rarely or inaccurately used. The focus of the SORRT program is to expand the patient's repertoire of retrieval strategies. This is done through three levels of training. The first level is "discrimination training." Here the patient is presented pairs of words auditorily. At various stages in this training procedure, the patient is asked to respond "yes" or "no" as to whether the words in a given pair rhyme, are synonyms, or are antonyms. The second level of training is "selective matching." At this level, the patient is required to select from among three alternatives the word that rhymes or is a synonym or antonym of a stimulus word. The third level, "expressive-generative training," requires the patient to produce a word that rhymes or is a synonym or antonym of a stimulus word. Logue and Dixon provide a detailed description of the SORRT program, along with data on the performance of fluent and nonfluent subjects, and three case reports demonstrating the program's effectiveness. What remain to be developed are criteria identifying those patients who are appropriate candidates for this program.

Another approach to facilitating word retrieval by mildly aphasic patients has been described by Linebaugh (1983). This approach, known as Lexical Focus, is predicated on the observation that many of the word retrieval errors of mildly aphasic persons represent verbal paraphasias. That is, the word produced in error is related to the desired word, the two frequently being members of a common superordinate category. The assumption is made, therefore, that the aphasic speaker was able to access the appropriate superordinate category (one of many factors involved in the organization of one's lexicon), but was unable to retrieve the specific lexical item desired. Lexical Focus is thus described by Linebaugh as designed to improve the aphasic patient's "lexical dexterity" (Darley et al., 1980).

In this approach, patients are asked to name as many items in a designated superordinate category as they can. To facilitate performance, patients are encouraged to employ "search strategies." For example, if they are to name as many fruits and vegetables as they can, the patients may be instructed to imagine they are walking through the produce section of a supermarket or looking in their refrigerator. When the patients' performances reach criterion on a broad superordinate category, they are asked to name as many items as they can in a narrower subcategory (e.g., fruits *and* vegetables/fruits *or* vegetables; sports/sports played with a ball). A third, yet narrower, subcategory (e.g., fruits/citrus fruits, berries; sports played with a ball/sports played with a ball and a stick) may be presented upon reaching criterion for the second level category. Linebaugh (1983) has provided a detailed description of the Lexical Focus procedure along with suggested categories and criteria.

The third approach derives from a 1979 study by Cooper and Rigrodsky that assessed the effects of verbal training on aphasic patients' explanations of conservation, i.e., the preservation of equivalent volume or weight despite irrelevant perceptual changes. The specific conservation tasks employed were (1) a liquid conservation task where two equivalent amounts of water in identical containers remain equivalent when the contents of one container are poured into a taller, thinner container, and (2) a weight conservation task where two identical balls of clay remain equivalent in weight when one is elongated.

For both tasks, nine aphasic subjects were required to explain verbally the continued equivalence of the two amounts of water or clay. The subjects' responses were judged for the inclusion of various concepts by which the continued equivalence could be explained, rather than linguistic accuracy or complexity. Following pretesting, the nine subjects underwent an experimental protocol, part of which included listening to possible explanations for the weight conservation task. These explanations were intended to serve as verbal models for the subjects. Comparisons of pre- and post-training explanations of conservation revealed significant improvement in the explanations for the weight task for which training had been provided, and a nonsignificant trend toward improvement in the liquid task. Cooper and Rigrodsky interpreted these findings as indicating that verbal modeling had a facilitating effect on the task which received training, with some generalization to the untrained task.

A Closing Admonition

Patients with mild aphasia frequently require intensive treatment to enable them to return successfully to their work. These patients are sometimes dismissed too casually because their needs are less obvious. The difference between success and failure can be tragic when the potential is so high.

Schuell, Jenkins, and Jiménez-Pabón
(*Aphasia in Adults*, 1964, p. 368)

As you conclude your reading of this chapter, it would be my desire that your interest in the mildly aphasic patient would be increased. Overall, the interest of aphasiologists in mild aphasia has grown since 1978, but it remains low as compared with other aspects of this disorder. As you read this chapter, did you notice the decrease in the number of relevant sources as you progressed from the section on Phenomenology to that on Treatment? Surely this disparity exists in all aspects of aphasiology, for description must precede application. But as clinicians, can we afford to be complacent in applying our available information? More to the point, can our mildly aphasic patients afford this complacency? As clinical scientists, we have the ability and responsibility to develop new treatment approaches and assess their efficacy. Would that we all might be challenged by the above words of Schuell and her colleagues, rather than haunted by them.

References

Basili, A. G., Diggs, C. C., & Rao, P. R. Auditory processing of brain-damaged adults under competitive listening conditions. *Brain and Language*, 1980, *9*, 362-371.

Berry, W. R. Testing auditory comprehension in aphasia: Clinical alternatives to the Token Test. In Brookshire, R. H. (Ed.), *Clinical Aphasiology: Conference Proceedings*. Minneapolis: BRK Publishers, 1976.

Borkowski, J. G., Benton, A. L., & Spreen, O. Word fluency and brain damage. *Neuropsychologia*, 1967, *5*, 135-140.

Brookshire, R. H. A token test battery for testing auditory comprehension in brain-damaged adults. *Brain and Language*, 1978, *6*, 149-157.

Brown, C. S., & Cullinan, W. L. Word-retrieval difficulty and disfluent speech in adult anomic speakers. *Journal of Speech and Hearing Research*, 1981, *24*, 358-365.

Chapey, R. A divergent semantic model of intervention in adult aphasia. In Brookshire, R. H. (Ed.), *Clinical Aphasiology: Conference Proceedings*. Minneapolis: BRK Publishers, 1977.

Cooper, L. D., & Rigrodsky, S. Verbal training to improve explanations of conservation with aphasic adults. *Journal of Speech and Hearing Research*, 1979, *22*, 818-828.

Darley, F. L., Helm, N. A., Holland, A., & Linebaugh, C. W. Techniques in treating mild or high-level aphasic impairment. In Brookshire, R. H. (Ed.), *Clinical Aphasiology: Conference Proceedings*. Minneapolis, BRK Publishers, 1980.

DeRenzi, E., Faglioni, P., & Previdi. Increased susceptibility of aphasics to a distractor task in the recall of verbal commands. *Brain and Language*, 1978, *6*, 14-21.

DeRenzi, E., & Ferrari, C. The Reporter's Test: A sensitive test to detect expressive disturbances in aphasics. *Cortex*, 1978, *14*, 279-293.

DeRenzi, E., & Vignolo, L. A. The Token Test: A sensitive test to detect receptive disturbances in aphasics. *Brain*, 1962, *85*, 665-678.

Elmore-Nicholas, L., & Brookshire, R. H. Effects of pictures and picturability on sentence verification by aphasic and nonaphasic subjects. *Journal of Speech and Hearing Research*, 1981, *24*, 292-298.

Golper, L. A. C., Thorpe, P., Tompkins, C., Marshall, R. C., & Rau, M. T. Connected language sampling: An expanded index of aphasic language behavior. In Brookshire, R. H. (Ed.), *Clinical Aphasiology: Conference Proceedings*. Minneapolis: BRK Publishers, 1980.

Goodglass, H., & Kaplan, E. *Boston Diagnostic Aphasia Examination*. Philadelphia: Lea & Febiger, 1972.

Holland, A. *Communicative Abilities in Daily Living*. Baltimore: University Park Press, 1980.

Katz, R. C., LaPointe, L. L., & Markel, N. N. Coverbal behavior and aphasic speakers. In Brookshire, R. H. (Ed.), *Clinical Aphasiology: Conference Proceedings*. Minneapolis: BRK Publishers, 1978.

Linebaugh, C. W. Treatment of anomic aphasia. In Perkins, W. H. (ed.), *Current therapy of communication disorders: Language handicaps in adults*. New York: Thieme-Stratton, 1983.

Linebaugh, C. W., Kryzer, K. M., Oden, S. E., & Myers, P. S. Reapportionment of communicative burden in aphasia. In Brookshire, R. H. (Ed.), *Clinical Aphasiology: Conference Proceedings*. Minneapolis: BRK Publishers, 1982.

Loban, W. *Language development: K through 12*. National Council of Teachers of English Report #18. Champaign, IL, 1967.

Logue, R. D., & Dixon, M. M. Word association and the anomic response: Analysis and treatment. In Brookshire, R. H. (Ed.), *Clinical Aphasiology: Conference Proceedings*. Minneapolis: BRK Publishers, 1979.

McNeil, M. R., & Prescott, T. E. *Revised Token Test*. Baltimore: University Park Press, 1978.
Porch, B. E. *Porch Index of Communicative Ability*. Palo Alto, CA: Consulting Psychologists Press, 1967.
Schuell, H., Jenkins, J. J., & Jiménez-Pabón, E. *Aphasia in adults*. New York: Harper & Row, 1964.
Shewan, C. M. *Auditory Comprehension Test for Sentences*. Chicago: Biolinguistics Clinical Institutes, 1980.
Shewan, C. M., & Canter, G. J. Effects of vocabulary, syntax, and sentence length on auditory comprehension in aphasic patients. *Cortex*, 1971, *7*, 209-226.
Tompkins, C. A., Rau, M. T., Marshall, R. C., Lambrecht, K. J., Golper, L. A. C., & Phillips, D. S. Analysis of a battery assessing mild auditory comprehension involvement in aphasia. In Brookshire, R. H. (Ed.), *Clinical Aphasiology: Conference Proceedings*. Minneapolis: BRK Publishers, 1980.
Ulatowska, H. K., Hildebrand, B. H., & Haynes, S. M. A comparison of written and spoken language in aphasia. In Brookshire, R. H. (Ed.), *Clinical Aphasiology: Conference Proceedings*. Minneapolis: BRK Publishers, 1978.
Ulatowska, H. K., Macaluso-Haynes, S., & North, A. J. Production of narrative and procedural discourse in aphasia. In Brookshire, R. H. (Ed.), *Clinical Aphasiology: Conference Proceedings*. Minneapolis: BRK Publishers, 1980.
Ulatowska, H. K., North, A. J., & Macaluso-Haynes, S. Production of narrative and procedural discourse in aphasia. *Brain and Language*, 1981, *13*, 345-371.
Waller, M. R., & Darley, F. L. Effect of prestimulation on sentence comprehension by aphasic subjects. *Journal of Communication Disorders*, 1979, *12*, 461-479.
Waller, M. R., & Darley, F. L. The influence of context on the auditory comprehension of aphasic subjects. In Brookshire, R. H. (Ed.), *Clinical Aphasiology: Conference Proceedings*. Minneapolis: BRK Publishers, 1978. (a)
Waller, M. R., & Darley, F. L. The influence of context on the auditory comprehension of paragraphs by aphasic subjects. *Journal of Speech and Hearing Research*, 1978, *21*, 732-745. (b)
Wertz, R. T. Treating mildly aphasic patients. In Brookshire, R. H. (Ed.), *Clinical Aphasiology: Conference Proceedings*. Minneapolis: BRK Publishers, 1978.
Wilcox, M. J., Davis, G. A., & Leonard, L. B. Aphasics' comprehension of contextually conveyed meaning. *Brain and Language*, 1978, *6*, 362-377.
Yorkston, K. M., & Beukelman, D. R. A system for assessing grammaticality in connected speech of mildly aphasic individuals. In Brookshire, R. H. (Ed.), *Clinical Aphasiology: Conference Proceedings*. Minneapolis: BRK Publishers, 1978.
Yorkston, K. M., & Beukelman, D. R. A system for quantifying verbal output of high-level aphasics. In Brookshire, R. H. (Ed.), *Clinical Aphasiology: Conference Proceedings*. Minneapolis: BRK Publishers, 1977.
Yorkston, K. M., & Beukelman, D. R. An analysis of connected speech samples of aphasic and normal speakers. *Journal of Speech and Hearing Disorders*, 1980, *45*, 27-36.
Yorkston, K. M., Beukelman, D. R., & Flowers, C. R. Efficiency of information exchange between aphasic speakers and communication partners. In Brookshire, R. H. (Ed.), *Clinical Aphasiology: Conference Proceedings*. Minneapolis: BRK Publishers, 1980.

Jennifer Horner

Moderate Aphasia

Treatment of the aphasic individual has, in past years, been governed by concepts of auditory stimulation (Duffy, 1981; Schuell, Jenkins, & Jiménez-Pabón, 1964), intermodality deblocking (Weigl & Bierwich, 1970), task continua facilitation (Rosenbek, Lemme, Ahern, Harris, & Wertz, 1973), cognitive retraining (Martin, 1981; Wepman, 1972) and operant methodology (Holland, 1972; LaPointe, 1977). With these models as background, the purpose of this chapter is to review recent studies describing deficits of the moderately impaired aphasic individual from a psycholinguistic perspective. Clinical implications of these descriptive investigations will be highlighted. Psycholinguistic treatment studies, though sparsely represented in recent literature, will be described.

Assessing Moderate Aphasic Impairment

A current view of diagnosis is: "Diagnosis in [a]phasia implies the effort to identify the configuration of deficits in a particular case with one of the dozen or so recognized syndromes. Secondarily, it implies the identification of the probable site of lesion, on the basis of established correlations between syndromes and their most frequent lesion sites" (Albert, Goodglass, Helm, Rubens, & Alexander, 1981, p. 17). Identifying "the configuration of deficits" requires both quantitative and

---

©College-Hill Press, Inc. All rights, including that of translation, reserved. No part of this publication may be reproduced without the written permission of the publisher.

qualitative description. To achieve a quantitative description, one must define the degree of impairment in a variety of language behaviors. To achieve a qualitative description, one must interpret the resultant profile with regard to the recognized aphasia syndromes (and with regard to normal language performance). Quantifying an aphasic deficit involves defining the deficit as mild, moderate, or severe. Qualifying an aphasic deficit involves making inferences about the mechanisms underlying the aphasia, and it is for this purpose that the psycholinguistic model is particularly helpful.

Moderate aphasia can be operationally distinguished from mild and severe aphasia as follows. *Mild aphasia* is usually characterized by a language pattern that shares more features with normal language than deviates from it. Anomia is usually a predominant feature. Communicative competence is usually well preserved in the sense that the individual is aware of his or her deficits and uses compensatory strategies (e.g., delay, circumlocution) to deliberately compensate for aphasic performance difficulties (see Linebaugh's chapter). *Severe aphasia* is characterized by a marked reduction in the repertoire of language forms, such as a reduced lexical dictionary or simplified syntactic rules. A patient with severe aphasia is no longer able to use language for successful communicative interchange (see Helm-Estabrooks' chapter). The language performance in *moderate aphasia* falls on standardized tests in defined ranges: e.g., 40 to 70th percentile on the *Porch Index of Communicative Ability* (Porch, 1967); 40.0 to 70.0 aphasia quotient on the *Western Aphasia Battery* (Kertesz, 1980), or rating of "2" or "3" on the 5-point severity scale of the *Boston Diagnostic Aphasia Exam* (Goodglass & Kaplan, 1972a). The moderately aphasic individual has a broad language repertoire, which argues against a "loss" of linguistic forms and rules. On the other hand, *language is fundamentally altered from normal with regard to its specificity, complexity, and organization.* In addition, the language of the moderately aphasic individual is affected by memory and vigilance limitations (Brookshire, 1978), and reduced awareness of response accuracy (Martin, 1974; Porch, 1981).

With this definition in mind, the purpose of this chapter is to review psycholinguistic studies regarding the lexical-semantic, morphosyntactic, phonologic, and pragmatic abilities of moderately aphasic individuals. This chapter will attempt to show why a qualitative psycholinguistic assessment —above and beyond a quantitative assessment—is imperative to a clinically adequate description of aphasic language.

Psycholinguistics

By way of introduction to the psycholinguistic literature, a general understanding of the goals of linguistics is in order. Simply, *linguistics* involves the study of the regularities of language structure. The branch of linguistics known as *psycholinguistics* involves the study of the psychological processes underlying language performance. The primary contribution of psycholinguistic research to aphasiology has been to enhance our understanding of the mechanisms underlying aphasic language disruption. While many of the findings of this research may apply to mild aphasia and severe aphasia, moderate aphasia has been most widely studied in this regard. According to Ulatowska (1979), recent contributions of linguistics to aphasiology are empirical, procedural, and theoretical in nature. Among the *empirical* contributions are the ideas that aphasic error types and patterns are uniform across aphasia types (e.g., Blumstein, 1973) and that aphasic deficits can be selective (Geschwind, 1965a), two points that speak to the regularity of language organization in the brain. From a *procedural* perspective, linguistics has contributed new approaches for analysis of aphasic speech and language. Recent applications include: transformational grammar (Myerson & Goodglass, 1972), case grammar (Tonkovich, 1979), phonological process analysis (Kearns, 1980), metalinguistic tasks (von Stockert, 1972), sentence verification procedures (Brookshire & Nicholas, 1980a, 1980b, 1981). From a *theoretical* perspective, models of markedness theory (Ulatowska & Baker, 1975), lexical-semantic organization (Caramazza & Berndt, 1978), phonology (Kean, 1977), and pragmatics (Davis & Wilcox, 1981; Holland, 1980) are representative of the breadth of the contribution of linguistics to aphasiology. Thus, evolving theories of linguistics have contributed significantly to our understanding of the psycholinguistic mechanisms underlying historically recognized aphasia syndromes. (See Berndt & Caramazza, 1981; Blumstein, 1981; Buckingham, 1981 for exemplary reviews.) Psycholinguistic principles can also be used to identify idiosyncratic compensatory aphasic behaviors as shown in a case study by Hand, Tonkovich, and Aitchison (1979).

Thus, diagnosis in aphasia requires both quantitative and qualitative assessment. The challenge to the clinician is to go beyond quantitative analyses that yield overall percentiles, quotients, and severity ratings within specific performance areas. The challenge to the clinician is to ferret out the systematic nature of language errors, and to develop a qualitative description of aphasic symptoms. The challenge to the clinician is to describe not only *what* is wrong and *how much* the behavior deviates from normal, but also to describe *why particular errors occur.*

Dissociation of Functions in Aphasia

Dissociation of functions is a basic concept underlying recent psycholinguistic research. Dissociation refers to the phenomenon of functional disconnection of higher cortical functions. On the one hand, a function (code, modality, process) may be *preserved but functionally disconnected* from related subsystems that normally contribute to the realization of a behavior. Weigl and Fradis (1977) called this a "transcoding deficit." On the other hand, a function may be *selectively impaired and thereby functionally disconnected* from its parent system. In short, two functions may be intact but noninteractive because of an impairment in the connecting pathway, or a function may be selectively impaired and therefore noncontributory to related systemic functions. The degree to which an intact dissociated function can be assessed by intact pathways, or the degree to which an impaired dissociated function can be facilitated through the process of pairing intact with impaired functions ("deblocking," Weigl & Bierwisch, 1970) may affect recovery of the impaired function. The recovered function (the reorganized behavior) may differ qualitatively from the original behavior, but if treatment is successful, the reorganized or substituted behavior will be adequate to its purpose. In this chapter, the functions of interest are purposeful oral-verbal communication behaviors.

The concept of dissociation of functions helps the student of aphasia understand how the varieties of aphasia are defined in terms of the relative preservation or impairment of behaviors such as naming, fluency, comprehension, and repetition (Albert et al., 1981; Benson, 1979a, 1979b; Kertesz, 1979). Furthermore, the concept of dissociation of functions provides a thread that ties together the psycholinguistic studies described in this chapter. The reader is advised to keep in mind the concept of dissociation and related assumptions. First, the lexical-semantic (or syntactic, or phonologic) system can be selectively impaired. Second, processes underlying lexical-semantic (or morphosyntactic, or phonologic) performance may be selectively impaired within each system. Third, the quality of aphasic errors reflects the pattern of dissociation among language functions. Fourth, by analyzing the relative impairment or sparing of performance intersystemically (e.g., by comparing lexical-semantic with morphosyntactic performances) or intrasystemically (e.g., by analyzing lexical-semantic ability in spontaneous speech versus confrontation naming), one can infer the nature of the psycholinguistic process disruption.

Marin, Saffran, and Schwartz (1976) suggest three clinical implications emanating from the dissociation of functions model. First, the brain-damaged individual is adaptive and will strive to accomplish his or her functions as best as he or she can. Second, the functional impairment can alter the ways in which intact processes emerge in behavior. Third, recovery of language does not represent the creation of new subsystems; rather, recovery of language implies a reorganization that emphasizes intact subsystems (p. 869).

To summarize, the dissociation model suggests that focal brain damage may selectively impair a language function and/or may selectively impair the various pathways of access to specific functions. Once a qualitative analysis is completed, the clinician can develop rationale for task selection. The clinician may choose to pair intact and impaired functions using deblocking procedures with the goal of improving the impaired function *per se*. The clinician may choose to train the patient to use intact functions to circumvent the deficient function. Or, the clinician may choose to train the patient to use intact functions to deliberately access an intact but behaviorally disconnected function.

Lexical-Semantic Disruption

The moderately impaired aphasic individual invariably presents some degree of word-finding difficulty. The recent literature suggests that lexical-semantic errors reflect one (or more) of the following problems: (1) incomplete *access* to the semantic properties of the intended word, (2) *impoverishment* of semantic associations within a semantic field, or (3) *lexical* disorganization (e.g., broadening or misalignment of semantic features or boundaries). The research has shown that lexical-semantic performance is affected by: (1) spontaneous (nonconstrained) versus semantically- or syntactically-constrained contexts, (2) by the semantic feature composition or markedness value of words, and (3) by lexical dimensions such as semantic category, word frequency and form class. The major conclusion of recent studies is that naming ability is not an all-or-none phenomenon but rather represents the end result of a variety of processes that may be impaired alone or in combination depending on the locus and/or extent of the aphasia-producing lesion. Some representative studies will be described.

Benson (1979c) has presented an excellent overview of the anomias and their neurologic correlates. By integrating past research (Geschwind, 1965b; Goodglass & Baker, 1976; Goodglass, Barton, & Kaplan, 1968; Goodglass, Kaplan, Weintraub, & Ackerman, 1976; Luria, 1966), Benson identified nine varieties of anomia. He identified "word production anomia," "semantic (nominal) anomia," "word selection (word dictionary) anomia," "category-specific anomia," "modality-specific anomia," and others. For the purpose of illustration, *word selection anomia* will be briefly contrasted with *semantic anomia*. Word selection anomia is described by Benson as a "pure anomic aphasia," i.e., with no other disturbance of production, comprehension, repetition, reading or writing. According to Benson, this patient fails to name objects on confrontation but readily demonstrates their use, proving that the individual recognizes the object but cannot produce the name (Benson, 1979c, p. 303). This is a one-way defect in that the patient is unable to select the correct word from the lexicon despite the ability to recognize it when spoken by another person. *Semantic anomia,* in contrast, occurs when the patient is both unable to retrieve the name and unable to recognize the word when it is either spoken or written. The patient with a word selection deficit is more likely to respond to phonetic and contextual cues than the patient with semantic anomia.

Benson describes the neurologic correlates of each clinical variety of anomia. He describes how visual, auditory, and tactile association areas converge on the angular gyrus, and, as such, the angular gyrus represents a polymodal "semantic field." Interference with polymodal association by damage to the angular gyrus is likely to cause semantic anomia. In contrast, word selection anomia is more likely to occur after a more specific lesion in the temporal-occipital function areas, wherein the "concept" is preserved but access to the lexical dictionary is impeded. Thus the distinction between a loss of words versus a problem of access appears to be clinically valid and lesion-specific.

Many factors influence the way in which words are represented (associated or organized) in the brain and subsequently how words are retrieved. Some influencing factors are: word frequency and picturability (Goodglass, Hyde, & Blumstein, 1969), grammatical class (Goodglass, Gleason, Bernholtz, & Hyde, 1972), and operativity (Gardner, 1973). Concept arousal and word retrieval depend not only on number and type of associations (Goodglass & Baker, 1976), but also on the ability of the individual to access intact representations (Milberg & Blumstein, 1981).

An innovative approach to the study of semantic disorganization is the "semantic features" model. In this model, certain features comprising a word are considered "defining features" (i.e., essential properties of a concept), and others are considered "characteristic features" (i.e., accidental properties, often referential or affective). Using a semantic categorization paradigm, Grober, Perceman, Kellar, and Brown (1980) noted that patients with anterior lesions observed semantic category boundaries defined by both "defining" and "characteristic" features, while patients with posterior lesions did not. The latter group based their categorization decisions on "characteristic" features only. (See also Zurif, Caramazza, Myerson, & Calvin, 1974.)

Also using a semantic features paradigm, Buckingham and Rekart (1979) analyzed types of anomic errors in light of their component features. Their findings suggested three possible reasons for the occurrence of semantic paraphasias: (1) unshared features of the target word and the paraphasic error are missing from the repertoire of semantic features; (2) shared features are more important than unshared features, causing the latter to lose their discriminatory effect, and/or (3) during an individual's search for an intended word, unshared features may be erroneously activated (Buckingham & Rekart, 1979, p. 206).

The effects of cues and contextual factors on naming performance have also been explored in recent psycholinguistic studies. Weigl and Bierwisch (1970) suggest that aphasic individuals do not have restricted access to a particular semantic field (category) but lack precision in selecting words within the chosen field. Marshall and Ewanowski (1976) confirmed this idea, finding that contextual information enhanced naming ability *if* the information unequivocally directed the aphasic individual to a particular semantic field. If the semantic field was correctly accessed, selection of a specific word within that field was enhanced. If the contextual information was nonspecific or ambiguous the likelihood of either a related or unrelated semantic error was increased. Wales and Kinsella (1981) further suggested that syntactic constraints can influence word retrieval, with content words more easily retrieved than functors. Pease and Goodglass (1978) studied the effect of six types of cues on naming, and discovered that regardless of type of aphasia, initial phoneme and context completion cues were most helpful, a finding supported by Podraza and Darley (1977). Looking at the influence of contextualization in a somewhat different way, Williams and Canter (1981) compared noun recall in response to pictures in isolation to noun recall in response to identical stimuli presented in composite pictorial form. In this study, Broca's aphasic patients were able to name pictures more readily when they were presented in isolation, while Wernicke's aphasic patients had greater success in the composite pictorial condition.

The markedness[1] value of words also affects accessibility of nouns. Drummond, Gallagher, and Mills (1981) compared word retrieval ability for adjectives controlled for semantic feature complexity and markedness. Marked adjectives were more easily retrieved on a sentence completion task than unmarked adjectives (though unmarked adjectives proved to be easier than marked adjectives on a recognition task). Adjectives defined as "less complex" in terms of the types of features comprising them—

TABLE 4-1
Semantic Disruption in the Adult: An Organization and Retrieval Model (Fedor, 1981).

MODEL:

    The mature semantic system organizes vocabulary on at least two levels; according to word meaning (Level I) and word sound (Level II). Organization mechanisms act with retrieval mechanisms at both levels when the system is functioning normally. In anomia, impairment may occur in either organization or retrieval mechanisms, at either level in the system.

ASSESSMENT:

    I. First Decision: Is the problem one of *organization* or *retrieval*?
    II. Second Decision: Is the problem at Level I (meaning) or Level II (sound)?

TREATMENT:

    A. Disorganization, Level I Tasks

        1. Categorization according to semantic relationships, e.g.,

            (a) Grouping contrast coordinates with target (*knife*, fork, spoon)
            (b) Grouping functional associates with target (*knife*, cut, spread)
            (c) Grouping superordinates with target (*knife*, utensils, silverware)

        2. Pair modalities, e.g.,

            Patient gestures while verbalizing target words.

    B. Disorganization, Level II Tasks

        1. Categorization according to phonologic relationships, e.g.,

            (a) Grouping words having same initial phoneme
            (b) Grouping words that rhyme

    Disorganization, Levels I or II Tasks (Compensatory)

        Teach use of *circumlocution, pause* and *indefinites* to replace neologisms and paraphasias.

C. **Retrieval, Level I Tasks. Cues are Facilitative.**
   1. Sentence completion tasks
      High Probability, e.g., "Eat soup with a _____."
      Low Probability, e.g., "There are many _____."
   2. Paired associate tasks

D. **Retrieval, Level II Tasks. Cues are Facilitative.**
   1. Produce target after initial sound/syllable cue.
   2. Produce target after initial letter name, written, and/or spoken.
   3. Produce target after cued with word that rhymes.

Retrieval, Levels I or II Tasks
1. Oral reading
2. Writing to dictation
3. Writing to picture-object confrontation

---

and corresponding perceptual dimensions coded by these features—were found to be easier than adjectives defined as "more complex." These findings suggest that semantic properties of words interact with task type, perceptual factors, and type of aphasia on word retrieval tasks. Findings regarding word retrieval at the sentence level are also of interest. Buckley and Noll (1981) evaluated the ability of aphasic adults to recall sentences. They found that operative nouns were more easily recalled than figurative nouns, dynamic verbs were more easily recalled than stative verbs, and high-probability words were more easily recalled than low-probability words.

While disruption of lexical-semantic abilities in aphasia is unquestionably a complex issue, the recent literature has contributed to our understanding of psycholinguistic dimensions relevant to the act of naming. Clinically, it is possible to control stimuli and stimulus contexts along these relevant dimensions to assess the type of anomia and to maximize a patient's success in using his or her lexical repertoire. Fedor (1981), for example, outlined a treatment approach based on organization and retrieval concepts described above and by others (Buckingham & Kertesz, 1974; Goodglass & Baker, 1976; Zurif et al., 1974). As outlined in Table 4-1, Fedor suggests specific treatment tasks depending on two decisions: (1) Is the naming problem one of organization or retrieval? and (2) Does the naming problem occur at the level of meaning (i.e., selecting from the lexical dictionary), or sound (i.e., mapping phonologic representations onto lexical choices)? (A discussion of the interaction of lexical and phonologic disorders is presented later.) When treating anomia, controlling the modality of performance, the intensity of stimulation, and the hierachical presentation of cues is important, as illustrated by Linebaugh and Lehner (1977) and Rosenbek, Green, Flynn, Wertz, and Collins (1977).

Returning to the idea of dissociation, a patient described by Hier and Mohr (1977) is of interest. In this patient, written naming was superior to oral naming—an oral-graphic dissociation. When treating such a patient, one would hope for, but not necessarily observe, generalization from the relatively spared ability (written naming) to the relatively deficient ability (oral naming). A methodology is available for identifying generalization effects, either across behaviors, across modalities, or across stimuli (LaPointe, 1978a). Rosenbek, Becher, Shaughnessy, and Collins (1979) recommend the use of single-case designs for identifying dissociations among behaviors and corresponding generalization effects in treatment. For example, Thompson and Kearns (1981) evaluated acquisition, generalization, and maintenance by an anomic patient for homogeneous lexical sets. In their patient, improvement in recall of treated lexical items did not generalize to untreated semantically related lexemes. In a study of an individual with conduction aphasia, Sanders, Davis, and Hubler (1979) studied generalization across modalities. Specifically, they treated naming ability and measured the effect on repetition ability. Similar performance in both areas during treatment led the authors to tentatively conclude that naming and repetition were not dissociated in their patient, but rather that naming and repetition were governed by interdependent mechanisms. Treatment generalization effects may be related to the form class of the stimuli. For example, retrieval of prepositions was a treatment goal for a chronic Broca's aphasic patient described by Fedor, Schafer, and Horner (1981). This patient was able to learn prepositions in three modalities treated in succession (gesture, oral-verbal, and graphic), but intermodality generalization was minimal, suggesting a three-way dissociation. It is clear that more single-subject studies are needed to identify dissociations of functions and to assess treatment generalization effects.

In summary, recent descriptions of lexical-semantic disruption suggest several clinical implications. Regarding definition of anomia, it is possible to differentiate at least three major types of lexical-semantic difficulty: (1) a problem of access to the semantic properties of words, (2) an impoverishment within a semantic field, or (3) a problem of lexical organization *per se*. The literature also suggests several relevant psycholinguistic dimensions a clinician may control when developing treatment tasks and cueing hierarchies: types of cues and contexts, semantic feature and markedness value, semantic category, word frequency, form class, imageability, and operativity and dynamicity of lexical items. Identification of dissociated functions may be critical to the success of treatment in terms of improvement on the criterion behavior as well as generalization across behaviors, modalities, and stimuli.

Morphosyntactic Disruption

The moderately aphasic individual often has difficulty expressing ideas at the sentence level. Recent research has shown that morphosyntactic performance by aphasic adults is affected by (1) spontaneous (non-constrained) versus constrained task formats, (2) modality of performance, and (3) the length, complexity, and grammatical topography of sentences. Recent advances in the study of morphosyntactic abilities are several. First, the definition of "sentence meaning" has been refined. Second, the concept of syntactic processing is broadened to include syntactic comprehension as well as syntactic production. Third, syntactic processing abilities in different types of aphasia have been distinguished. Fourth, the influence of phonology on syntactic realization is better understood. Finally, the idea that the abilities of the intact minor hemisphere may be used to restore functional language has been proposed. Representative literature will be cited to illustrate these advances.

Recent literature suggests that aphasia-producing lesions may selectively impair the syntactic system independently of the lexical system. To clarify this issue of lexical-syntactic dissociation, Caramazza and Berndt (1978) describe the essential differences between lexical and sentence meaning. They state that lexical meaning and sentence meaning differ in the way they are represented semantically. Three distinctions can be made. First, lexical meaning is fixed, while sentence meaning is novel. Second, the lexicon is acquired through several separate dimensions: phonologic, syntactic, semantic, and (in literate adults) graphemic, while sentence meaning is usually acquired primarily through the auditory modality. Third, words have meaning in isolation, while sentences have meaning only by virtue of word combinations, i.e., sentence meaning involves a "combinatorial operation" wherein a finite set of rules is applied recursively to produce an unlimited number of sentence types. Thus, novelty, the mode of acquisition, and combination rules distinguish sentence meaning from word meaning and help explain why lexical-syntactic dissociations can occur.

Several studies confirm the concept of lexical-syntactic dissociation. Using an anagram "sentence ordering task" von Stockert (1972) observed that an individual with Broca's aphasia performed well when sentence construction depended on major lexical items. Individuals with Wernicke's aphasia, in contrast, performed well when sentence construction (via constituent ordering) depended on the syntactic relations conveyed by grammatical morphemes. It appears from this and subsequent studies (e.g., Gallagher, 1981; Heilman & Scholes, 1976; Rothi, McFarling, & Heilman, 1982) that lexical knowledge is spared and syntactic knowledge is impaired in nonfluent aphasia while the reverse is true in fluent aphasia. This lexical-syntactic processing dissociation has been identified in the comprehension as well as in the production abilities of Broca's and Wernicke's aphasic patients (Gallagher, 1981; Saffran, Schwartz, & Marin, 1980; Zurif & Caramazza, 1976). The idea that lexical-syntactic processing strategies are similar in receptive and expressive modalities supports the psychological reality of a syntactic processing mechanism. Our understanding of "agrammatism" has been enhanced by these recent notions.

The idea that prosodic-phonologic factors influence syntactic processing is another concept that has been recently described. The importance of prosodic features to nonfluent (Broca's) aphasic language was recognized by Goodglass (1968). He proposed a "stress-saliency" hypothesis to explain the preservation or loss of functors in sentences. The term "saliency" refers to informational load, affective tone, and increased intonational emphasis. Goodglass suggested that "...a basic feature of Broca's aphasia is the increased difficulty mobilizing the speech output system which requires a stressed element to put it into action" (1976, p. 252). The stress-saliency hypothesis accounts in part for the telegraphic form of Broca's aphasic speech as well as the effortful and interrupted delivery of speech, notably at phrase boundaries.

Kean (1977) extended this phonologic interpretation of agrammatism. She defined a "phonologic word" as: ". . . the strings of segments marked by boundaries which function in the assignment of stress to a word" (p. 22). As such, the realization of segmental (phoneme) and suprasegmental (stress and intonation) features are inseparable during speech. In Kean's model, affixes and functors are deemed not to be "phonologic words" because, by definition, ". . . they do not carry stress or affect the stress pattern of the sentence" (p. 23). In short, Kean interprets agrammatism to be a phonologic disorder primarily characterized by *phonological simplification of sentences.* The findings of Swinney, Zurif, and Cutler (1980) support Kean's model. They suggest that normal adults use stress in sentence comprehension and production for two purposes: (1) to distinguish among word classes, and (2) to locate high information words.

They suggest that in Broca's aphasia, a deficiency in the assignment of stress accounts for an impaired ability to distinguish substantive (open class) words from function (closed class) words. Because functors are unstressed, difficulties for this class of words ensue in Broca's aphasia. For example, processing of prepositions by agrammatic aphasic individuals is impaired as described in both historical and more recent literature (Friederici, 1981; Mack, 1981; Seron & Deloche, 1981). This current view of the interaction of phonologic-prosodic form with syntactic form represents a significant departure from more traditional models that represent grammatical rules and phonological rules as distinct psycholinguistic entities.

Recent literature also contributes to treatment of aphasic syntactic deficits. In 1972, Goodglass, Green, Bernholtz, and Hyde developed a "Story Completion Task," whereby a variety of increasingly complex phrase and sentence types, as defined by transformational rules, are elicited. Helm-Estabrooks, Fitzpatrick, and Barresi (1981) recently developed a *Syntax Stimulation Program (SSP)* for eight sentence types using this story completion paradigm. Briefly, this approach involves presentation of stories designed to elicit sentences in a hierarchy of difficulty. Two levels of response difficulty are addressed: the first requires the patient to produce a delayed repetition of the target response; the second requires the patient to complete the given story with a self-retrieved target response. All stories are accompanied by line drawings depicting the associated story. Measureable gains in sentence formulation by a chronically agrammatic individual suggest the *SSP* to be an efficacious syntax program.

In 1979, Tonkovich studied the language of a Broca's aphasic individual using Fillmore's case grammar. Fillmore's conception of syntax is that the verb is the core of a sentence and that nouns in sentences assume specific "case relations" to the verb depending on their functions in sentences. For example, the word *table* in the following sentences assumes different cases depending on the context: (1) The *table* fell (objective case); (2) The vase fell from the *table* (source case); (3) She put flowers on the *table* (locative case), etc. (Tonkovich, 1979, p. 245). Tonkovich found that in Broca's aphasia agentive and objective cases were more robust than instrumental, source, or goal cases; semantically similar cases such as source and goal were likely to be confused; and semantically redundant forms were likely to be omitted or in error. As an extension of Fillmore's model, Loverso, Selinger, and Prescott (1979) developed a "verb as core" treatment for aphasic syntactic deficits. In this approach, verbs are used as the pivot-stimuli and wh-questions are provided as cues to elicit sentences of the "actor-action-object" type, both graphically and verbally. Standardized test-retest measures showed this "verbing strategy" to be an effective approach to remediation of sentence formulation deficits.

Finally, a "minor-hemispheric mediation" approach to aphasia treatment has recently been proposed (Horner, 1983; Horner and Fedor, 1983). The underlying assumptions of this model are: (1) under appropriate stimulus conditions, the minor hemisphere can be tapped to mediate language recovery, and (2) the potential for aphasia recovery can be enhanced through systematic pairing of linguistic behaviors with ideographic stimuli, subserved by the domimant and minor hemispheres, respectively. Specific treatment tasks for moderately impaired aphasic individuals presenting either Broca's or Wernicke's aphasia are outlined using three general types of ideographic stimuli: prosodic-affective, visual-spatial-holistic, and rudimentary linguistic behaviors.

In summary, current psycholinguistic notions about syntactic disruption in aphasia were presented. First, syntactic processing may be selectively impaired, suggesting a dissociation from other psycholinguistic functions. Second, syntactic comprehension appears to parallel syntactic production. Third, phonology interacts with syntactic disruption in nonfluent aphasia. Treatment approaches have been described, or suggested, by recent advances. Among these, a "minor hemispheric mediation" approach to treatment of moderate aphasia has been proposed.

Phonologic Disruption

The moderately aphasic individual often suffers an impairment in the phonologic realization of utterances. Phonology encompasses not only the selection and sequencing of phonemes in the creation of words, but also the prosodic ("stress-saliency") dimensions of speech operating at the sentence level. Recent studies of aphasic phonologic disorders suggest that phonologic realization varies as a function of (1) propositional-automatic-imitative constraints, (2) phoneme type, (3) prosodic features, (4) overall speech fluency, and (5) lexical and syntactic features. Representative studies will be reviewed.

Selection and sequencing of sounds is no longer viewed as merely a surface manifestation of language. Phonology is recognized as a rule-governed linguistic system in its own right. Analyses of phonologic errors in aphasia suggest that the psycholinguistic mechanisms governing selection and sequencing of sounds interact in a dynamic if not predictable fashion with lexical-semantic and syntactic subsystems. Furthermore, traditional substitution, omission and distortion analyses are being replaced by distinctive feature, markedness and phonological process analyses of aphasic phonologic disruption.

Kellar and Roch Lecours (1980) and Shewan (1980) discussed two aspects of phonologic production. The first aspect is the internal representation that constitutes the plan for phoneme realization; errors at this level are "phonemic" errors. The second aspect is the internal monitor for speech, which involves organizing the motor commands for sound production *per se*; failures at this level are "phonetic" errors. Conceived as such, aphasic speech sound errors may result from a defect of the "phonological-articulatory" process, i.e., at either the phonemic level, the phonetic level, or both. The important point here is that *common linguistic principles* are likely to influence *both* phonemic and phonetic errors (Goodglass, 1975). This conclusion is drawn in part from Blumstein's early study (1973) in which she found that phonologic error patterns in Broca's, Wernicke's, and Conduction aphasia were *qualitatively* similar. For all three subject groups, two-thirds of phoneme errors differed from the target by one distinctive feature and unmarked-for-marked substitutions outnumbered marked-for-unmarked substitutions 2 to 1. Further analyses revealed differences among the aphasia types: In Broca's aphasia, phonologic processing appeared to operate at the syllabic level, while in Wernicke's and Conduction aphasia, phonologic processing appeared to operate at the level of phrases and sentences. To discern error patterns researchers suggest it is necessary to use stimuli controlled for type of phoneme and phoneme word-position, and to elicit speech in a variety of contexts: self-initiated, automatic, and imitative speech (Burns & Canter, 1977). Furthermore, it is essential that analyses account for the fluent or nonfluent nature of the presenting aphasia (Roch Lecours & Rouillon, 1976).

Recent studies document the interaction of phonology with syntax (see Kean, 1977) and phonology with lexicon. The latter is addressed in recent studies of neologistic jargon aphasia. O'Connell (1981) suggests that neologisms have several sources. A neologism may be: (1) a complex phonemically paraphasic distortion of a correctly retrieved word, (2) a two-stage error where faulty semantic retrieval undergoes phonological disruption, or (3) the product of recombinations of units from surrounding utterances to "fill in" for intended words (O'Connell, 1981, p. 301). O'Connell's first explanation is consistent with a "conduction theory" (Kertesz & Benson, 1970) which suggests that neologisms result from an excessive accumulation of phonemic paraphasias, such that the intended utterance is no longer recognizable. O'Connell's second and third explanations derive from a "masking theory" (Buckingham, 1979) wherein phonologic distortions appear to "fill anomic gaps." A "level of activity notion" proposed by Farmer and O'Connell (1979) suggests that phonemic paraphasias and neologisms reflect an overaroused language system in which selection of both lexical and phonemic units are compromised.

The coincidence of phonologic and lexical-semantic disruption appears to be related to site and extent of lesion. Cappa, Cavallotti, and Vignolo (1981) correlated lesion sites identified by CT scan with prevalence of lexical versus phonemic errors in fluent aphasia. Phonemic errors (phonemic paraphasias, phonemic groping [conduites d'approche], neologisms, and phonemic jargon) correlated with lesions near the sylvian fissure. Lexical errors (circumlocution, verbal paraphasia, semantic jargon) correlated with lesions distant from the sylvian fissure.

Of special interest in recent literature is an innovative application of "phonological process" analysis to description of acquired neurogenic phonologic disorders. Kearns (1980) defines this approach: "Phonological analysis procedures attempt to generate rules which relate phonetic errors to underlying forms and to intended sounds. An important component of the analysis procedure is the incorporation of environmental (contextual) considerations into the rule derivation" (Kearns, 1980, p. 187). Kearns evaluated a moderately aphasic-apraxic adult and identified several general error trends using the "phonological process" analysis. In terms of *syllable structure processes,* final consonant deletion and cluster reduction were observed. In terms of *phonemic substitution processes,* stopping and fronting occurred frequently. The third process, *assimilation,* was also observed. Kearn's study recommends the phonological process approach to the study of phonologic disruption and, potentially, to the development of treatment rationale.

In summary, it is now recognized that phonology is governed by psycholinguistic rules, and that phonology interacts in aphasia syndromes with syntactic and lexical-semantic performance. Although phonologic errors manifest somewhat differently in fluent and nonfluent aphasia syndromes, the commonalities and differences are not yet fully understood. As psycholinguistic principles governing phonologic disruption evolve, it is hoped that corresponding treatment approaches can be developed. Current research suggests that phonologic treatment rationale will necessarily include considerations of prosodic contour, fluency of speech, phonologic contextual influences, and lexical and syntactic constraints as well as the distinctive feature and markedness composition of phonologic error profiles.

Pragmatic Disruption

The final area of concern in this chapter is the area of pragmatic abilities of the moderately impaired aphasic individual. Recent literature emphasizes the need for evaluation of communicative competence as a function complementary to linguistic competence and the importance of incorporating pragmatic considerations in the treatment of aphasic individuals. Representative literature will be reviewed.

By way of introduction to pragmatics, it is necessary to understand the various ways in which meaning is conveyed through language. Meaning can be conveyed by (1) word in isolation (conveying both referential and descriptive meaning), (2) words in relation to other words (semantic fields, features, and networks), (3) words in sentences, and (4) relations among sentences (Lesser, 1978; Schachter, 1976). In the broader perspective of "language pragmatics," the study of meaning involves investigations into how one's communicative intentions are mapped onto linguistic form. Pragmatic rules govern how language is used in social contexts (Bates, 1976) to convey a variety of intentions: requesting, asserting, questioning, ordering, arguing, advising, and warning (Searle, 1969). An individual's use of language based on an understanding of how language works in social interactions is termed "communicative competence" (Holland, 1977, p. 171). Major advances have been made in recent years in the study of pragmatics and communicative competence in aphasia.

One premise of these studies is that functional communication by aphasic adults is not related to the accuracy of utterances but rather to "getting a message across" through the use of both linguistic and paralinguistic behaviors. Studies have found that aphasic adults are limited in the variety of speech acts which they use (Wilcox & Davis, 1977), and are below normal in the proportion of communicative attempts to communicative successes (Holland, 1978). Holland (1977) and Ulatowska, Haynes, Hildebrand, and Richardson (1977) agree that some moderately aphasic individuals are extremely "functional" depending on their use of compensatory strategies. It appears that linguistic competence and communicative competence interact in ways not completely predictable by the overall severity of aphasia.

Studies of comprehension suggest that aphasic individuals who are able to use extralinguistic cues such as contextually conveyed meaning tend to perform better in "real-life situations" than one might expect from their performance on standard aphasia batteries (Stachowiak, Huber, Poeck, & Kerschensteiner, 1977; Wilcox, Davis, & Leonard, 1978). Studies of expression suggest that patients who use a variety of compensatory strategies (e.g., nonverbal signs) are able to convey their intentions, despite linguistic failures (Prinz, 1980).

Chapey and her associates have contributed to our understanding of aphasic communicative competence by studying divergent semantic behavior. Chapey (1977) suggests that aphasic patients may have both convergent and divergent linguistic difficulties. She suggests that many aphasic individuals are functionally deficient in situations that require the use of divergent semantic strategies, i.e., information-getting, problem solving, and persuasion. Chapey, Rigrodsky, and Morrison (1977) further suggest that aphasic individuals are unable to "proliferate" ideas on a topic both in terms of the number and the variety of relevant ideas. Divergent language also involves a "judgment ability," i.e., the ability to evaluate the adequacy of messages and revise them depending on the pragmatic intentions and the demands of the situation. Chapey and Lubinski (1979) found aphasic patients to be below normal in overall semantic judgment scores and suggest that divergent and convergent behaviors are distinct abilities for aphasic individuals. The rationale, principles, and stages of divergent semantic therapy are described by Chapey (1981).

The most notable advances in the area of pragmatics include the development of a test, *Communicative Abilities in Daily Living (CADL)* by Holland (1980) and the development of a treatment approach, *Promoting Aphasics Communicative Effectiveness (PACE)* by Davis and Wilcox (1981). Holland's test has the unique purpose of assessing the "functional communication" of aphasic adults. It provides the clinician with a valuable means of measuring communicative behavior in natural contexts, which may then be compared with the patient's language impairment. Ten functional categories are evaluated using the *CADL* (See Table 4-2).

Regarding treatment, Prinz (1980) advised: "It is incumbent on the clinician to emphasize the patient's communicative assets by providing a conversational setting designed to elicit a variety of pragmatic intentions and the appropriate use of strategies to realize these intentions" (p. 71). Davis (1980) and Davis and Wilcox (1981) attempt to incorporate parameters of natural conversation in aphasia treatment. This treatment approach: (a) emphasizes the use of language in context, (b) controls structural aspects of face-to-face conversation and (c) stimulates the use of nonverbal as well as verbal channels to convey messages. The main goal of the *PACE* approach is the communication of messages, not linguistic accuracy or complexity. Four interdependent principles of *PACE* are:

1. There is an exchange of new information between the clinician and the patient.
2. The patient has a free choice as to which communicative channels he or she may use to convey new information.
3. The clinician and the patient participate equally as senders and receivers of messages.
4. Feedback is provided by the clinician in response to the patient's success in conveying a message. (Davis & Wilcox, 1981, p. 180).

TABLE 4-2
Ten Categories of Performance on the CADL (Holland, 1980).

1. Reading, writing, and using numbers to estimate, calculate, and judge time
2. Speech acts
3. Utilizing verbal and nonverbal context
4. Role playing
5. Sequenced and relationship-dependent communicative behavior
6. Social conventions
7. Divergencies
8. Nonverbal symbolic communication
9. Deixis
10. Humor, absurdity, metaphor

Thus, recent studies of pragmatics and divergent semantic behavior have served to broaden our view of aphasic communicative impairments. Several conclusions from the literature are: (1) the variety of speech acts used by aphasic individuals may be depressed; (2) the contexts in which language is used may be restricted; (3) the adequacy of conveying intentions reflects the interaction of both linguistic competence (divergent and convergent aspects) and communicative competence and (4) communicative competence in part reflects the patient's ability to use alternate (i.e., nonlinguistic) communication channels. In general, studies suggest that communicative competence and linguistic competence are not synonymous functions. In an aphasic individual, overall language competence may not always predict his "communicative competence."

In summary, several clinical guidelines from the study of pragmatics are: (1) evaluate communicative competence in a variety of communicative contexts (e.g., *CADL*); (2) control the variety of pragmatic functions (intentions) of speech acts; (3) emphasize communication adequacy over linguistic accuracy; (4) use spontaneous compensatory strategies to enhance communicative effectiveness and/or train the patient in the use of alternate behaviors; (5) train flexibility in the choice of communicative channels (verbal and/or nonverbal); and (6) treat both convergent and divergent semantic abilities.

Summary

Treatment of aphasic individuals requires an appreciation for the nature of language disorganization following focal brain damage. Descriptive psycholinguistic studies have enhanced our appreciation for how linguistic subsystems can be disrupted and/or dissociated, how linguistic subsystems interact with one another, and how aphasic deficits influence the way intact functions emerge in behavior. The clinician's task is not only to describe the degree of language impairment but also to assess the qualitative features of language impairment. The prevalent theme expressed in this chapter is that the psycholinguistic approach to aphasia is particularly well-suited to this qualitative diagnostic purpose. The literature reviewed in this chapter focused on lexical-semantic, morphosyntactic, phonologic, and pragmatic studies of the moderately aphasic individual. From this review it became apparent that an understanding of psycholinguistic mechanisms operating in aphasic language, notably "dissociation of functions," is necessary if aphasia clinicians are to render well-reasoned and effective treatment. Perhaps through a heightened appreciation for the psycholinguistic intricacies of aphasic language we may help our patients realize their full communicative potential.

Note

[1] "Among related categories which differ in markedness, we define the unmarked member as compared to the marked member as: 1) conceptually and/or formally simpler, and therefore more natural, 2) usually statistically more frequent, 3) usually acquired earlier in the process of language development." (Ulatowska & Baker, 1975, p. 153).

Acknowledgment

Funded, in part, by the Axe-Houghton Foundation, New York, NY. My appreciation to Dr. Craig Linebaugh for his review of this chapter.

References

Albert, M. L., Goodglass, H., Helm, N. A., Rubens, A. B., & Alexander, M. P. *Clinical aspects of dysphasia*. New York: Springer-Verlag Wien, 1981.

Bates, E. Pragmatics and sociolinguistics in child language. In D. Morehead & A. Morehead (Eds.), *Directions in normal and deficient child language*. Baltimore: University Park Press, 1976.

Benson, D. F. *Aphasia, alexia, and agraphia*. New York: Churchill Livingstone, 1979. (a)

Benson, D. F. Aphasia. In K. M. Heilman & E. Valenstein (Eds.), *Clinical neuropsychology*. New York: Oxford University Press, 1979, 22-58. (b)

Benson, D. F. Neurologic correlates of anomia. In H. Whitaker & H. A. Whitaker (Eds.), *Studies in neurolinguistics* (Vol. 4). New York: Academic Press, 1979, 293-328. (c)

Berndt, R. S., & Caramazza, A. Syntactic aspects of aphasia. In M. T. Sarno (Ed.), *Acquired aphasia*. New York: Academic Press, 1981, 157–182.

Blumstein, S. E. *A phonological investigation of aphasic speech*. Hague: Mouton, 1973.

Blumstein, S. Phonological aspects of aphasia. In M. T. Sarno (Ed.), *Acquired aphasia*. New York: Academic Press, 1981, 129–156.

Brookshire, R. H. Auditory comprehension and aphasia. In D. F. Johns (Ed.), *Clinical management of neurogenic communicative disorders*. Boston: Little, Brown & Company, 1978, 103–128.

Brookshire, R. H., & Nicholas, L. E. Verification of active and passive sentences by aphasic and nonaphasic subjects. *Journal of Speech and Hearing Research*, 1980, *23*, 878–893. (a)

Brookshire, R. H., & Nicholas, L. E. Sentence verification and language comprehension of aphasic persons. In R. H. Brookshire (Ed.), *Clinical Aphasiology: Conference Proceedings, 1980*. Minneapolis: BRK Publishers, 1980, 53–63. (b)

Brookshire, R. H., & Nicholas, L. E. Comprehension of spoken active and passive sentences by aphasic and nonaphasic subjects. In R. H. Brookshire (Ed.), *Clinical aphasiology: Conference Proceedings, 1981*. Minneapolis: BRK Publishers, 1981, 108–114.

Buckingham, H. W. Linguistic aspects of lexical retrieval disturbances in the posterior fluent aphasias. In H. Whitaker & H. A. Whitaker (Eds.), *Studies in neurolinguistics*, (Vol. 4). New York: Academic Press, 1979, 269–292.

Buckingham, H. W. Lexical and semantic aspects of aphasia. In M. T. Sarno (Ed.), *Acquired aphasia*. New York: Academic Press, 1981, 183–214.

Buckingham, H. W., & Kertesz, A. A linguistic analysis of fluent aphasia. *Brain and Language*, 1974, *1*, 43–62.

Buckingham, H. W., & Rekart, D. M. Semantic paraphasia. *Journal of Communication Disorders*, 1979, *12*, 197–209.

Buckley, C. E., & Noll, J. D. Lexical parameters affecting sentence recall by aphasic adults. In R. H. Brookshire (Ed.), *Clinical aphasiology: Conference proceedings, 1981*. Minneapolis: BRK Publishers, 1981, 96–104.

Burns, M. S., & Canter, G. J. Phonemic behavior of aphasic patients with posterior cerebral lesions. *Brain and Language*, 1977, *4*, 492–507.

Cappa, S., Cavallotti, G., & Vignolo, L. A. Phonemic and lexical errors in fluent aphasia: Correlation with lesion site. *Neuropsychologia*, 1981, *19*, 171–178.

Caramazza, A., & Berndt, R. S. Semantic and syntactic processes in aphasia: A review of the literature, *Psychological Bulletin*, 1978, *85*, 898–918.

Chapey, R. A divergent semantic model of intervention in adult aphasia. In R. H. Brookshire (Ed.), *Clinical Aphasiology: Conference Proceedings, 1977*. Minneapolis: BRK Publishers, 1977, 257–264.

Chapey, R. Divergent semantic intervention. In R. Chapey (Ed.), *Language intervention strategies in adult aphasia*. Baltimore: Williams & Wilkins, 1981.

Chapey, R., & Lubinski, R. Semantic judgment ability in adult aphasia. *Cortex*, 1979, *15*, 247–256.

Chapey, R., Rigrodsky, S., & Morrison, E. M. Aphasia: A divergent semantic interpretation. *Journal of Speech and Hearing Disorders*, 1977, *42*, 287–295.

Davis, G. A. A critical look at PACE therapy. In R. H. Brookshire (Ed.), *Clinical Aphasiology: Conference Proceedings, 1980*. Minneapolis: BRK Publishers, 1980, 248–257.

Davis, G. A., & Wilcox, M. J. Incorporating parameters of natural conversation in aphasia treatment. In R. Chapey (Ed.), *Language intervention strategies in adult aphasia*. Baltimore: Williams & Wilkins, 1981, 169–193.

Drummond, S. S., Gallagher, T. M., & Mills, R. H. Word retrieval in aphasia: An investigation of semantic complexity. *Cortex*, 1981, *17*, 63–82.

Duffy, J. R. Schuell's stimulation approach to rehabilitation. In R. Chapey (Ed.), *Language intervention strategies in adult aphasia*. Baltimore: Williams & Wilkins, 1981, 105-140.

Farmer, A., & O'Connell, P. Neuropsychological processes in adult aphasia: Rationale for treatment. *British Journal of Disorders of Communication*, 1979, *14*, 39-49.

Fedor, K. H. *Semantic disruption in the adult: An organization and retrieval model*. Paper presented to the North Carolina Speech-Language-Hearing Association. Asheville, 1981.

Fedor, K. H., Schafer, N., & Horner, J. *Transcoding across three modalities in Broca's aphasia*. Paper presented to the American Speech-Language-Hearing Association. Los Angeles, 1981.

Friederici, A. D. Production and comprehension of prepositions in aphasia. *Neuropsychologia*, 1981, *19*, 191-200.

Gallagher, A. J. Syntactic versus semantic performance of agrammatic Broca's aphasics on tests of constituent-element-ordering. *Journal of Speech and Hearing Research*, 1981, *24*, 217-223.

Gardner, H. The contribution of operativity to naming capacity in aphasic patients. *Neuropsychologia*, 1973, *11*, 213-220.

Geschwind, N. Disconnexion syndromes in animals and man. *Brain*, 1965, *88*, 237-294, 585-644. (a)

Geschwind, N. The varieties of naming errors. *Cortex*, 1965, *3*, 97-112. (b)

Goodglass, H. Studies on the grammar of aphasics. In S. Rosenberg & J. Koplin (Eds.), *Developments in applied psycholinguistic research*. New York: Macmillan, 1968.

Goodglass, H. Phonological factors in aphasia. In R. H. Brookshire (Ed.), *Clinical Aphasiology: Conference Proceedings, 1975*. Minneapolis: BRK Publishers, 1975, 28-44.

Goodglass, H. Agrammatism. In H. Whitaker & H. A. Whitaker (Eds.), *Studies in neurolinguistics* (Vol. 1). New York: Academic Press, 1976, 237-260.

Goodglass, H., & Baker, E. Semantic field, naming and auditory comprehension in aphasia. *Brain and Language*, 1976, *3*, 359-374.

Goodglass, H., & Kaplan, E. *The Boston Diagnostic Aphasia Exam*. Philadelphia: Lea & Febiger, 1972. (a)

Goodglass, H., & Kaplan, E. *Assessment of aphasia and related disorders*. Philadelphia: Lea & Febiger, 1972. (b)

Goodglass, H., Barton, M. I., & Kaplan, E. Sensory modality and object-naming in aphasia. *Journal of Speech and Hearing Research*, 1968, *3*, 257-267.

Goodglass, H., Hyde, M. R., & Blumstein, S. Frequency, picturability and availability of nouns in aphasia. *Cortex*, 1969, *5*, 104-119.

Goodglass, H., Kaplan, E., Weintraub, S., & Ackerman, N. The tip-of-the-tongue phenomenon in aphasia. *Cortex*, 1976, *12*, 145-153.

Goodglass, H., Gleason, J. B., Bernholtz, N. A., & Hyde, M. R. Some linguistic structures in the speech of a Broca's aphasic. *Cortex*, 1972, *8*, 191-212.

Grober, E., Perceman, E., Kellar, L., & Brown, J. Lexical knowledge in anterior and posterior aphasics. *Brain and Language*, 1980, *10*, 318-330.

Hand, C. R., Tonkovich, J. D., & Aitchison, J. Some idiosyncratic strategies utilized by a chronic Broca's aphasic. *Linguistics*, 1979, *17*, 729-761.

Helm-Estabrooks, N., Fitzpatrick, P. M., & Barresi, B. Response of an agrammatic patient to a syntax stimulation program for aphasia. *Journal of Speech and Hearing Disorders*, 1981, *46*, 422-427.

Heilman, K. M., & Scholes, R. J. The nature of comprehension errors in Broca's conduction and Wernicke's aphasics. *Cortex*, 1976, *12*, 258-265.

Hier, D. B., & Mohr, J. P. Incongruous oral and written naming. Evidence for a subdivision of Wernicke's aphasia. *Brain and Language*, 1977, *4*, 115-126.

Holland, A. L. Case studies in aphasia rehabilitation using programmed instruction. *Journal of Speech and Hearing Disorders*, 1972, *37*, 3–21.
Holland, A. L. Some practical considerations in aphasia rehabilitation. In M. Sullivan & M. S. Kommers (Eds.), *Rationale for adult aphasia therapy*. Omaha: University of Nebraska, 1977, 167–180.
Holland, A. L. Functional communication in the treatment of aphasia. In L. J. Bradford (Ed.), *Communication disorders: An audio journal for continuing education* (Vol. 3). New York: Grune & Stratton, 1978.
Holland, A. L. *CADL: Communicative abilities in daily living*. Baltimore: University Park Press, 1980.
Horner, J. Broca's aphasia: Facilitation and reorganization. In W. H. Perkins (Ed.), *Current therapy of communication disorders*. New York: Thieme-Stratton, 1983.
Horner, J., & Fedor, K. H. Minor hemisphere mediation in aphasia treatment. In H. Winitz (Ed.), *Treating language disorders: For clinicians by clinicians*. Baltimore: University Park Press, 1983.
Kean, M. L. The linguistic interpretation of aphasic syndromes: Agrammatism in Broca's aphasia, an example. *Cognition*, 1977, *5*, 9–46.
Kearns, K. P. The application of phonological process analysis to adult neuropathologies. In R. H. Brookshire (Ed.), *Clinical Aphasiology: Conference Proceedings, 1980*. Minneapolis: BRK Publishers, 1980, 187–195.
Kellar, E., & Roch Lecours, A. Sequences of phonemic approximations in aphasia. *Brain and Language*, 1980, *11*, 30–44.
Kertesz, A. *Aphasia and associated disorders: Taxonomy, localization, and recovery*. New York: Grune & Stratton, 1979.
Kertesz, A. *Western Aphasia Battery*. London, Canada: University of Western Ontario, 1980.
Kertesz, A., & Benson, D. Neologistic jargon: A clinicopathological study. *Cortex*, 1970, *6*, 362–386.
LaPointe, L. L. Base-10 programmed-stimulation: Task specification, scoring and plotting performance in aphasia therapy. *Journal of Speech and Hearing Disorders*, 1977, *42*, 90–105.
LaPointe, L. L. Aphasia therapy: Some principles and strategies for treatment. In D. F. Johns (Ed.), *Clinical management of neurogenic communicative disorders*. Boston: Little, Brown & Co., 1978, 129–190. (a)
LaPointe, L. L. Multiple baseline designs. In R. H. Brookshire (Ed.), *Clinical Aphasiology: Conference Proceedings, 1978*. Minneapolis: BRK Publishers, 1978, 20–39. (b)
Lesser, R. *Linguistic investigations of aphasia*. New York: Elsevier, 1978.
Linebaugh, C., & Lehner, L. Cueing hierarchies and word retrieval: A therapy program. In R. H. Brookshire (Ed.), *Clinical Aphasiology: Conference Proceedings, 1977*. Minneapolis: BRK Publishers, 1977, 19–31.
Loverso, F. L., Selinger, M., & Prescott, T. E. Applications of verbing strategies to aphasia treatment. In R. H. Brookshire (Ed.), *Clinical Aphasiology: Conference Proceedings, 1979*. Minneapolis: BRK Publishers, 1979, 229–238.
Luria, A. R. *Higher cortical functions in man*. New York: Basic Books, 1966.
Mack, J. L. The comprehension of locative prepositions in nonfluent and fluent aphasia. *Brain and Language*, 1981, *14*, 81–92.
Marin, O. S. M., Saffran, E. M., & Schwartz, M. F. Dissociations of language in aphasia: Implications for normal function. *Annals of the New York Academy of Science*, 1976, *280*, 868–884.
Martin, A. D. A proposed rationale for aphasia therapy. In B. Porch (Ed.), *Clinical Aphasiology: Conference Proceedings, 1974*. Albuquerque, NM, 1974, 79–94.

Martin, A. D. An examination of Wepman's thought centered therapy. In R. Chapey (Ed.), *Language intervention strategies in adult aphasia*. Baltimore: Williams & Wilkins, 1981, 141-154.
Marshall, T. D., & Ewanowski, S. J. *The effects of linguistic context on the word finding abilities of aphasic adults*. Paper presented to the American Speech-Language-Hearing Association, Houston, 1976.
Milberg, W., & Blumstein, S. E. Lexical decision and aphasia: Evidence for semantic processing. *Brain and Language*, 1981, *14*, 371-385.
Myerson, R., & Goodglass, H. Transformational grammars of aphasic patients. *Language and Speech*, 1972, *15*, 40-50.
O'Connell, P. F. Neologistic jargon aphasia: A case report. *Brain and Language*, 1981, *12*, 292-302.
Pease, D. M., & Goodglass, H. The effects of cueing on picture naming in aphasia. *Cortex*, 1978, *14*, 178-189.
Podraza, B.L., & Darley, F. L. Effect of auditory prestimulation on naming in aphasia. *Journal of Speech and Hearing Research*, 1977, *20*, 669-683.
Porch, B. *The Porch Index of Communicative Ability*. Palo Alto, CA: Consulting Psychologists Press, 1967.
Porch, B. E. Therapy subsequent to the *PICA*. In R. Chapey (Ed.), *Language intervention strategies in adult aphasia*. Baltimore: Williams & Wilkins, 1981, 283-296.
Prinz, P. M. A note on requesting strategies in adult aphasics. *Journal of Communication Disorders*, 1980, *13*, 65-73.
Roch Lecours, A., & Rouillon, F. Neurolinguistic analysis of jargonaphasia and jargonagraphia. In H. Whitaker & H. A. Whitaker (Eds.), *Studies in neurolinguistics* (Vol. 2). New York: Academic Press, 1976, 95-144.
Rosenbek, J., Becher, B., Shaughnessy, A., & Collins, M. Other uses of single-case designs. In R. H. Brookshire (Ed.), *Clinical Aphasiology: Conference Proceedings, 1979*. Minneapolis: BRK Publishers, 1979, 311-316.
Rosenbek, J., Green, E., Flynn, M., Wertz, R. T., & Collins, M. Anomia: A clinical experiment. In R. H. Brookshire (Ed.), *Clinical Aphasiology: Conference Proceedings, 1977*. Minneapolis: BRK Publishers, 1977, 103-111.
Rosenbek, J. C., Lemme, M. L., Ahern, M. B., Harris, E. H., & Wertz, R. T. A treatment for apraxia of speech in adults. *Journal of Speech and Hearing Disorders*, 1973, *38*, 462-472.
Rothi, L. J., McFarling, D., & Heilman, K. M. Conduction aphasia, syntactic alexia, and the anatomy of syntactic comprehension. *Archives of Neurology*, 1982, *39*, 272-275.
Saffran, E. M, Schwartz, M. F., & Marin, O. S. M. The word order problem in agrammatism. II. Production. *Brain and Language*, 1980, *10*, 263-280.
Sanders, S. B., Davis, G. A., & Hubler, V. A study of the interdependence of word retrieval and repetition in conduction aphasia. In R. H. Brookshire (Ed.), *Clinical Aphasiology: Conference Proceedings, 1979*. Minneapolis: BRK Publishers, 1979, 270-277.
Schachter, J. Some semantic prerequisites for a model of language. *Brian and Language*, 1976, *3*, 292-304.
Schuell, H., Jenkins, J., & Jiménez-Pabón, E. *Aphasia in adults*. New York: Harper & Row, 1964.
Searle, J. R. *Speech acts*. London: Cambridge University Press, 1969.
Seron, X., & Deloche, G. Processing of locatives "in," "on," and "under" by aphasic patients: An analysis of the regression hypothesis. *Brain and Language*, 1981, *14*, 70-80.
Shewan, C. M. Phonological processing in Broca's aphasics. *Brain and Language*, 1980, *10*, 71-88.

Stachowiak, F. J., Huber, W., Poeck, K., & Kerschensteiner. Comprehension in aphasia. *Brain and Language*, 1977, *4*, 177-195.

Swinney, D. A., Zurif, E. B., & Cutler, A. Effects of sentential stress and word class upon comprehension in Broca's aphasics. *Brain and Language*, 1980, *10*, 132-144.

Thompson, C. K., & Kearns, K. An experimental analysis of acquisition, generalization and maintenance of naming behavior in a patient with anomic aphasia. In R. H. Brookshire (Ed.), *Clinical Aphasiology: Conference Proceedings, 1981*. Minneapolis: BRK Publishers, 1981, 35-45.

Tonkovich, J. D. Case relations in Broca's aphasia: Some considerations regarding treatment. In R. H. Brookshire (Ed.), *Clinical Aphasiology: Conference Proceedings. 1979*. Minneapolis: BRK Publishers, 1979, 239-247.

Ulatowska, H. K. Application of linguistics to treatment of aphasia. In R. H. Brookshire (Ed.), *Clinical Aphasiology: Conference Proceedings. 1979*. Minneapolis: BRK Publishers, 1979, 317-323.

Ulatowska, H. K., & Baker W. D. On a notion of markedness in linguistic systems: Application to aphasia. In R. H. Brookshire (Ed.), *Clinical Aphasiology: Conference Proceedings. 1975*. Minneapolis: BRK Publishers, 1975, 153-164.

Ulatowska, H. K., Haynes, S. M., Hildebrand, B. H., & Richardson, S. M. The aphasic individual: A speaker and listner, not a patient. In R. H. Brookshire (Ed.), *Clinical Aphasiology: Conference Proceedings. 1977*. Minneapolis: BRK Publishers, 1977, 198-213.

von Stockert, T. R. Recognition of syntactic structure in aphasic patients. *Cortex*, 1972, *8*, 323-334.

Wales, R., & Kinsella, G. Syntactic effects in sentence completion by Broca's aphasics. *Brain and Language*, 1981, *13*, 301-307.

Weigl, E., & Bierwisch, M. Neuropsychology and linguistics: Topics of common research. *Foundations of language*, 1970, *6*, 1-18.

Weigl, E., & Fradis, A. The transcoding processes in patients with agraphia to dictation. *Brain and Language*, 1977, *4*, 11-22.

Wepman, J. Aphasia therapy: A new look. *Journal of Speech and Hearing Disorders*, 1972, *37*, 203-214.

Wilcox, M. J., & Davis, G. A. Speech act analysis of aphasic communication in individual and group settings. In R. H. Brookshire (Ed.), *Clinical Aphasiology: Conference Proceedings. 1977*. Minneapolis: BRK Publishers, 1977, 166-174.

Wilcox, M. J., Davis, G. A., & Leonard, L. B. Aphasics' comprehension of contextually conveyed meaning. *Brain and Language*, 1978, *6*, 362-377.

Williams, S. E., & Canter, G. On the assessment of naming disturbances in adult aphasia. In R. H. Brookshire (Ed.), *Clinical Aphasiology: Conference Proceedings. 1981*. Minneapolis: BRK Publishers, 1981, 155-165.

Zurif, E. G., & Caramazza, A. Psycholinguistic structures in aphasia: Studies in syntax and semantics. In H. Whitaker & H. A. Whitaker (Eds.), *Studies in neurolinguistics* (Vol. 1). New York: Academic Press, 1976, 261-292.

Zurif, E., Caramazza, A., Myerson, R., & Calvin, J. Semantic feature representation for normal and aphasic language. *Brain and Language*, 1974, *1*, 167-187.

Nancy Helm-Estabrooks

Severe Aphasia

Severe Aphasia Defined

The diagnosis of severe acquired aphasia indicates that an individual no longer is able to use the primary (verbal expression and comprehension) and secondary (writing and reading comprehension) language modalities for successful communicative interchange. Such an individual may earn an aphasia severity rating of 0 or 1 on the Boston Diagnostic Aphasia Examination (Goodglass & Kaplan, 1972a, 1972b) with a score of 0 indicating "no usable speech or auditory comprehension" and a score of 1 indicating "all communication is through fragmentary expression, great need for inference, questioning, and guessing by the listener. The range of information which can be exchanged is limited, and the listener carries the burden of communication."

An aphasia severity rating should be based on both conversational and expository speech samples, and the patient's ability to produce or comprehend written messages. The reason for this is that certain syndromes may affect only verbal production or auditory comprehension while other language areas and pathways remain intact. The patient with aphemia, for example, may be unable to communicate verbally, but have normal writing, auditory, and reading comprehension skills (Albert, Goodglass, Helm, Rubens, & Alexander, 1981). Aphemia and pure word deafness, a syndrome which affects only auditory process, are not truly aphasic syndromes because language per se is not impaired. Patients with these

©College-Hill Press, Inc. All rights, including that of translation, reserved. No part of this publication may be reproduced without the written permission of the publisher.

disorders may be misdiagnosed as having severe aphasia if reading and writing skills are not considered.

Encompassing Syndromes

The term severe aphasia is a quantitative one insofar as it refers to a significant degree of language impairment. Although this term most typically is associated with the syndrome called *global aphasia*, other aphasic syndromes and conditions can quantitatively be classified as severe. Among these are: severe *Broca's aphasia*, severe *Wernicke's aphasia*, and mixed *transcortical aphasia*. Added to these distinct syndromes are the cases of nonclassifiable severe aphasia, that is, patients whose language profiles do not coincide with those of specific aphasia syndromes. All such classes of patients may earn similar low scores on the BDAE aphasia severity rating. Qualitatively, however, they may be quite distinguishable both in terms of behavior and site of brain lesions. Likewise, although the common clinical goal for these patients is to regain functional communication skills, the treatments will vary qualitatively among patients, so that a prescriptive approach cannot be followed. Instead, the clinician must approach each severely aphasic patient as an individual who brings to language tasks a unique set of spared and impaired skills. These assets and deficits can be identified, described, and understood in such a way that the spared neurobehavioral features serve as a means for regaining or circumventing those which *appear* lost.

This chapter addresses the treatment of severe aphasia. It does not offer prescriptions. Rather, it suggests a *qualitative* approach to the most devastating of human social problems. This approach will be illustrated through case studies of patients, all of whom were diagnosed quantitatively as having severe aphasia, but who were qualitatively quite different and thus were treated according to their individual neurobehavioral profiles and not according to a diagnostic label.

The Qualitative Approach To Severe Aphasia

Perhaps no other aphasic condition requires quite so careful a diagnostic evaluation as severe aphasia. This statement may appear incongruous to clinicians who would point out that severely aphasic patients will perform poorly in all language modalities and, therefore, will earn poor scores on many of the standardized measures of aphasia. The rhetorical question for them becomes, "What's to test?" "They can't do *anything*." It may *never* be the case, however, that severely aphasic patients can do "nothing," but only careful assessment will reveal the exact nature of the patient's retained skills. In addition to standardized testing, assessment will require nonstandardized administration of standardized assessment tools and administration of informal tests. Above all, it will require that the clinician describe the patients' response to each test item, rather than simply scoring those responses. As noted above, the severely aphasic patient, by definition, will have low scores on language tests. Merely confirming that fact is not only uninteresting, it contributes nothing to the treatment plan, particularly if one is to use retained skills as a rehabilitative springboard.

It is axiomatic that aphasia therapy should begin where the patient has the greatest chance of success. With severely aphasic patients, identification of the patients' strengths presents a significant challenge. To meet that challenge, we may have to call upon colleagues, such as neuropsychologists, and other allied health and medical personnel, as well as family members.

Examples of all of the above will serve to clarify the qualitative approach to severe aphasia.

Noting the Nature of the Response

With the possible exception of the Porch Index of Communicative Abilities multidimensional scoring system (Porch, 1971), a simple score earned on a test is not particularly informative and contributes little to the treatment plan. In the case of severe aphasia, it is important to know *what* the patient did when he or she failed to perform correctly. For example, a hypothetical patient may have given the following responses during administration of the Boston Diagnostic Aphasia Exam (BDAE): Instead of repeating the word "chair" correctly, he said "I don't know." When asked to point to the picture *cactus*, he pointed to *hammock*. Instead of writing his whole name, he wrote the first three letters then began to perseverate on the third. Realizing his errors, he threw down the pen. When asked to match the written word *circle* to its geometric representation, he matched it instead to *square*.

Rather than assigning scores of zero to each of these responses, the clinician should record or describe each unique response, because these and similiar pieces of information are crucial to understanding the patient's assets and deficits. In the above example, the first response tells us that the patient has some capacity for meaningful speech (he said "I don't know"). The second response tells us that he knows or appreciates that "cactus" is an object and not a letter or color (semantic categories also represented on the test card). The third response indicates that he recognizes when he is writing inappropriate letters and is appropriately frustrated (he threw down his pen when he began to perseverate), and the final one, wherein he matched the word *circle* with a square, suggests that he may have a form of "deep dyslexia," in which a close semantic reading error is made (Marshall & Newcombe, 1973).

Given this and similar pieces of qualitative information regarding the patient's performance, the clinician is ready to explore the effects of a nonstandardized administration of the same tasks.

Non-Standardized Administration of Standardized Tests

While the patient described above earned low scores on a standard administration of the BDAE, nonetheless he offered a rich variety of responses. The clinical question now becomes, "What will happen to the patient's performance if I change X?" Some examples of the way one might approach this question are offered below.

Auditory Comprehension

Instead of pointing to the BDAE picture of the *cactus*, the patient pointed to *hammock*. If an audiogram has already established an adequate level of speech reception, the BDAE task itself can be altered to investigate auditory comprehension further. In the standardized format, word discrimination is tested with two cards (7" x 10") with 18 items each, offered one at a time. These items are divided into three semantic categories (card 1 = objects, letters, colors; card 2 = actions, geometric forms, and numbers). It is possible, given this array, that visual scanning, visual discrimination, or figure/ground problems may complicate the assessment of auditory comprehension for single words. If, however, the individual components of the pictures are cut out and placed farther apart on a dark background, the patient's performance on this task may change. This point was demonstrated quite dramatically with a 63-year-old patient. At the time of hospital discharge, four months following onset of a stroke, he earned a score of 46/72 on the BDAE word-discrimination subtest. Approximately three months later, he was readmitted after a second stroke and found to have a score of 27/72, indicating that his auditory comprehension problems were now in the severe range. When this BDAE subtest was readministered using the cut-up stimuli, however, he earned a score of 47/72, indicating that the new stroke had not exacerbated his previously moderate auditory comprehension deficit. Instead, it appeared to have caused visual-spatial or visual discrimination problems which interfered with his ability to select pictured stimuli from a composite card. Thus, a nontraditional administration of this standardized auditory comprehension test contributed valuable information which could be used in designing a treatment plan.

Writing

The hypothetical patient described earlier was unable to write his name because of perseveration problems. Typically, writing skills are tested with the BDAE by offering the patient an unlined 8½" x 11" piece of paper placed lengthwise. This allows us to assess visual field neglect and inability to maintain the horizontal plane. Perseveration after the first few correctly formed letters is not an uncommon phenomenon. If such a patient is allowed to "window-write," however, this phenomenon may cease to occur. In "window-writing," the clinician cuts a small square opening in an index card, places the card on unlined paper, and instructs the patient to write the first letter of the target word in the opening, or window. The card is then moved to allow for the next letter. The patient is unable to see the previous letter and, thus, is not "pulled" to that letter. In the case of a long word, the clinician may have to remind or show the patient what letter(s) he or she has already written, as the "windown-writing" process is a somewhat slow and laborious one, and the patient may forget what has gone before. This approach does allow us, however, to sort out what may be a visual "pull" form of perseveration from a spelling problem or motor perseveration, an important distinction when planning treatment.

Reading

The BDAE tests the comprehension of printed words by asking patients to look at a word and then point to its pictured representation on one of the two composite cards described above. Our hypothetical patient pointed to *square* after reading "circle," thus showing a semantic appreciation of the target word. Given that the BDAE pictures are black line drawings on a white background, figure/ground problems rather than "deep dyslexia" possibly underlie such an error. The visual problem may be circumvented by coloring in the line drawing and thus allowing a fairer assessment of the ability to comprehend written words. We recently saw a patient who could not match unshaded line drawings to real objects at better than chance level. Once the drawings were shaded in, his performance was 100%, and he went on to successfully complete a program of Visual Action Therapy (Helm-Estabrooks, Fitzpatrick, & Barresi, 1982).

These examples serve to illustrate how nonstandardized administration of standardized tests may provide the clinician with valuable diagnostic and treatment-planning information. Another important source of information comes from the administration of nonstandardized or informal tests.

Informal Tests

Severely aphasic patients sometimes have retained ability to understand and execute "whole body" commands, that is, commands carried out using axial pathways (Geschwind, 1967; Johnson, Sahoske, Grembowski, & Rubens, 1976), yet few, if any, formal aphasia tests assess this ability. Any clinician who is expected to treat a patient with severely impaired auditory comprehension, therefore, must construct an informal test of whole-body commands such as "stand up," "turn around," "bend over," "stand like a boxer," "take a bow." As Johnson et al. have suggested, the preserved ability to follow axial commands may serve as basis for treating severe aphasia.

Similarly, clinicians are advised to test both limb and facial praxis skills in severely aphasic patients. Degradation of these skills often co-occurs with severe language problems (DeRenzi, Pieczuro, & Vignolo, 1966; Liepman, 1905). Just as facial apraxia may interfere with speech production, limb apraxia may interfere with the execution of symbolic gestures and/or writing. Thus, severe apraxia may effectively block outgoing communication pathways and require specific therapeutic intervention.

Another valuable source of information not assessed by standardized tests relates to the patient's ability to communicate *nonvocally* in a natural setting. Experienced clinicians know that some patients can earn poor scores on formal tests of aphasia but seem to interact quite successfully in their daily environments. Realizing how important this information is for both planning and assessing the effects of therapy, our staff developed a simple nonvocal communication scale to be rated by family members, nursing staff, and other members of the rehabilitation team. It meets none of the requirements for a standardized test, but it does meet a clinical need.

Finally, informal tests can be used to delineate further a skill already evaluated by a standardized test. For example, the hypothetical patient described above earned a score of 0/10 on the BDAE subtest of word repetition, but he clearly said "I don't know" for *chair*. Can he now repeat the phrase "I don't know"? Our ongoing study of a treatment approach called Voluntary Control of Involuntary Utterances (Helm & Barresi, 1980), shows that severely aphasic patients, indeed, may repeat their real word stereotypes and involuntary verbalizations. Furthermore, patients can often correctly read these utterances aloud, despite failure to read BDAE subtest words aloud. This preserved ability can serve as a basis for treatment, as will be demonstrated in a case study to follow.

Obtaining Critical Information from Others

The nonvocal communication scale mentioned above is rated by a variety of people who interact with the severely aphasic patient. These people also may serve as a good source of information regarding the patient's verbal successes and failures. Holland (1982) has shown that even severely aphasic patients (according to standardized test results) may communicate successfully, using a variety of verbal strategies in settings outside the language-therapy room. This kind of information can be incorporated into the treatment plan. For example, we treated a globally aphasic patient who, according to the nursing staff, drew a toilet and a bottle of milk of magnesia when they failed to understand his verbal and gestural attempts to tell them he was constipated. We then discovered that when this patient was allowed to depict target messages graphically, his ability to verbalize these messages improved dramatically. Perhaps the best example of the use of drawing for rehabilitation of severe aphasia is seen in the work of Van Eeckhout, Pillon, Signoret, and Lhermitte (1981). By encouraging a former cartoonist with a right hemiplegia and global aphasia to express himself through left-hand drawing, these investigators were able to develop a rehabilitation program which has resulted in two published books for aphasic patients (Lorant, Van Eeckhout, & Sabadel, 1980; Van Eeckhout & Sabadel, 1982). It should be noted that during the process of working on left-handed drawing the patient began to show recovery of verbal skills.

While informal observations made by our colleagues may offer valuable cues as to the patient's capacity for and mode of communication, their formal observations may prove even more valuable. For example, we used Visual Action Therapy in an attempt to treat one nonglobal, but severely aphasic patient, who failed to respond to any of several verbal/auditory treatment methods. With Visual Action Therapy he progressed rapidly to the final step of Level I. This step requires the patient to look at two objects, and watch while both are hidden for a few seconds. The clinician then returns one object to the patient's view and the patient must gesturally represent the object which remains hidden. This particular patient was unable to remember which item remained hidden. We conferred with the neuropsychologist, who informed us that the patient had performed poorly on tests of both verbal and nonverbal short-term memory. A check of his CT (computerized tomographical) scan showed two left-hemisphere lesions, one of which involved the middle temporal gyrus extending into the inferior temporal gyrus. Horel (1978) suggests that this area may play a role in human memory. These neuropsychological and CT scan findings appeared sufficient to explain the patient's failure to respond to any of our treatment approaches and he was discharged.

As this case demonstrates, knowledge of lesion localization is of more than academic interest to the speech/language pathologist. The site and extent of the brain lesion may be crucial to planning the treatment approach. Another example of the value of CT scan information for aphasia rehabilitation is a study which retrospectively examined the relationship between lesion sites and response to Melodic Intonation Therapy (Helm, Naeser, & Kleefield, 1980). Two of the four patients who responded poorly to MIT had small right hemisphere lesions in addition to a significant left hemisphere lesion. Although they were able to complete the Melodic Intonation Therapy program, their conversational speech did not improve. This information can be used to help determine whether future patients are candidates for this particular treatment approach. Furthermore, this finding lends some credance to the notion that Melodic Intonation Therapy exploits intact right hemisphere functions such as appreciation of melody (Kimura, 1964) and intonation (Blumstein & Cooper, 1974) for purposes of aphasia rehabilitation (Helm-Estabrooks, 1983b).

Thus, lesion localization is an important part of the diagnostic evaluation and treatment plan and, whenever possible, the speech-language pathologist should request and receive this or other neurological information. Just as it is necessary to identify preserved areas of performance, it is necessary, when treating severely aphasic patients, to identify preserved areas of the brain.

Treating Severe Aphasia: Five Case Studies

Global Syndromes

Individuals with global aphasia are severely impaired in their ability to perform through any language modality. In addition, global aphasic patients may have oral/facial and limb apraxia as part of their symptom complex. Classically, global aphasia is associated with a large left hemisphere lesion which destroys the cortical frontotemporo parietal language zones and extends deeply into the white matter (Albert, Goodglass, Helm, Rubens, & Alexander, 1981). Recent research using CT scan localization techniques and BDAE test results, however, show that a relatively smaller, and mostly subcortical, lesion involving the internal capsule and putamen may undercut the primary language zones and produce a global aphasia (Naeser, Alexander, Helm-Estabrooks, Levine, Laughlin, & Geschwind, 1982).

Case I: Global Aphasia

Neurobehavioral Characteristics. Patient A was a 56-year-old right-hemiparetic male, 3-months post onset of a left hemisphere stroke when we first saw him. Administration of the Boston Diagnostic Aphasia Examination showed him to have a severe aphasia, earning a severity rating of .5 for his ability to converse and describe the "Cookie Theft" picture. His verbalizations were restricted to "good," "no," "I don't know," and "okay." His overall auditory comprehension Z score was −1.0 standard deviation away from the norm for aphasic patients. Of the four BDAE auditory comprehension subtests, his relatively worse performance was on word discrimination, earning only 17 out of 72 points. He had no ability to name items verbally, or to produce automatized verbal sequences. He repeated 3/10 words, but could not repeat sentences. By contrast, he wrote 20 numbers, 9 letters, and the words "key" and "chair" in a written confrontation naming task. His symbol discrimination was excellent. He matched all 10-letter/word stimuli to their differently written counterparts, e.g., matching block printing to cursive script. Reading comprehension was less spared, with earned scores of 4/10 on word/picture matching and 3/10 on sentences and paragraphs.

A's overall PICA score was 7.07. He earned 7.41 on gestural subtests, 4.25 on verbal subtests, and 7.23 on graphic subtests. He refused to produce pantomimes for subtests II and III, and his comprehension of verbs and nouns was 6.9 and 5.5, respectively.

Praxis examination showed him to have severe facial, but only moderate limb apraxia. Neuropsychological testing indicated relatively good visual skills. On the "parietal lobe" battery, he earned 9.5/13 for drawing, 8/10 for constructing block designs, and 12/12 for reproducing stick designs. CT scanning showed a subcortical, putaminal lesion. A was concerned, cooperative, alert, and motivated.

Course of Treatment. A's test results indicated good visual and matching skills (10/10 word discrimination, 15 on PICA subtest VIII, and good block and stick designs) and only moderate limb apraxia. On the basis of these preserved skills, A was entered into a course of Visual Action Therapy (VAT). This method trains patients to produce symbolic hand gestures for hidden items. VAT has been described elsewhere (Helm-Estabrooks, 1983 (a); Helm-Estabrooks, Fitzpatrick, & Barresi, 1982).

Following a one-month, completed course of VAT (approximately 20 sessions), A earned an overall PICA score of 9.25, with 10.6 gestural, 6.68 verbal, and 9.16 graphic scores.

Because he was now producing more spontaneous speech, A was entered into a course of Voluntary Control of Involuntary Utterances described below in association with another case.

Unclassifiable Severe Aphasia

Perhaps 60% of the aphasic population can be classified into specific aphasia syndromes (M. Alexander, personal communication). For example, the syndrome known as global aphasia is associated with severe impairment of all language modalities, yet some patients have severely restricted verbal and written output but relatively more intact auditory and reading comprehension skills. While not truly *globally* aphasic, nonetheless, these patients are *severely* aphasic. Because the clinician often is called upon to rehabilitate such patients, two cases will be described here.

Case II: Unclassifiable Severe Aphasia

Neurobehavioral Characteristics. Patient B was a 55-year-old, right-hemiplegic male who was two months beyond a left hemisphere stroke when we first saw him. On the basis of conversational and expository speech, he was assigned an aphasia severity rating of .5. He had no "running" speech but, instead, produced occasional utterances such as "oh," "yes," "no," and the nonsense-stereotype "oh-win-ee-oh." His overall auditory comprehension score was − .25 standard deviation from the mean for aphasic individuals. He had marked oral/facial, and limb apraxia. He produced no verbal naming, repetition, automatized speech, oral reading, singing, or rhythms.

Islands of preserved language ability were: good auditory comprehension of nouns, verbs, and one- and two-stage commands; good comprehension of written language (8/10 for word/picture matching, 8/10 for sentences and paragraphs); ability to write the names of 9/10 items in a written confrontation-naming task. Examination of his incorrect verbal responses showed that he said "who" when asked to blow, and "I go" when asked to repeat "I got home." He also said "mama" and "thanks" during the test for verbal agility.

His untimed Wechsler Adult Intelligence Scale performance IQ was 108. CT scanning showed a patchy cortical lesion in Wernicke's area with a more complete lesion in the white matter deep to Wernicke's area. The largest portion of the lesion involved the anterior supermarginal gyrus, corona radiata, and periventricular white matter lateral to the body of the lateral ventricle. There was no lesion in or deep to Broca's area. He was alert, cooperative, appropriately concerned, frustrated, and eager to work.

Course of Treatment. Although B was unable to read any BDAE words aloud, clinical experience with other patients suggested that B might be able to read words orally that he had produced spontaneously in other contexts. This proved to be the case. When presented with *oh, mama, thanks, I go, you, no,* and *who,* he read these aloud. Importantly, we knew from his good BDAE reading comprehension scores that this oral reading was not an automatic, meaningless exercise for him. To the original list, we then added words with emotional value, such as *love* and *die.* In keeping with the findings of Landis, Graves, and Goodglass (1982), we have found that some severely aphasic patients are able to read such words far better than emotionally neutral words. B was no exception. He easily read "love" and "die." Each word then was printed separately on 3" x 5" cards for self-practice. His reading list soon consisted of many emotion-laden words, including *fun, hit, lucky, ouch, shame, bull,* and *kiss.* Some of these were chosen by the clinician and some were spontaneous words newly uttered by B. This treatment approach, which we call Voluntary Control of Involuntary Utterances (VCIU), has been described elsewhere (Helm-Estabrooks, 1983a). Briefly, the patient determines the practice lexicon in VCIU, although the clinician begins the treatment process of offering words which the patient has been heard to say or is thought to be capable of reading aloud. If, instead of producing the target word, the patient says another real word, then the original stimulus word is set aside and the "error" word is offered for oral reading. In order to qualify as a practice word (the 3" x 5" word cards are given to the patient for self-practice), the patient must have read the target word aloud correctly and with ease, that is, without articulatory or paraphasic struggle. In addition to oral reading, responsive naming or exercises for the target words are incorporated into the treatment session. For example, to elicit the word "love," the clinician may ask "what is the opposite of hate?"

Within approximately four months, B had a list of 267 words and short phrases which he could read aloud and use in conversation. Most were highly functional, for example, *buddy, care, dime, beer, dirty, more, nice, warm, Dottie, sis, where is it? I'm hot, I don't care, I love you, I'm cold.*

Although his BDAE verbal scores rose significantly during this period, they did not reflect the extent of his functional communication. And, interestingly enough, although he could read 267 of his self-determined words and phrases, he read aloud only one of the BDAE words and none of the sentences upon retesting.

Case III: Unclassifiable Severe Aphasia

Neurobehavioral Characteristics. Patient C was a 55-year-old male referred to us two months following onset of a left hemisphere stroke which left him with right hemiplegia and severe aphasia. His conversation and expository speech output consisted of the nonsense-stereotype "dee-oh-ah." Although he appeared to have good comprehension for personally relevant conversational material, he earned an overall BDAE score of -1.0 standard deviation for auditory comprehension. A score lower than this would be consistent with a diagnosis of global aphasia, given his other language deficits. He had no ability to name or produce automatized verbal sequences. He repeated two words but no sentences and orally read only one word. He wrote his name and a few numbers and letters. All reading skills were severely compromised. His best BDAE performance was to sing popular songs with good melody and word approximations and to perform rhythmic tapping.

He had severe oral/facial apraxia earning 0/30 points on our praxis exam. Gestural limb praxis skills were moderately intact with an earned score of 32/60.

C's WAIS performance IQ was 83, while his "parietal lobe" drawings were assigned 9/13 points. He lost only one point on a test of his ability to copy stick designs.

A CT scan showed a lesion in the anterior limb of the left internal capsule which extended forward beyond the frontal horn, and anteriorly and superiorly to involve white matter. He was alert and cooperative but very frustrated by his speech problems.

Course of Treatment. A summary of C's preserved skills showed that he could break out of his verbal stereotype and produce real words when he sang familiar songs such as "I've Been Working on the Railroad." He had good visual/spatial skills and fair ability to produce representational gestures to command and upon imitation.

We decided upon a combined treatment approach which would capitalize on all of his intact skills. During a trial of Melodic Intonation Therapy, he was asked, first, to listen to the intoned phrase "I am fine" and then slowly sing it in unison with the clinician, who helped him tap it out syllable by syllable. He then repeated it correctly, and finally was able to produce this phrase in response to a probe question. Because this was the first time in 2 months that C had produced meaningful speech, he began to cry after hearing himself intone "I am fine." His family was equally emotional when his performance was repeated at bedside during visiting hours. C was enrolled in a simultaneous course of Melodic Intonation Therapy (Sparks, Helm, & Albert, 1974; Sparks & Holland, 1976) and Visual Action Therapy for improving limb gestures. He completed Limb/VAT in 15 sessions and was evaluated with the PICA. (At the same time he also had received 15 sessions of Melodic Intonation Therapy). His overall PICA score was 8.11, with a gesture score of 10.9, a verbal score of 4.47, and a graphic score of 6.83. On the ward he had been heard to utter multisyllable words such as "tomorrow" spontaneously, and phrases such as "I did" and "this morning." Because of his persistent oral/facial apraxia, he was entered into a course of Facial/VAT which was developed for training oral/facial praxis items (Helm-Estabrooks & Albert, 1980). Following along the same task hierarchy used for Limb/VAT, the oral/facial program trains patients to represent hidden items, (flower, whistle, cup, razor, chapstick, kaleidoscope, straw, and lollipop) with gestures which involve the face or oral apparatus.

C completed the Facial/VAT program in 31 sessions. PICA re-evaluation showed an overall score of 10.25, with a gestural score of 12.4, a verbal score of 11.4, and a graphic score of 6.6. Significantly, his verbal score had improved 6.93 points with a combination of Face/VAT and MIT.

Four months after admission, C's overall BDAE auditory comprehension Z score was at nearly zero, an improvement of one standard deviation. Furthermore, he now showed some verbal naming skills, improving these scores by more than one full standard deviation.

Severe Wernicke's Aphasia

Unlike global or other nonfluent aphasias, Wernicke's aphasia is characterized broadly as fluent, that is, the patient's speech output has good prosody, good articulation, normal or greater than normal phrase length, and a full range of grammatical forms. The presence of literal, verbal, and neologistic paraphasias, however, make this output difficult or impossible to understand. Furthermore, the patient with Wernicke's aphasia may have several auditory-comprehension problems so that communication through the auditory/verbal mode is drastically compromised. In addition, the written output of Wernicke's patients often mirrors their verbal output, while reading may or may not be as impaired as auditory comprehension (Heilman, Rothi, Campanella, & Wolfson, 1979).

Case IV: Severe Wernicke's Aphasia

Neurobehavioral Characteristics. Patient D was a 51-year-old non-hemiparetic male who was admitted to our service two months following a stroke. He was alert and cooperative, but apparently unconcerned about his fluent paraphasic speech output. His conversation and BDAE "Cookie Theft" description were rated .5 on the Aphasia Severity Rating Scale. His speech had normal prosody, phrase length, and articulation, but was very paraphasic. His speech contained verbal, literal, and neologistic errors and thus was fluent but without information. In addition, he had obviously severe auditory comprehension problems and earned an overall auditory comprehension Z score of −1.5. He earned no points for oral naming, reading, automatized speech, or repetition. His best oral reading performance was the word "class" for *chair*. Examples of his repetition errors are as follows: *chair* was repeated as "chess," *You know how* was repeated as "Let us doubt him," *hammock* was "To may who it were." Singing and rhythmic tapping were impaired. He often appeared confused by the tasks and required special care in establishing "set."

He demonstrated good comprehension of "whole body" commands.

D's WAIS performance IQ was 77. He reproduced 9/10 stick designs to memory on the Boston "parietal lobe" test. It was noted that D was unable to supplement his impaired verbal output with meaningful gestures. Despite the absence of hemiparesis, he used vague, nonrepresentational gestures. The CT scan showed a left-hemisphere lesion which had almost completely isolated Wernicke's area.

Course of Treatment. Despite his severe Wernicke's aphasia, D had good visual memory (he recalled 9/10 stick designs) and moderately intact visual recognition (7/10 scored on BDAE symbol/word recognition). He produced *real word* approximations for *chair* in repetition ("class") and oral reading ("chess").

Based on the findings, we chose to enroll him in a course of Visual Action Therapy to improve his ability to establish "set" for structure tasks, to become aware of task expectations, to increase his critical skills, and to encourage production and use of representational gestures. (The tendency of Wernicke's patients to use copious, but nonspecific gestures was described by Cicone, Wapner, Foldi, Zurif, & Gardner, 1979). Furthermore, it was thought that the use of this silent method might lead to better self control of D's "press of speech."

D completed Limb/VAT in 10 sessions and Face/VAT in 6 sessions. By this time, he was producing closer verbal approximations in naming, e.g., "hand" for *glove*. He now orally read 5/10 BDAE words. Repetition still was severely impaired.

It was decided that a modified VCIU approach now might offer him better control of his verbal output. Beginning with the BDAE words which he had correctly read aloud and adding others, we employed the following procedure: (1) D read the word aloud; (2) D repeated the word after the clinician without seeing the printed word; (3) D chose the target word upon hearing it from an array; (4) D used the word in a confrontation of responsive naming task.

Approximately 3½ months following admission, D left the hospital to resume management of his own small neighborhood grocery store after several 3-day weekend passes showed him capable of carrying out the tasks necessary for that job.

Case V: Severe Wernicke's Aphasia

Neurobehavioral Characteristics. Patient E was a 55-year-old nonhemiparetic male transferred to our medical center 2 months after sustaining a left temporal/parietal contusion with significant intracerebral hemorrhaging. Administration of the Boston Diagnostic Aphasia Examination showed that E was alert but not well oriented and had great difficulty attending to tasks. He demonstrated great "press" of neologistic fluent speech, and his auditory comprehension deficits immediately became obvious in conversation. He seemed aware of his difficulty with language tasks, quickly becoming annoyed and obstinate about testing. Despite this, he remained polite, using phrases like "thank you" and "excuse me." Perseveration was prominent on those tasks which were attempted.

Due to his reluctance and the severity of his problem, he earned no points on BDAE subtests beyond 3/8 points for automatized speech, 2/10 for word repetition, and 2 points for good ability to produce a familiar tune.

He also could produce correct runs of words in song and showed an obvious fondness for music.

Within the first 2 weeks of evaluation, he became preoccupied with hospital discharge and showed increased paranoid tendencies. By the 3rd week he refused both testing and treatment.

When presented at Aphasia Round one month after admission, he showed improved conversational turn-taking, good use of nonvocal communication skills such as gestures and facial expressions, some runs of clear speech, and a tendency to get the first few items correct when a new task was introduced.

Course of Treatment. Following Aphasia Rounds, E's case was reviewed for possible re-introduction of treatment. Because he now refused to enter the treatment room, we decided instead to sit down with him in the hall, TV room, or bedside in a casual and friendly way. Because he was able to respond to the first few items correctly when new tasks were introduced, we decided to employ four different tasks during short (10-15 minute sessions) several times a day. Because he associated the BDAE tester with his frustration and failure, two other speech-language pathologists were designated as his therapists.

Based on his performance strengths, the treatment tasks were (1) repetition of words he used correctly in speech, (2) verbal identification of popular taped songs, (3) verbal identification of photographed faces associated with music, particularly jazz, and (4) singing songs while reading the lyrics.

Within 2 weeks of this approach, E had experienced sufficient success to participate willingly in more typical 30-minute therapy sessions carried out in a treatment room. He also began attending the twice-weekly, hour-long aphasic group meetings. Two months later, re-evaluation showed that his overall BDAE auditory comprehension score had improved by nearly 2 standard deviations and that his aphasia severity rating for conversation was 2, indicating that he shared the burden of communication with the examiner. At that time, he was introduced to the Helm-Elicited Language Program for Syntax Stimulation (Helm-Estabrooks, 1981), originally developed for use with agrammatic patients (Helm-Estabrooks, Fitzpatrick, & Barresi, 1981). This program, which uses a story-completion format to elicit examples of eleven syntactic constructions, has subsequently proven useful with paragrammatic patients. After a brief introduction to HELPSS, E was discharged from the hospital with pictured stimuli. This allows the program to be carried out via daily calls in which the verbal story stimuli are presented by the clinician. Several other patients have been treated successfully in this way, thereby allowing early hospital discharges for patients who are unable to attend clinic-based outpatient therapy sessions. This format particularly favors nonhemiparetic patients who have no need for physical and occupational therapy.

Summary

This chapter has addressed the treatment of severe aphasia defined here as a disorder of both primary (verbal expression and comprehension) and secondary (writing and reading comprehension) language skills. Several classifiable aphasic syndromes, including global aphasia and Wernicke's aphasia, as well as nonclassifiable syndromes, may generally be labelled as forms of severe aphasia because they seriously compromise the patient's ability to communicate effectively. It is proposed, however, that successful management of these patients will be based upon a careful qualitative analysis of the individual's performance on standardized and experimental language and neuropsychological tests, as well as neurological findings.

An understanding of the qualitative approach to treatment will enable the clinician to determine which method(s) make the best use of an individual patient's retained skills for purposes of re-integrating or circumventing his or her areas of communication deficits.

This qualitative approach, illustrated through five case studies of patients with differing forms of severe aphasia, has shown how the unique language, neuropsychological, and neurological findings of each case led to individualized rehabilitation programs which incorporated both established and custom-made treatment methods.

References

Albert, M., Goodglass, H., Helm, N, Rubens, A., & Alexander, M. *Clinical aspects of dysphasia*. New York: Springer-Verlag, 1981.

Blumstein, S., & Cooper, W. Hemispheric processing of intonation contours. *Cortex*, 1974, *10*, 146–150.

Cicone, M., Wapner, W. Foldi, N., Zurif, E., & Gardner, H. The relationship between gesture and language in aphasic communication. *Brain and Language*, 1979, *8*, 324–439.

DeRenzi, E., Pieczuro, A., & Vignolo, L. Oral apraxia and aphasia. *Cortex*, 1966, *2*, 50–73.

Geschwind, N. The apraxias. In E. W. Straus & R. M. Griffith (Eds.), *Phenomenology of will and action*, pp. 91–102. Pittsburgh: Duquesne University Press, 1967.

Goodglass, H., & Kaplan, E. *Assessment of aphasia and related disorders*. Philadelphia: Lea & Febiger, 1972. (a)

Goodglass, H., & Kaplan, E. *Boston Diagnostic Aphasia Examination*. Philadelphia: Lea & Febiger, 1972. (b)

Heilman, K., Rothi, N., Campanella, D., & Wolfson, S. Wernicke's and global aphasia without alexia. *Archives of Neurology*, 1979, *36*, 129-133.

Helm, N., & Barresi, B. Voluntary Control of Involuntary Utterances: A treatment approach for severe aphasia. In R. H. Brookshire (Ed.), *Clinical Aphasiology: Conference Proceedings*. Minneapolis: BRK Publishers, 1980.

Helm, N., Naeser, M., & Kleefield, J. CT scan localization and response to melodic intonation therapy. Academy of Aphasia Annual Meeting, South Yarmouth, MA, October, 1980.

Helm-Estabrooks, N. *Helm Elicited Language Program for Syntax Stimulation*. Austin, TX: Exceptional Resources, 1981.

Helm-Estabrooks, N. Approaches to testing subcortical aphasias. In W. H. Perkins (Ed.), *Current therapy of communication disorders*. New York: Thieme-Stratton, 1983. (a)

Helm-Estabrooks, N. Exploiting the right hemisphere fore language rehabilitation: Melodic intonation therapy. In E. Perceman (Ed.), *Cognitive processing in the right hemisphere*. New York: Academic Press, Inc., 1983. (b)

Helm-Estabrooks, N., & Albert, M. *Visual Action Therapy for Global Aphasia*, Veterans Administration Merit Review Grant, 1980.

Helm-Estabrooks, N., Fitzpatrick, P., & Barresi, B. Response of an agrammatic patient to a syntax stimulation program for aphasia. *Journal of Speech and Hearing Disorders*, 1982, *46*, 422-427.

Holland, A. L. Observing functional communication of aphasic adults. *Journal of Speech and Hearing Disorders*, 1982, *47*, 50-56.

Horel, J. A. The neuroanatomy of amnesia. *Brain*, 1978, *101*, 403-445.

Johnson, M., Sahoske, P., Grembowski, C., & Rubens, A. Preservation of responses requiring whole body movements in severe aphasia. Paper presented to American Speech and Hearing Association Convention, Houston, 1976.

Kimura, D. Left-right differences in the perception of melodies, *Quarterly Journal of Experimental Psychology*, 1964, *15*, 335-358.

Landis, J., Graves, R., & Goodglass, H. Aphasic reading and writing: Possible evidence for right hemisphere participation. *Cortex*, 1982, *18*, 105-112.

Liepmann, H. Die lenke Hemisphare und das Handeln, *Munch. Med. Wschr.*, 1905, *2*, 2375-2378.

Lorant, G., Van Eeckhout, P., & Sabadel. *L'Homme qui ne savant plus parler*. Paris: Nouvelles Editions Baudinière, 1980.

Marshall, R. C., & Newcombe, F. Patterns of paralexia: A psycholinguistic approach. *Journal of Psycholinguistic Research*, 1973, *2*, 175-199.

Naeser, M., Alexander, M., Helm-Estabrooks, N., Levine, H., Laughlin, S., & Geschwind, N. Aphasia with predominately subcortical lesion sites, *Archives of Neurology*, 1982, *39*, 2-14.

Porch, B. E. *Porch Index of Communicative Ability*. Palo Alto, CA: Consulting Psychologist Press, 1971.

Sparks, R., Helm, N., & Albert, M. Aphasia rehabilitation resulting from melodic intonation therapy. *Cortex*, 1974, *10*, 303-316.

Sparks, R., Holland, A. Method: Melodic intonation therapy for aphasia, *Journal of Speech and Hearing Disorders*, 1976, *41*, 287-297.

Van Eeckhout, P., Pillon, B., Signoret, J., & Lhermitte, F. The application of drawings to the rehabilitation of an aphasic patient. Paper presented at Symposium on Aphasia Therapy, Eramus University, Rotterdam, The Netherlands, October 1981.

Van Eeckhout, P., & Sabadel. *Histoires Insolites Pour Faire Parler*. Paris: Medecine et Sciences Internationales, 1982.

Penelope Starratt Myers

Right Hemisphere Impairment

Introduction

There has long existed an intuitive knowledge among speech-language pathologists that right hemisphere-damaged patients do not communicate adequately. Clinicians working with this population on motor-speech disorders or on reading and writing deficits have observed that their patients appear to manage well on a superficial level, but experience problems with more sophisticated communication demands. Yet, the precise nature of their problems remained elusive, and the idea of treating the disorders was not seriously entertained until very recently. In the last 5 to 10 years, research with brain-damaged, split-brain, and normal subjects using new and sophisticated techniques has generated enough data to shed new light on the role of the right hemisphere (RH) in the fully functioning brain. Clearly, the most significant advance in RH communication disorders has been a more precise delineation of the deficits themselves. Rather than merely drawing inferences from the well-known litany of RH perceptual deficits, it has now become possible to extract some of the unifying themes that carry through from a basic perceptual level to the higher order cognitive one. Clinically, this knowledge has helped refine intuition and anecdotal evidence into systematic data-based judgement.

This chapter will explore the nature of the perceptual and cognitive deficits associated with RH damage, and the ways in which they relate to each other to create communication impairments. Read the following discussion with several notes of caution in mind. First, this area of study is in its infancy and, despite significant advances, much less is known about the operations of the right than the left hemisphere. Second, in some aspects, the RH is more diffusely organized and is not as neatly packaged as the left (Goldberg & Costa, 1981; Semmes, 1968). Very few localization studies on RH communication disorders have been done, and many more are needed to account for variables such as site, size, and depth of lesion, degree of handedness, age, sex, and education level of the patient. Not all RH patients will experience all of the problems described below.

Finally, adequate diagnostic tools and therapy materials do not exist in published form at this time. Guidelines for assessment and treatment are provided throughout this chapter (for more detail, see Myers, 1982). Research bearing directly on the efficacy of specific techniques has yet to be done, so the therapist is cautioned accordingly.

The long list of impairments associated with RH disease can be broken down into four major categories: (1) lower-order perceptual problems, which include left-sided neglect and various visuospatial deficits; (2) problems with affect and prosody; (3) linguistic disorders; and (4) higher-order perceptual and cognitive deficits, including those impairments that result in general communicative inefficiency.

Many of the disorders in each category are related to those in other areas and can exert a cumulative effect on communication. For speech pathology, the advances in knowledge about the last two areas holds special significance. Most of the lower-order perceptual disorders in the first category have been well known for the past 40 years, but new work in this area has had an impact on our understanding of the communication deficits experienced by RH patients. Although therapy procedures have not been developed for working on prosodic impairments and affect, there has been a heightened interest in their effect on communication in RH patients. Each of the four categories will be discussed separately below.

Section I: Lower-Order Perceptual Deficits

The act of perception incorporates several simultaneous processes. At its most basic level, it involves the recognition or discrimination of a stimulus. On a higher level, perception involves certain associative operations so that the stimulus is not only recognized, but understood. Extracting meaning from sensory information on this higher level requires that the perceiver take into account the external context in which the stimulus is embedded, and that he integrate it with certain internal associations. The notion of "pure perception" is too simplistic to explain this nonverbal or preverbal process. There probably is no such thing as "pure perception," since no stimulus is truly isolated or truly neutral. Perception is thus both a discriminatory and an interpretive act. Breaking it down into lower and higher order operations is somewhat artificial, but serves as a useful organizational tool for purposes of discussion. The disorders discussed in this section, then, reflect deficits in basic perceptual processes, but have an effect on higher-order perception as well. They are grouped together here as lower-order perceptual disorders to lay the foundation for a discussion of their impact on communication in Section IV.

The lengthy list of visuospatial disorders associated with RH disease usually includes deficits in the following abilities: (1) visual discrimination; (2) visual memory; (3) visual integration; (4) visual imagery; (5) facial recognition (prosopagnosia); (6) topological and geographic orientation; (7) visuoconstructive deficits (constructional apraxia); (8) spatial orientation; and (9) neglect of the left half of space (see Joynt & Goldstein, 1975 for an excellent review). Many of these deficits affect the patient's ability to regain independence and care for himself. In the early months post onset he may, for example, forget how to get back to his room, have difficulty remembering familiar faces, or be unable to groom himself properly.

Neglect

Almost all of these disorders will be significantly heightened if the patient also suffers from neglect of the left half of space. Unlike homonymous hemianopsia, which prevents the patient from seeing the left side, left-sided neglect inhibits his ability to conceive of and, therefore, act on or respond to input from the left. It is usually seen in cancellation tasks, in which the patient is asked to cross out randomly spaced figures on a page, or in copy drawing, as well as from behavioral observation. The left-neglect patient will draw objects, such as a flower, with extraneous detail on the right and omissions on the left. In copying a clock face, the patient may include all the numbers on the right and leave the left side blank. Sometimes neglect is accompanied by denial of illness or the patient's refusal to recognize his or her paretic extremities as his or her own (anosognosia). In addition, the patient may appear inattentive and unresponsive. Although spatial neglect has been found in lesions of the left hemisphere (LH), it has been most closely associated with lesions in the right temperoparietal and occipitoparietal areas (Critchley, 1953; Fredericks, 1963; Heilman, 1979; Heilman & Watson, 1977; LeDoux, 1978).

The exact nature of the disorder is unclear and numerous theories have been proposed to explain it. (See Bisiach, Luzzatti, & Perani, 1979; Heilman, 1979, for more detail and further references.) In the early 20th century, the notion of an internal representation of the body or "body schema" was introduced by H. Head (1920), and was later invoked by a number of researchers to explain unilateral neglect (Brain, 1941; Critchley, 1953; Gerstman, 1942). The main problem with this explanation is that it fails to account for the full range of symptoms associated with neglect, including the fact that it extends to the entire left half of space. Another early theory proposed that neglect was caused by a lack of synthesis in the flow of information to one hemisphere (Denny-Brown, Myers & Horenstein, 1952).

More recently, Heilman and his associates have proposed that neglect is a deficit in attention and a breakdown in the orienting response (Heilman, 1979; Heilman & Valenstein, 1972; Watson, Heilman, Cauthen, & King, 1973). Their theories are based on work done with animals (Watson, Miller, & Heilman, 1977; Watson et al., 1978) and with RH patients. As Heilman explains it, the orienting response is an alerting mechanism that prepares or alerts the organism to sensory stimulation and reduces the threshold to incoming stimuli. Heilman (1979) states that "Lesions which induce the unilateral neglect syndrome produce a unilateral reduction of arousal. Because one hemisphere is hypoaroused, it cannot prepare for action and it is therefore akinetic" (p. 284). In a detailed account of the anatomical and physiologic basis of the theory, he designates three cortical regions (inferior parietal lobule, dorsilateral frontal lobe, and the cingulate gyrus), their interconnections, and their connections to the brain stem reticular formation as the critical areas involved in orienting, attention, and trimodal association.

Other researchers take issue with the purely physiologic approach. Bisiach and his colleagues (1979, 1981) see neglect as a disorder affecting the internal representation of the spatial schema of all incoming stimuli. In one study, for example, they found their RH subjects made errors of omission in their verbal descriptions of the left half of a familiar scene—in this case, the cathedral square in Milan—regardless of the orientation they were asked to assume in recalling the image. Their results indicated that the patients' internal concept of, or representation of, the scene was as flawed as their response to real, externally presented stimuli.

It may seem superfluous for speech pathologists to become involved in the theoretical debate over the causes of neglect. Yet, there are several reasons why they should. First, patients with neglect usually present the most severe disorders in visuospatial perception and communication. Second, speech pathologists are called on to treat reading and writing disturbances that are a direct result of neglect (Collins, 1976; LaPointe & Culton, 1969; Metzler & Jelinek, 1976; Stanton et al., 1979, 1981). Finally, since neglect has a very definite impact on the recovery of independence in daily activities, speech pathologists may be consulted by other members of a rehabilitation team about ways to overcome the effects of neglect in a number of tasks. Yorkston (1981), for example, reports a fairly typical request for intervention in helping a left-neglect patient learn to transfer from wheelchair to bed. In such cases, she suggests breaking tasks into small steps and orienting the patient through a series of verbal cues. Each of the steps in the transfer was preceded by an anticipatory question ("How well did you do on this step?") and followed by a review question ("How well did you do?"). Although the task had to be broken down initially into 27 steps, the number was eventually reduced, and the patient was able to transfer successfully. Diller and Weinberg (1977) suggest that retraining of this type is possible with neglect patients via awareness training, small steps, and intensive repetition. Stanton et al. (1981) advocate a verbal cueing strategy accompanied by mass practice for retraining reading skills. It appears that such a strategy can be successful, though not necessarily generalizable.

The implicit assumption in verbal cueing strategies is that the language system can be used to help the patient orient and attend to the left half of space. the degree to which one supports such a strategy partly reflects one's concept of neglect. If one believes it is the result of inattention, one would anticipate that verbal cues, vigilance training, and constant repetition first by the clinician, then by the patient, would be successful. If, on the other hand, one subscribes to a more representational theory, one might want to make more use of other modalities and tasks (such as tactile exploration) as a means of helping the patient refine his internal concept of space. Most of the work on neglect, of course, is aimed at compensation rather than recovery, and most speech pathologists use a combination of strategies. Other professionals (physical and occupational therapists) work on neglect as well, so it is wise to coordinate efforts and program type with them.

Although some of the more disruptive aspects of the syndrome (denial of illness and hemispatial neglect) abate somewhat, flatness of affect and attenuated responsiveness may persist over time (Heilman, 1979). Flat affect and impaired prosody will be discussed in Section II. Neglect is a collection of symptoms and is not really a lower-order perceptual deficit, but because it is implicated in a number of the visuospatial disorders explored below, an understanding of its course and behavioral manifestations is critical at the outset to any discussion of RH patients.

Visuospatial Deficits

Although visual discrimination disorders are often associated with RH disease, the discrimination of such attributes as size or curvature has not been found to be significantly impaired in any brain damaged group (Benton, 1979). Bisiach, Nichelli, and Spinnler (1976) did find significant deficits in the perception of length, and figure-ground disorders have been found in both aphasic and right parietal populations (Russo & Vignolo, 1967; Weinstein, 1964).

Spatial orientation deficits have also been found in patients with RH lesions. For example, Ratcliff (1979) found right posterior patients significantly impaired compared to left posterior subjects in performing a mental rotation task. Benton, Hannay, and Varney (1975) found severe impairments in the ability to determine the directional orientation of visually presented lines. In addition, RH patients are often impaired in the ability to orient to geography, either in map reading, maze solving, or in describing familiar routes (Benton, 1979). Neglect of the left side may make a significant contribution to failure in such tasks. It has also been suggested that impaired topological orientation is affected by the ability to maintain an internal spatial representation. Butters and Barton (1970) found parietal lobe patients, especially those with RH damage, were impaired in three tasks requiring them to shift or reverse perspective in thought, and they suggested that the ability to perform reversible operations in space (i.e. dressing) is associated with a deficit in imaging processes.

Although the ability to read a map or find one's way home does not impact directly on communication skills, the idea that these disorders reflect a deficit in internal visuospatial representation does. The list of visual processing deficits associated with RH disease almost always includes a reference to impaired "visual imagery" or "visual image making." The implications of such deficits for communication are far reaching, but for the practitioner, the problem with these terms is, what do they mean? What exactly is a visual image, and why has it become associated with RH damage?

In part, the connection between the two is based on the idea that thinking involves more than words, and since the LH is dominant for language, the RH must be dominant for nonverbal thought. Visual images have been conceived as a construct for nonverbal thought by many people thoughout history. Much of the recent work in visual imagery has been undertaken in psychological experiments using a paired-associate learning (PAL) paradigm (Bugeleski, 1968, 1970; Bower, 1970; Paivio, 1969, 1971; Rowher, 1970). In such experiments, subjects learn lists of word pairs and are then asked to report the second word of a pair in a recall experiment. The investigators look at the mnemonic power of various types of words (abstract vs. concrete, for example) and various strategies used in the recall task. It has been found that the generation of an internal picture or image is an effective strategy, and that the more concrete a word, the more "highly imageable" it is. Based on work of this type, proponents of the Dual Coding Theory (Paivio, 1971) claim that there is a dual coding system in which verbal processes and nonverbal imagery represent the two alternate systems. Extending these results to the area of hemisphere asymmetry, some researchers have suggested that the RH, specialized for visuospatial input, is dominant for visual imagery coding. And, because concrete words are more readily imaged in a PAL task, some assume that the RH is more adept with concrete input and visual imagery (West, 1977, 1978). Hence, speech pathologists are cautioned in lecture halls, symposia, and workshops that the RH patient may have a deficit in visual imagery, without a clear understanding of what this means in the abstract, or what it means for the patient.

The work done in PAL tasks envisions images as a sort of "mental picture" in the "mind's eye" or as a "sensory-like datum" (Paivio, 1969; Weber & Bach, 1979). It is important to note, however, that many researchers take issue with this view (see Pylyshn, 1973, for an excellent review and counterpoint). It would be a mistake to extrapolate this rather narrow view of images as tools in a PAL task to represent the sum total of our experience of images. As Myers (1980) points out, "The assumption that images are mental pictures specialized to depict concrete events denies the essential complexity and multidimensional aspects of imagery" (p. 69). She goes on to say:

> Rather than a picture or recording that bears some structural relation to raw sensory data, an image is a non-verbal confluence of emotion, intellect and sensation. An image is a simultaneous integration of multiple dimensions and levels of perceived (i.e. interpreted) experience. It represents a synthesis of internal (to the perceiver) and external events free of time and space limitations. Thus the word "home" may evoke a single image which in one instant of time captures knowledge of multiple and possibly conflicting aspects of all the homes one has known across temporal boundaries. These qualities make possible the feeling that one has recalled the essence of an experience. It is these same qualities that make it difficult to transfer complex images directly into words. (p. 69).

It is also these same qualities that suggest a more powerful connection between the RH and imagery, but that makes its discussion out of place in a section on lower-order perception. The issue will be raised again, but the reader is cautioned to remember that there is no direct evidence to indicate that RH patients actually do suffer from a deficit in image making. Most of the claims are based on inference and, when they are made, the reference is usually to images in the most narrow sense of the word—i.e., as ideographic reconstructions.

Facial recognition disorders (prosopagnosia) have sometimes been linked to a deficit in visual recall or the recall of images. Many people, however, think of prosopagnosia as less of a defect in matching external stimuli to internal images or in discrimination of discrete attributes than as the inability to integrate them simultaneously. Prosopagnosia is often found in patients with bilateral lesions, but it has been associated specifically with RH lesions as well (Benton & Van Allen, 1968; DeRenzi, Faglioni, & Spinnler, 1968; DeRenzi & Spinnler, 1966; Warrington & James, 1967). Isolated case reports in the literature are often arresting. Among the most dramatic was Charcot's patient who could not recognize his own face in the mirror. Myers (1978) discusses a patient, 20 years post onset, who had trained himself to use specific visual and auditory cues (hair color, vocal features, etc.) to recognize his clients at work, members of his own family, and the characters in a television drama. The disorder may be socially embarrassing or isolating for the patient. Family and friends unaware of prosopagnosia as a distinct deficit may assume that the patient is suffering from general confusion. Current treatment in our profession is generally restricted to increasing family and patient awareness, and providing suggestions for using analytic cues as a means of compensation.

Benton and Van Allen (1968) refer to prosopagnosia as a form of "simultagnosia" or a deficit in synthesizing disparate elements into a meaningful composite. Other visual integration deficits have been found in RH patients. Newcombe and Russell (1969), for example, found RH subjects significantly impaired in visual closure tasks, and Warrington and James (1967) found that their performance on a task involving the perception of incomplete figures was significantly worse than that of their LH subjects. In fact, many of the visuospatial skills in the intact RH are thought to reflect a facility for synthesizing sensory input (Bogen, 1969; Galin, 1974, Ornstein, 1977; Sperry, 1968; Zaidel, 1978). Myers (1979) and Myers and Linebaugh (1980) found RH patients severely impaired on a test specifically designed to assess visual integration, *The Hooper Visual Organization Test* (Hooper, 1958). Out of a possible 30 points the mean for the RH subjects in the latter study was 9.88, compared to 23.2 for the normal controls.

Finally, various visuoconstructive deficits have been found in RH patients, though they have also been reported frequently in LH patients. Performance, of course, depends on task demands (block design, visual sequential memory, copy drawing, spontaneous graphic production) and the degree to which the subject relies on, or can rely on, verbal strategies in task execution. In RH patients the collection of constructive disorders is usually referred to as constructional apraxia, and will often impair graphic performance.

Reading and Writing Deficits

Reading and writing disturbances in this population are often noted clinically. Treatment for these deficits has a longer history in our profession than does treatment for any other type of RH communication disorder (motor speech problems excepted). Before providing treatment, it is obviously important to distinguish between perceptually based deficits and those that are linguistic in nature. The perceptual deficits in reading may reflect impaired scanning and tracking as well as left-sided neglect. LaPointe and Culton (1969) have described a treatment program they used with a single neglect case. Their program included copy-drawing drills, drawing from memory, and tactile tracing. As previously mentioned, Stanton et al. (1981) advocate a verbal cueing strategy, and had success using it with two RH neglect patients. In addition, clinicians have used standard cues such as a red line drawn down the left side of the page to help remind the patient to attend to the left. Myers (in press) has outlined a systematic series of tasks for both reading and writing deficits that are perceptually based.

Writing disturbances in RH patients generally include omission of strokes and graphemes as well as perseveration. Metzler and Jelinek (1976), for example, found that their 20 subjects were significantly impaired compared to normal controls on a number of graphic tests. The writing deficits in their experimental group included: spelling errors (usually due to perseverated or omitted graphemes); perseveration of strokes, graphemes, syllables, and words; omissions of words and strokes; failure to dot *i's* and cross *t's*; and extra capitalization. Treatment involving drills in copying and tactile exploration may be effective. Increasing the patient's awareness of errors is almost always a necessary first step.

This concludes the section on lower-order perceptual disorders. As stated earlier, many of these deficits will be affected by, and have an effect on, higher-order processing and production in the complex process of communication.

Section II: Affect and Prosody

Among the disorders most commonly ascribed to RH damage are deficits in affect and prosody. RH patients may lack the normal range of facial expression (flat affect), and speak in a monotone because the prosodic features of their speech are attenuated. Unlike anterior aphasic patients, who can be painfully aware of and depressed by their disorder, many RH patients evince little or no response to their impairments. Some RH patients with neglect may even deny illness altogether, making it difficult to motivate them in the rehabilitation process. Their minimization of their problems led Hecaen (1962) to use the term "indifference reaction" to characterize this constellation of symptoms, and led others to investigate the possible connection between the RH and the mediation of emotion. This is one of the most important and difficult questions in this area. Does the flat affect found in some RH patients reflect an underlying emotional attenuation? Or is it simply a superficial deficit in the ability to adequately express experienced affective states? The answer has far-reaching implications for the rehabilitation of this population, and much of the research reported in this section addresses the issue directly or indirectly. The solution to the puzzle has not been found, but recent research has helped link some of the pieces together.

Experimental evidence of the flat emotional responses in RH patients is well documented. Gianotti (1972), for example, found that the response to failure among 160 left- and right-hemisphere patients differed significantly. Left hemisphere (LH) patients tended to display catastrophic reactions (heightened anxiety, tears, refusal to complete the task), while RH patients either joked about, or appeared relatively unaffected by, the stress of failure. Furthermore, physiologic measurements of RH patients demonstrate hypoarousal to pain and to emotionally laden stimuli. Using a measure of a galvanic skin response (GSR), Heilman, Schwartz, and Watson (1978) found that RH subjects with left neglect demonstrated significantly lower GSR's to pain than did either the LH or non-neurologically impaired control group. Recently, Morrow, Vrtunsk, Kim, and Boller (1981) discovered a difference in GSR's in response to emotional and neutral slides. Their LH and RH groups had significantly smaller GSR's than normal controls, and GSR's in the RH subjects were significantly smaller than those in the LH group. The LH and control group had a significantly larger response to emotional (vs. neutral)slides, while the RH group produced almost no GSR at all to either type of slide.

RH superiority in reacting to emotionally laden auditory and visual stimuli has been found in normal subjects. Various dichotic studies have shown a left ear (RH) advantage in evaluating the emotional tone of recorded voices (Carmon & Nachson, 1973; Haggard & Parkinson, 1971; King & Kimura, 1972). In a review of dichotic studies investigating prosodic features, particularly intonational contour, Zurif (1974) concluded that "the ear advantage is determined less by the acoustic correlates of a linguistic property than by the use to which those correlates must be put. Thus, when the acoustic parameters of intonational contour...must be processed or matched independently of their linguistic medium, they become tied to the right hemisphere. In contrast, when these same parameters are used in the service of linguistic decisions, they are focused upon and utilized by the language mechanisms of the left hemisphere" (p. 395). Among the problems posed in dichotic studies investigating asymmetry for affective and prosodic elements is the difficulty in separating out the various features which are present as a result of the linguistic nature of the stimuli.

Visual studies with normal subjects using tachistoscopic presentation pose different limitations. The stimuli are presented to one visual half-field while the subject fixates on a central point. Thus, the input goes to only one hemisphere. Stimulus duration is circumscribed by normal lateral eye movement and generally can only be displayed for approximately 40 to 60 msec. Despite this limitation, tachistoscopic studies have advanced our knowledge about the role of the RH in responding to affective input. Numerous studies have tested asymmetry for facial recognition and, in recent years, have looked at the perception and discrimination of faces with emotional expressions. Generally, the results of these experiments have supported the view that facial recognition is faster or more accurate with a left visual-field (RH) presentation (Geffin, Bradshaw, & Wallace, 1971; Hilliard, 1973; Jones, 1979; Klein, Muscovitch, & Vigna, 1976; Leehey & Cahn, 1979; Rizzolatti, Umilita, & Berlucchi, 1971). Galper and Costa (1980), however, offer a good argument against what they term the "simplistic view" that the RH is the "sole mediator" of facial recognition. Numerous variables, such as the field dependence or independence of the subject, the sex of the subject, or the sex of the depicted face can play a role (Rapaczynski & Ehrlichman, 1979; Strauss & Muscovitch, 1981). A right visual-field (LH) superiority has been found, for example, in the recognition of the faces of famous people (Marzi & Berlucchi, 1977).

In an effort to better understand the role of the RH in both face recognition and the mediation of emotion, several people have used emotional faces as a variable (Hansch & Priozzollo, 1980; Strauss & Moscovitch, 1981; Suberi & McKeever, 1977). In general, the results of these studies have been consistent with a RH superiority in face and expression recognition, and in the recall of affective visual input.

Diamond and his colleagues (1976) were able to overcome the time limitation imposed on stimuli in tachistoscopic methods by using opaque contact lenses with off center slits which are designed to send visual input to a single half-field. Thus, they were able to show three films (a Tom and Jerry cartoon, a travelogue, and a surgical operation) to 14 right-handed normal subjects. The subjects rated the films on a nine-point scale as humourous, pleasant, unpleasant, or "horrific." No significant differences were found between the hemispheres on the first two ratings, but differences were found for the judgment of "unpleasant" on all films. In the left visual-field condition, the subjects tended to find more unpleasant features than in either the right visual-field or free vision conditions. The authors suggest that "each hemisphere has its own distinct emotional vision of the world" and that "each makes a unique contribution to the whole" (p. 692). They add that the right visual-field condition and free vision condition so closely resembled each other that it appears the RH response is more latent, or is perhaps suppressed in the intact brain by the LH.

Dekosky, Heilman, Bowers, and Valenstein (1980) looked at the ability of unilaterally brain damaged patients to discriminate emotional input in free vision. In six different tasks, their 27 subjects were required either to name the emotion depicted in a scene or face, or to discriminate between two faces or emotions (same or different). The RH subjects were significantly worse than the LH and normal control group in naming the emotional scenes, discriminating between neutral faces, and discriminating between emotions depicted in facial expressions. All nine of the RH subjects had neglect. The authors also report a tendency for the RH patients to be more impaired than the LH group in tasks where they had to either name or choose the accurate facial emotion.

Facial recognition, facial expression, detection of commonality of emotion between pictured emotional scenes and verbally described emotional situations were all investigated in a study by Cicone, Wapner, and Gardner (1980). Aphasic, RH, frontal leucotomy, and normal controls served as subjects. The RH group demonstrated reduced emotional sensitivity with verbal as well as visual stimuli. In discussing the quality of the RH responses, the authors explain that while many RH subjects were able to infer emotions correctly, they had difficulty applying this "inferential process" to the task. They state, "These observations suggest, at least in the case of some right hemisphere patients, a general impairment of the ability to apply inferential processes realistically to the external environment" (p. 156).

The degree to which recognizing a facial expression or emotion depends on facial recognition skills remains unclear. The results of the Dekosky study did not demonstrate them as separate abilities in brain damaged subjects. In the Cicone et al. study, only the RH and frontal leucotomy subjects had trouble in the facial recognition task. However, the correlation between scores on that test and those on the emotional expressions test was very low. And, some studies using normal subjects have indicated an independence between facial recognition skills and the recall of emotional faces (Ley & Bryden, 1979).

Another source of inquiry into the nature of emotional representation and its possible alteration as a result of RH disease has been in the area of auditory processing using right brain damaged subjects. Heilman, Scholes, and Watson (1975) have used the term "auditory affective agnosia" to describe the impaired ability to right parietal patients with neglect to discriminate and comprehend affectively toned sentences. Using a group of LH patients with lesions corresponding to those in the RH group, they found that neither group was impaired in comprehending the meaning of the tape-recorded stimulus sentences. The RH group, however, was significantly worse than the LH group in comprehending the mood (happy, sad, angry, or indifferent) of the speaker. In 1977, Tucker, Watson, and Heilman extended the study to further clarify the findings. In one task, subjects had to determine whether or not two identical neutral sentences were said with the same or different emotion (in 16 trials) and had to judge the mood of the speaker in an additional 16 trials. Their RH subjects, performing at a level no better than chance, were significantly more impaired on these tasks than the LH group. These results are at odds with the findings of Schlanger, Schlanger, and Gerstman (1976), although only three of their 20 subjects had temporoparietal lesions and it is uncertain whether or not they had neglect.

To find out if discrimination of affect extended to production of emotional tone, Tucker et al. (1977) designed a second experiment in which they asked their subjects to listen to tape-recorded sentences in which the speaker's tone was neutral. The sentences were followed by a mood marker (happy, sad, angry, or indifferent) and subjects were asked to repeat the sentence with the indicated emotional overlay. Their sentences were taped and evaluated for mood by three judges. Again, the RH group did not perform above the level of chance.

Rather than looking at deliberate emotional expression produced on command, Buck and Duffy (1981) designed a study investigating the production of spontaneous expression among four groups of subjects: aphasic, RH, parkinsonian, and normal controls. The subjects were shown affective slides that were divided into four categories including landscapes, unusual configurations, people familiar to the patient, and unpleasant scenes. The subjects' reactions were videotaped as they watched the slides. Naive judges were asked to: (a) guess the nature of the slide by categorizing the facial expression of the subject, and (b) rate the overall expressiveness of the subject. The judges gave significantly lower expressiveness ratings to RH and parkinsonian subjects, compared with aphasic and control patients. There were no significant differences in ability to categorize facial expression (and, hence determine the nature of the slide) between the aphasic and control groups. But the judges were significantly less accurate in judging the emotional reactions of the RH and parkinsonian groups.

In fact, no significant differences were found between the last two groups. The authors concluded that the power of a nonverbal message "arising spontaneously" from the affective state of the patient may not be disrupted by LH damage, but may be impaired by RH damage.

The prosodic features on nonaffective messages can also be disturbed in RH damage (Weintraub, Mesulam, & Kramer 1981; Ross & Mesulam, 1979). More precise documentation and analysis of prosodic deficits have been undertaken recently. Kent and Rosenbek (in press) used spectographic analysis to study the prosodic disturbances associated with various sites of lesion. In the RH group, their results revealed a reduction in acoustic energy in higher and midfrequency regions, and nasalization occurring with inadequate oral articulation. Like parkinsonian dysarthria, the RH subjects had a normal (or faster) rate, less than normal energy in frequencies above 500 Hz, and reduced acoustic contrast, so that they were perceived as speaking in a monotone with indistinct articulation and a mild to moderate hypernasality. Ross (1981) proposed a model of prosodic production and comprehension in which the anterior RH subserves the production of prosody, and the posterior RH is crucial to the comprehension of prosodic and affective speech. Damage to the anterior area, he suggests, creates a motor "aprosodia" characterized by poor expression, but good comprehension of affective speech. Damage to the posterior region, on the other hand, would lead to a more severe defect in receptive prosodic disturbances. His findings regarding the posterior RH are at odds with those of Tucker et al. (1977), who found their posterior patients impaired in production, as well as in comprehension of intonation pattern. More localization studies investigating the possible dissociation between prosodic expression and reception are needed.

The experimental evidence to date suggests a strong RH involvement in processing and producing prosodic and affective features of messages. It is interesting to note that exaggerated intonational contour has been used successfully in the treatment of anterior aphasia utilizing a technique called melodic intonation therapy (Sparks, Helm, & Albert, 1974). Research has also supported clinical reports of flat affect, impaired comprehension of emotional tone, and disturbed or attenuated prosody in some RH patients. Therapy for these disorders, beyond counselling the patient and family, is almost nonexistent. There is good reason for this. We still do not know if the patient's flat affect reflects a deeper emotional deficit or if it is an impairment superimposed over an intact emotional structure. Ferreting out the patient's internal emotional state from its outward projection is tricky business. One of the few investigations that has attempted to look at the subjective experience of emotion in RH patients is an unpublished study by Enders (1979). She gave the Lorr Feeling and Mood

Scale to RH, LH, and non-neurologically impaired controls and did not find significant differences among the groups on self-ratings of anger, energy, cheerfulness, anxiety, depression, or friendliness. She points out, however, that the results of the study did not always correspond to some of the subjective reports of attenuated feelings of anger from the RH patients.

More work investigating emotional responsiveness in RH patients is needed. Research with normal subjects suggests a significant role for the RH, not only with prosody and emotional expressiveness, but also in the internal affective state. We must be careful, however, about making automatic assumptions regarding the effect of cortical brain damage on what appear to be functions of the same area in the intact brain. The lack of responsiveness noted in RH patients may be caused by other factors besides emotion. These will be explored in Section IV. Still, we must beware of treating the symptoms without a more thorough grasp of the cause. It may be possible to retrain patients to express affect by improving prosodic and nonverbal features of their messages, for example, or by training them to recognize and comprehend the meaning of affective material. The latter poses less risk, and would probably be helpful to the overall receptive skills of patients. But the former task, while helping patients communicate better on one level, may mask a deeper deficit with which we are not equipped to deal.

Section III:
Linguistic Deficits

Right hemisphere communication disorders clearly fall outside the continuum of aphasic-like behaviors. However, some RH patients do demonstrate deficits on pure linguistic tasks. Auditory and visual processing demands, and syntactic complexity appear to play a role in the linguistic problems discussed below. Performance on more sophisticated communication tasks can be attributed to the higher-order cognitive and perceptual problems covered in Section IV.

Because standardized diagnostic batteries designed specifically for RH patients have not yet been developed, many clinicians use aphasia tests as part of their assessment. These tests may serve as useful tools, but should be administered with caution. The test stimuli are not generally sophisticated or divergent enough to reveal higher-level deficits. Scoring systems are generally inadequate in accounting for the full range of RH communication behavior. Often, for example, the patient's extraneous comments noted by the clinician in the margin of the test will be more revealing than the scores themselves. Depressed scores may be less a result of linguistic problems than of impaired visuospatial skills or neglect (see Section I). A complex visual array of target and foils may result in delayed responses as the patient searches for an adequately understood target item.

With these cautionary notes in mind, several researchers have used aphasia batteries to look at RH performance on linguistic tasks. Deal, Deal, Wertz, Kitselman, and Dwyer (1979) compared the performance of RH subjects with that of aphasic subjects on the *Porch Index of Communicative Abilities* (PICA) (Porch, 1967) to see if there were similarities. Their retrospective study of 111 RH subjects revealed that while the RH subjects did make errors, the PICA was probably not the best instrument to use with this population. Some subjects, for example, had more difficulty on tasks considered easier for aphasic patients, and had less difficulty on subtests considered harder for aphasic patients.

Subtests of the *Boston Diagnostic Aphasia Examination* (BDAE) (Goodglass & Kaplan, 1967) have been used by a number of researchers. Myers (1978) found that the mean scores of her 8 subjects on the 18 subtests of the BDAE were above the cut-off level for aphasia. However, the range of reported scores demonstrated that some patients fell below the norm in word discrimination, comprehension of complex ideational material, animal naming (word fluency), oral sentence reading, word recognition and word-picture matching. Using the same test, Adamovich and Brooks (1981) found significant differences between their 5 RH subjects and 5 normal controls on several BDAE subtests. Scores on word discrimination, body part identification, and complex ideational material were lower in the experimental group. The authors point out that errors on numbers and letters made a significant contribution to the low scores on the word discrimination test. Complex ideational errors were thought to be a function of linguistic complexity and length. Body part identification errors may have been less the result of comprehension deficits than of impaired right-left discrimination, or of anosognosia, though the authors do not comment on this.

In the verbal expression subtests of the BDAE, Adamovich and Brooks's subjects were significantly impaired compared with controls on automatic sequencing and in responsive naming. The authors point out that the errors on the visual confrontation-naming subtest tended to be on naming items that were visually similar to the target items. They suggest that visual integration deficits as revealed by the *Hooper Visual Organization Test* (Hooper, 1958) in their experimental group may have been a contributing factor. It is interesting to note, however, that in a study using both the latter tests, Myers and Linebaugh (1980) found their 12 RH subjects were significantly impaired on the Hooper test, but had near perfect scores in the visual confrontation-naming subtest of the BDAE. Out of a possible 105 points, the mean for the RH subjects on this test was 97.

To further investigate naming, Adamovich and Brooks used the *Boston Naming Test* (Kaplan, Goodglass, & Weintraub, 1976) and found significantly lower scores in their RH group compared with controls. On the Word Fluency Measure (Borkowski, Benton, & Spreen, 1967), they also found their RH group had consistently lower scores than controls. Milner (1974) also found that word fluency tasks reveal RH deficits. Such an impairment in this population may partly reflect impaired control over available linguistic information. The animal-naming subtest of the BDAE in the Myers (1978) study showed that the RH subjects tended to use random strategies reflecting impaired use of associations.

Auditory comprehension disorders have been noted in tests other than the BDAE. McNeil and Prescott found that linguistic complexity was a factor in the impaired RH performance on the *Revised Token Test (RTT)* (McNeil & Prescott, 1978). Their results are consistent with those found by Adamovich and Brooks on the same test. In the latter study, the authors did not find significant differences between normal control and RH groups on two auditory memory tasks, and they concluded that complexity (embedding), rather than length, was the major factor in the impaired performance of the RH group on the RTT.

Factors other than linguistic complexity or verbal memory may play a role in the impaired performance of RH patients on the auditory comprehension tests listed above. In a study investigating recognition memory for verbal and nonverbal material, Riege, Metter, and Hanson (1980) found a double dissociation in stroke patients by task demands. Test stimuli in the auditory portion of the experiment included words (verbal) and bird calls (nonverbal). Subjects were asked to signal recognition of 10 previously presented test items which were randomly embedded in a list of 40 items. On the verbal portion of the test, they found that aphasic subjects were significantly impaired, but RH subjects performed as well as controls. However, the reverse was true on the nonverbal tasks. RH subjects were significantly impaired and aphasic subjects were not. These results were consistent across the long-term and the short-term memory conditions.

While this finding suggests that RH patients do not have deficits in word recognition and recall, it further demonstrates that auditory memory is not a unilateral function. The bird calls in this study were patterns of notes, and it is thought that the RH may be more adept with pattern recognition. Only a few years ago it was popular to associate the RH with musical abilities. Now it is recognized that musical performance and recognition, like language, is a complex behavior. Variables include intensity, duration, pitch, temporal sequencing, rhythm, and more. Generally, results of various studies have shown that the LH is more specialized for detecting temporal order (Carmon & Nachson, 1971; Halperin, Nachson, & Carmon, 1973; Mills & Rollman, 1980), duration and rhythm (Gordon, 1978). (See Gates & Bradshaw (1977) for a thorough review.) The RH has been associated with the detection of pitch. Milner (1962), for example, found that right temporal lobectomy patients were impaired in timbre and melody recognition. Shapiro, Grossman, and Gardner, (1981) found subjects with lesions in the right anterior, right central areas, and left central areas were significantly impaired in detecting phrasing and rhythm errors, while right anterior and right central patients were impaired in pitch recognition.

Sidtis (1980) states that the perception of pitch, timbre, and interval relationships between chords is partly determined by the harmonic composition of the tone. Reviewing the sometimes conflicting results of dichotic studies with normal subjects, he observes: "their results suggest that auditory function of the right hemisphere is specialized for the analysis of harmonic information" (p. 322). Sidtis sees harmonic information as the unifying factor in pitch perception. His study was designed to examine its role in eliciting hemisphere asymmetries for pitch discrimination in normal subjects. His results with the 96 right-handed subjects supported his hypothesis and he concludes: "It should also be noted that while complex pitch perception is an important expression of the right hemisphere's capacity for harmonic information processing, this function is likely to play a role in a wide range of auditory perception" (p. 328).

These findings are consistent with the studies demonstrating RH deficits in the detection of prosodic features and mood (see Section II). On complex and lengthy material, it may be that the examiner's phrasing and intonation patterns are not detected by the subject, or that the effort to discriminate them may interfere with overall comprehension of lengthy and complex test items. Thus, overall acoustic dimensions of the test stimuli may be as much a factor as linguistic embedding.

Phonemic discrimination, on the other hand, does not appear to play a role in linguistic comprehension tasks in RH patients. In a recent study Gianotti, Caltagirone, Miceli, and Masullo (1981) gave tests of semantic and phonemic discrimination to 50 RH and 39 control subjects. The performance of the RH group on word-to-picture matching (semantic) was significantly worse than that of controls, while there were no significant differences on the phonemic discrimination test.

In the same study, RH subjects were found not to be impaired in the ability to match printed words to pictures. These findings are consistent with those of Rivers and Love (1980) on a similar task, and with the findings in the Adamovich and Brooks (1980) study. In the latter, the authors report that, while single word reading was not impaired, their RH group was significantly worse than controls in the Sentence and Paragraph subtest of the BDAE. Performance deteriorated as stimulus length increased.

Other comprehension and expression deficits on tasks involving complex material are probably less a function of disorders in linguistic processing per se, than in extralinguistic and higher cognitive operations. These problems will be addressed in Section IV. When deficits are found that are thought to be purely linguistic in nature, most clinicians use the standard stimulation techniques used in aphasia therapy (Adamovich, 1981; Myers, 1982).

Section IV: Higher Cognitive Impairments

Although RH patients may demonstrate some language impairments as measured by aphasia tests, these deficits tell only a small part of the story. The true extent of RH communication disorders is apparent only when the patient is engaged in more sophisticated and open-ended communication tasks. The less concrete and the more complex the task, the more likely the patient will manifest the following deficits: (1) difficulty in organizing information in an efficient, meaningful way; (2) a tendency to produce impulsive answers that are rife with tangential and related, but unnecessary, detail; (3) difficulty in distinguishing between what is important and what is not; (4) problems in assimilating and using contextual cues; (5) a tendency to overpersonalize external events; (6) a tendency to lend a literal interpretation to figurative language; and (7) a reduced sensitivity to the communicative situation and to the pragmatic or extralinguistic aspects of communication (Myers, 1982).

Less than 10 years ago, the best we could do in describing these symptoms was to characterize RH speech as bizarre, inappropriate, confused, or confabulatory. While we recognized that the term "aphasic-like behavior" was wholly inadequate in describing what we observed, we were not able to be very specific in explaining why. Research in this area has sought a more precise delineation of the disorders and, in the last 5 or 6 years, has significantly advanced our understanding of the nature of RH communication impairments on this higher level. As a result, some unifying themes are beginning to emerge. Two of the most prominent are that RH patients appear to have difficulty in organizing information, and a deficit in relating to contextual cues.

In extensive interviews with 20 RH patients, Myers (1979) noted that when responding to open-ended questions, many patients could address, but not answer, the question. They seemed unable to structure the information at hand in a meaningful way. It appeared that they were not able to isolate and integrate relevant items and, that they catalogued random facts, rather than providing the interpretation of events called for by the question. Noting this same tendency, Gardner and Hamby (1979) designed a pilot study looking at the role of the RH in organizing information for communication. Their work was later refined into a more extensive investigation into the ability of RH subjects to manage complex linquistic material (Wapner, Hamby & Gardner, 1981). In both studies, RH subjects and controls were presented with several tasks, one of which was to retell auditorily presented stories which emphasized either spatial, emotional, or noncanonical (unexpected or nonsensical) elements. The retold stories of the RH group, particularly in those with noncanonical endings, demonstrated that the RH subjects seemed to be uncertain about what was important and what was incidental. Gardner and Hamby explained that their patients seemed "unable to isolate, and to appreciate the relations among, the key points of the story. The basic schema—the major episodes organized in an hierarchically-appropriate manner—seems disturbed." They suggested that "the basic scaffolding of the story has not been satisfactorily assimilated. And, without this organizing principle, patients cannot even judge which details, or parts, matter."

Delis, Wapner, Gardner, and Moses (in press) studied this organizing principle directly by asking 10 RH and 10 intact controls to arrange mixed-up sentences into meaningful paragraphs. The paragraphs fell into three categories conveying primarily spatial, temporal, or categorical components. The RH group was significantly impaired relative to controls on all three paragraph types. Further analysis revealed that the RH subjects organized the temporal paragraphs with significantly more accuracy than the spatial ones, and arranged the latter with significantly more accuracy than the categorical ones. The effects of fatigue, memory, and attention were ruled out in the experiment. It is interesting to note that one of their subjects who achieved a verbal IQ of 148 (99.9th percentile) on the *Wechsler Adult Intelligence Scale* scored a mean of only 38.12% in this study, compared to an overall mean for all RH subjects of 49.82%. This fact lends further support to the notion that even when linguistic information is readily available, RH patients may still have difficulty organizing it into a meaningful pattern. This may partly account for the rambling inclusion of tangential detail so characteristic of RH responses to divergent questions.

In the Wapner et al. (1981) study, it was noted by the authors that their RH subjects had no difficulty using phonology and syntax in retelling narratives. But they also point out that while normal controls usually paraphrased the stories, 10 of the 15 RH subjects repeated segments verbatim without recoding them—another sign of difficulty in interpreting events.

Two studies (Myers, 1979, Myers & Linebaugh, 1980) looked at this deficit in interpreting events by asking subjects to reach conclusions about pictured material. In the latter study 12 RH subjects and 12 normal controls (age and education matched) were asked not to describe—but to explain—what was happening in the Cookie Theft picture from the *Boston Diagnostic Aphasia Examination.* Subject responses were analyzed for content in the following manner: a list of concepts used by normal speakers in describing the picture was obtained from a study by Yorkston and Beukelman (1980). The list was then divided into interpretive and literal concepts. Literal concepts were operationally defined as those that had meaning separate from the context of the depicted events. Interpretive concepts were defined as those whose meaning was derived from the context of events in the picture. Thus, "woman" was considered literal, while "mother" was considered interpretive. Three judges rated the response transcripts and the results demonstrated that the RH subjects had significantly fewer interpretive concepts, compared with controls. The experimental group tended to itemize isolated bits of information—such things as cups and saucers, curtains, and so on—which did not further a description of the action. Where a control subject might explain that the little girl was reaching up for a cookie, the typical RH patient might say that she had her arm up. The connection between her arm, the boy reaching into the jar, and handing a cookie to her went unnoticed. Thus, the RH group often missed the relationships among the elements of the picture, and, consequently, failed to infer meaning from those relationships.

As was noted in Section I, the subjects in this study were also significantly impaired relative to controls in a test of visual integration. The authors suggested that this deficit in visual synthesis on a low order perceptual level may extend to a deficit in integration on a higher level. Their subjects had difficulty in extracting the critical bits of information, and in apprehending the relationships among them. Thus, they failed to make the best use of contextual cues in deriving the meaning of the depicted events.

Rivers and Love (1980) found the same pattern on a series of visual processing tasks presented to normal controls, LH and RH groups. Their RH subjects had no significant difficulty in giving word definitions, or in a word-reading test, but were significantly worse than controls in utilizing sentence clues to substitute a real for a nonsense word. In another one of the seven tasks in their study, subjects were asked to make up a story based on the events depicted in a series of three sequential pictures. According to the authors, the RH responses in this task indicated "a reduced ability to use fully the information contained in the sequences of three pictures to tell complete stories." (p. 360)

That this deficit in responding appropriately to contextual clues extends beyond visually presented stimuli is evident from both the Gardner and Hamby and the Wapner et al. studies, since their subjects were required to listen to auditorily presented narratives. In addition, Metzler and Jelinek (1976) found their RH subjects had problems in retelling the auditorily presented quicksand paragraph from *The Minnesota Test for Differential Diagnosis of Aphasia* (Schuell, 1957). Their subjects had significantly more irrelevancies than controls.

Impaired use of contextual clues may have been an indirect factor in another study. Wapner and Gardner (1980) looked at the ability of 47 brain-damaged patients and 10 normal controls to process various types of linguistic and nonlinguistic symbols. The symbols included such things as trademarks, traffic signs, and symbols associated with numbers. The subjects had to choose one of four pictures in which the target symbol was correctly displayed. That is, they had to demonstrate an understanding of the symbol by finding the picture that showed it in its correct context. The results demonstrated that both the RH and LH groups were significantly impaired relative to controls, but that the two brain-damaged groups did not differ significantly from each other in overall success rate. However, the RH group relied more heavily on linguistic cues, and their performance deteriorated as these cues were faded. Their performance was inferior to the LH group, for example, in the pictorial trademarks test—they tended to choose the "unrelated" foil more often. The results of this study suggest that, without linguistic cues, RH subjects may have more difficulty than LH ones in determining what sort of traffic sign is most appropriately displayed in front of a school, or where the Playboy bunny belongs. The RH group may have had problems not only in understanding the symbols, but in processing the contextual cues that were intended to help them in the task.

Nonlinguistic symbols have presented problems for RH patients in other studies. Gardner and Denes (1973) looked at aphasic patients' responses to connotative versus denotative material and included six RH subjects in the experimental population. The denotative section of the study required subjects to match a spoken target word to one of four pictures. The connotative task was derived from an adaptation of Osgood's pictorial semantic differential test (Osgood, 1960). Subjects had to point to one of two sets of geometric forms or expressive lines drawn in such a way as to "capture an aspect of connotation of the particular word" (p. 186). The authors noted that the behavior of the RH group on the connotative task was very different from that of the aphasic subjects. In general, the RH subjects protested against the task. Two of the six refused several times to take this part of the test. The scores of the three who did take it were lower than that of the average anterior aphasic patient. It may be that the difficulty in the RH group stemmed directly from a problem in handling connotative material, as the authors suggest. Or it may be that the novelty of the task disrupted their performance, just as other RH subjects found it difficult to relate to the unexpected or noncanonical elements in the previously reported research.

Clinical observations that RH patients tend to be literal-minded, to miss nuance and subtlety, to overlook intended and connotative meanings has been supported in several studies. Winner and Gardner (1977) asked aphasic and RH subjects to match a metaphoric sentence to its appropriate interpretation depicted in one of four pictures. Aphasic subjects chose significantly more metaphoric (correct) pictures than the RH subjects. The most frequent error choice in the RH group was a literal depiction of the metaphor. When asked to explain the meaning of the metaphors, most RH subjects gave an accurate interpretation and appeared unaffected by the dissociation between their verbal explanations and their picture choices.

Myers and Linebaugh (1981) investigated patients' comprehension of connotative language by looking at their understanding of common idiomatic expressions. RH, LH, and control subjects were presented with two-sentence stories, each of which ended with a common idiom. The outcome of the story could only be determined through an accurate interpretation of the idiom. The five response categories varied according to literal vs. accurate depiction of the idiom, and according to correct or incorrect context or setting of the story events. A final foil depicted the opposite outcome of the story. The results showed that the RH group made significantly more errors than either controls or aphasic subjects, and that, while they selected the correct context significantly more often than the wrong one, they selected the literal depiction of the idiom significantly more often than the appropriate one.

These findings appear, at first, to be at odds with the findings of Stachowiak, Huber, Poeck, and Kerschensteiner 1977),who looked at text comprehension in aphasic, RH, and normal controls. Subjects were asked to choose one of five pictures that most closely matched a six-sentence story read aloud to them. The story stimuli contained an idiom, and one of the foil pictures showed a literal depiction of the idiom. However, the idiom was used only as a means of making the material redundant, since it was itself defined in the third sentence of each story. Thus, the thrust of the study was comprehension of text, rather than of metaphoric language, and RH and control subjects performed without significant differences on the task.

Gardner, King, Flamm, and Silverman (1975) suggested that humorous material fuses both the cognitive and affective aspects of communication. With this in mind, they designed a study in which RH, LH, and control subjects had to pick out the most humorous picture from a set of four. Both right and left brain-damaged populations were significantly impaired in their ability to pick out the cartoon pictures, and there were no significant differences in their performances relative to one another. More recently, Wapner et al. (1981) looked at subjects' ability to choose the correct punchline from a set of four, after listening to the body of the joke. The four choices included endings that were: (1) appropriate and funny; (2) appropriate and straightforward, but not funny; (3) sad; and (4) a nonsequitur that did not flow from the body of the joke. The RH subjects chose endings in the fourth category three times as often as controls. In addition, they often confabulated, as they had in other parts of the study, to explain a link between their choice of a nonsequitur and the joke. And, when these same subjects were presented with a cartoon picture series, they responded in a serious, rather than amused way, to the cartoons, demanding explanations for what other subject groups found funny.

Taken together, this research adds to data-based evidence to support several clinical observations, such as the oft-noted failure of RH patients to appreciate humor (their own or other peoples'), as well as failure to appreciate the connotative aspects of communication. RH patients often appear unresponsive to intended meaning and to extralinguistic cues, while the opposite pattern has been found in aphasic patients (see Wilcox, Davis & Leonard, 1978). Their overall impairment in apprehending and using contextual information to derive meaning may partly explain their insensitivity to the pragmatic aspects of communication—they seem unable to fully appreciate the speaker's intentions, purpose of the exchange, or their listener's needs. In addition, the results reported in this section suggest RH patients have difficulty in tasks that require them to extract and isolate key elements, see the relationships among them, integrate them into an overall structure, and draw inferences based on those relationships.

How should we treat these disorders? Should we attempt to treat them at all? Clearly, treatment of communication deficits of any type is within the purview of speech and language pathologists. But we must be cautious. The research reported in this setion represents only a beginning. From trial treatment we can continue to expand our knowledge base. Myers (1982) offers specific suggestions for presenting the patient with material that requires him to associate, interpret, and derive meaning from context. Adamovich (1981) has suggested another approach based on theories of cognitive development. And there will doubtless be others. Those working directly with this population should be religious in keeping data, and should recognize the obligation they have to share that information in the form of single-case or group studies.

Speech pathologists have been well trained to work with communicatively impaired people, but few have had formal training in working with the symptoms described here. Only by educating ourselves through clinical experience and by keeping abreast of the rapidly expanding literature on the RH will we be able to apply our formal training to the needs of this population.

Summary

We have travelled what may seem like a long journey across several landscapes, exploring lower-order perceptual impairments, neglect, prosodic and affective deficits, and higher-order language impairments, and the effect of each on RH communication. These disorders may appear to be discrete entities, but, for several reasons, it would be a mistake to assume they are wholly distinct from one another. First, many patients, particularly those with extensive lesions, will be impaired to some extent in each area. Second, while aphasia disrupts a certain system or class of behaviors (language), RH damage appears to disturb a less specific, more generalized response to experience itself. If perception is understood as involving the ability to both discriminate and interpret at the same time, then the link between lower-order perception and the management of complex material is apparent. At no stage of perception does man act as a mere sensory recorder. He constantly weighs and relates the fragments of external and internal experience into a personal unique whole. He derives meaning from events by filtering out the irrelevant, extracting what seems critical, and by relating those chosen elements into a pattern. Thus, experience is interpreted through an almost instantaneous operation which is performed prior to verbalization. To perceive is to know something directly, without subjecting it to analysis. The perceiver is not passive, but is an active participant allowing his internal associations and knowledge to guide him. An impairment in perception, as it is described here, would impair the ability to grasp the essense of events, or to experience a sense of connectedness with the outside world. It is not surprising that RH patients, then, have difficulty utilizing and responding to all the extralinguistic or pragmatic aspects of communication, or that the linguistic system itself is inadequate in helping them derive meaning from on-going events. To understand and accurately communicate experience clearly requires the participation of both sides of the brain.

Much has been made of the differing processing styles of the two intact hemispheres. Originally, they were thought to differ according to stimulus type-linguistic versus nonlinguistic. Research with brain-damaged, split-brain (in particular), and normal subjects refined this notion. Currently, it is popular to assign propositional, linear, sequential, and analytic or feature detection capabilities to the LH. The RH is thought to be more adept at apprehending the gestalt, in detecting patterns without feature analysis, and in appropositional, simultaneous, synthetic, integrative processing (Bogen, 1969; Gazzaniga, 1970; Ornstein, 1977; Zaidel, 1978; Patterson & Bradshaw, 1975; Cohen, 1973). Experimental data support this hypothesis, though not definitively. And it can be related to some extent to some of the deficits described in this chapter.

New evidence, however, constantly refines our understanding of the roles of the two hemispheres and their cooperation in complex tasks. Recent neuroanatomical and cytoarchitectural data support the view that the RH is more adept with complex input. Reviewing the evidence, Goldberg and Costa (1981) suggest that the RH has greater neuronal capacity to deal with informational complexity, has more associative cortex, has more intraregional connections, and has a greater ability to process many modes of representation within a single cognitive task. The LH, they explain, has more sensory and motor representation, has more interregional connections, and is superior in tasks which require fixation upon a single mode of representation (p. 148).

The thrust of their argument is that the LH is adept with descriptive systems (language, mathematics, and other coded behaviors), while the RH is pivotal in managing novel tasks for which no descriptive system exists. A descriptive system, as they define it, is one which "implies any set of discrete units of encoding or rules of transformation that can be successfully applied to the processing of a certain class of stimuli" (p. 151). Reliance on a routinized descriptive system, they explain, puts demands on the LH, while the RH appears to have more facility for utilizing associative areas of the cortex and for cross-modal integration.

This hypothesis, based on evidence too extensive to cite here, supports, but also extends and enriches, our earlier understanding of how the two hemispheres operate alone and in concert. It also helps us conceive of what may occur with unilateral brain damage.

Many of the deficits outlined in this chapter appear to affect experiential processing or operations that do not rely on routinized codes—i.e. assimilating contextual cues, distinguishing what is important from what is not, perceiving relationships, interpreting events. RH patients appear impaired on tasks in which they cannot rely on language or any other descriptive system to provide clues about their experience. They do not deal well with novel or unexpected situations or stimuli. The rules that operate on the pragmatic aspects of communication are not as neatly defined or coded as are the rules governing language itself. And so it may be that the inappropriate behaviors of the RH patient represent, in part, difficulty in managing situations in which he cannot apply an objective routine or code, or may represent an excessive reliance on descriptive systems that do not apply to the situation at hand.

This speculation is offered as a way of helping to conceptualize and weave together the multiple aspects of RH communication disorders. The differing capacities of the two hemispheres is of interest to people in a wide range of fields. The clinician working with this population should read widely, and be cautious in accepting any simple notion of hemisphere asymmetry. The capacities of the RH, and the impact of damage in that hemisphere on communication, is a story that is just beginning to unfold.

References

Adamovich, B. L. Treatment of right hemisphere damaged patients: A panel presentation. A. Davis (Moderator), In R. H. Brookshire (Ed.), *Clinical Aphasiology: Conference Proceedings.* Minneapolis: BRK Publishers, 1981.

Adamovich, B. L., & Brooks, R. L. A diagnostic protocol to assess the communication deficits in patients with right hemisphere damage. In R. H. Brookshire (Ed.), *Clinical Aphasiology: Conference Proceedings.* Minneapolis: BRK Publishers, 1981.

Benton, A. L. Visuoperceptive, visuospatial, and visuoconstructive disorders. In K. M. Heilman & E. Valenstein (Eds.), *Clinical neuropsychology.* New York: Oxford University Press, 1979.

Benton, A. L., Hannay, J., & Varney, N. R. Visual perception of line direction in patients with unilateral brain disease. *Neurology,* 1975 *25,* 907-910.

Benton, A. L., & Van Allen, M. W. Facial recognition in patients with cerebral disease. *Cortex,* 1968, *4,* 344-358.

Bisiach, E. Capitani, E., Luzzatti, C., & Perani, D. Brain and conscious representation of outside reality. *Neuropsychologia,* 1981, *19,* 543-551.

Bisiach, E., Luzzatti, C., & Perani, D. Unilateral neglect, representational schema and consciousness. *Brain,* 1979, *102,* 609-618.

Bisiach, E., Nichelli, P., & Spinnler, H. Hemispheric functional asymmetry in visual discrimination between univariate stimuli: An analysis of sensitivity and response criterion. *Neuropsychologia,* 1976, *14,* 335-342.

Bogen, J. The other side of the brain. II. *Bulletin of the Los Angeles Neurological Society, 34,* 1969.

Borkowski, J. G., Benton, A. L., & Spreen, O. Word fluency and brain damage. *Neuropsychologia, 1967, 5,* 135-140.

Bower, J. H. Imagery as a relational organizer in associative learning. *Journal of Verbal Learning and Verbal Behavior,* 1970, *9,* 529-533.

Brain, W. R. Visual disorientation with special reference to lesions of the right cerebral hemisphere. *Brain,* 1941, *64,* 244-272.

Bugeleski, B. R. Images as mediators in one-trail paired-associate learning, II. *Journal of Experimental Psychology,* 1968, *77,* 328-334.

Bugeleski, B. R. Words and things and images. *American Psychologist, 25,* 1970.

Buck, R., & Duffy, R. J. Non-verbal communication of affect in brain-damaged patients. *Cortex,* 1981, *6,* 351-362.

Butters, N., & Barton, M. Effect of parietal lobe damage on the performance of reversible operations in space. *Neuropsychologia,* 1970, *8,* 205-214.

Carmon, A., & Nachson, I. Ear asymmetry in perception of emotional and non-verbal stimuli. *Acta Psychologia,* 1973, *37,* 351-357.

Cicone, M., Wapner, W., & Gardner H. Sensitivity to emotional expressions and situations in organic patients. *Cortex,* 1980, *16,* 145-158.

Cohen, G. Hemispheric differences in serial verses parallel processing. *Journal of Experimental Psychology,* 1973, *97,* 349-356.

Collins, M. The minor hemisphere. In R. H. Brookshire (Ed.), *Clinical Aphasiology: Conference Proceedings.* Minneapolis: BRK Publishers, 1976.

Critchley, M. *The parietal lobes.* London: Edward Arnold, 1953.

Deal, J., Deal, L., Wertz, R., Kitselman, K., & Dwyer, C. Right hemisphere PICA percentiles: Some speculations about aphasia. In R.H. Brookshire (Ed.), *Clinical Aphasiology: Conference Proceedings.* Minneapolis: BRK Publishers, 1979.

Delis, D.C., Wapner, W., Gardner, H., & Moses, J. The contribution of the right hemisphere to the organization of paragraphs. *Cortex,* in press.

Dekosky, S., Heilman, K., Bowers, D., & Valenstein, E. Recognition and discrimination of emotional faces and pictures. *Brain and Language,* 1981, *9,* 206-214.

Denny-Brown, D., Myers, J. S., & Horenstein, S. The significance of perceptual rivalry resulting from parietal lesion, *Brain,* 1952, *75,* 443-471.

DeRenzi, E., & Spinnler, H. Facial recognition in brain damaged patients, *Neurology,* 1966, *16,* 145-152.

DeRenzi, E., Faglioni, P., & Spinnler, H. Performance of patients with unilateral brain damage on face recognition tasks. *Cortex,* 1968, *4,* 17-34.

Diamond, S. J. Differing emotional responses from right and left hemispheres. *Nature,* June, 1976, 261.

Diller, L., & Weinberg, J. Hemi-inattention in rehabilitation: The evolution of a rational remedial program. In E. A. Weinstein & R. P. Friedland (Eds.), *Advances in neurology* (Vol. 18). New York: Raven Press, 1977.

Enders, M. Emotional responses in subjects with cerebral hemisphere damage. Rehabilitation Research and Training Center Grant #16-P-56803/3, The George Washington University Medical Center, Washington, D.C., unpublished study, 1979.

Fredericks, J. A. M. Constructional apraxia and cerebral dominance. *Psychiatria, Neurologia, Neurochirurgia,* 1963, *66,* 522-530.

Galin, D. Implications for psychiatry of left and right cerebral specialization, *Archives of General Psychiatry,* 1974, *31,* 572-583.

Galper, R. E., & Costa, L. Hemispheric superiority for faces depends on how they are learned. *Cortex,* 1980, *16,* 21-38.

Gardner, H., & Denes, G. Connotative judgements by aphasic patients on a pictorial adaptation of the semantic differential. *Cortex,* 1973, *9,* 183-96.

Gardner, H., King, P., Flamm, L., & Silverman, J. Comprehension and appreciation of humorous material following brain damage. *Brain,* 1975, *98,* 399-412.

Gardner, H., & Hamby, S. The role of the right hemisphere in the organization of linguistic materials. Paper presented to the International Neuropsychology Symposium, Dubrovnik, Yugoslavia, June, 1979.

Gates, A., & Bradshaw, J. L. The role of the cerebral hemispheres in music. *Brain and Language*, 1977, *4*, 403-31.

Gazzaniga, M. *The bisected brain.* New York: Appleton-Century-Crofts, 1970.

Geffin, G., Bradshaw, J. L., & Wallace, G. Interhemispheric effects on reaction time to verbal and non-verbal visual stimuli. *Journal of Experimental Psychology*, 1971, *87*, 415-422.

Gerstman, J. The problem of imperception of disease and of impaired body territories with organic lesions. *Archives of Neurology and Psychiatry*, 1942, *48*, 890-913.

Gianotti, G. Emotional behavior and hemispheric side of lesion. *Cortex*, 1972, *8*, 41-55.

Gianotti, G., Caltagirone, C., Miceli, G., & Masullo, C. Selective semantic-lexical impairment of language comprehension in right-brain-damaged patients. *Brain and Language*, 1981, *13*, 201-211.

Goodglass, H., & Kaplan, E. *The Boston Diagnostic Aphasia Examination.* Philadelphia: Lea & Febiger, 1967.

Goldberg, E., & Costa, L. Hemispheric differences in the acquisition and use of descriptive systems. *Brain and Language*, 1981, *14*, 144-173.

Gordon, H. Left hemisphere dominance for rhythmic elements in dichotically-presented melodies. *Cortex*, 1978, *14*, 58-69.

Haggard, P., & Parkinson, A. M. Stimulus and task factors as determinents of ear advantages. *Quarterly Journal of Experimental Psychology*, 1971, *23*, 168-177.

Halperin, Y., Nachson, I., & Carmon, A. Shift of ear superiority in dichotic listening to temporally patterned nonverbal stimuli. *Journal of the Acoustical Society of America*, 1973, *53*, 46-50.

Hansch, E. C., & Priozollo, F. J. Task relevant effects on the assessment of cerebral specialization for facial emotion. *Brain and Language*, 1980, *10*, 51-59.

Head, H. *Studies in neurology.* London: Oxford University Press, 1920.

Hecaen, H. Clinical symptomatolgy in right and left hemisphere lesions. In V. B. Mountcastle (Ed.), *Interhemispheric relations and cerebral dominance.* Baltimore: Johns Hopkins University Press, 1962.

Heilman, K. M., & Valenstein, E. Frontal lobe neglect in man. *Neurology*, 1979, *22*, 660-664.

Heilman, K.M., Scholes, R., & Watson, R. T. Auditory affective agnosia. *Journal of Neurology, Neurosurgery, and Psychiatry*, 1975, *38*, 69-72.

Heilman, K. M., & Watson, R. T. The neglect syndrome: A unilateral defect in the orienting response. In S. Harnad (Ed.), *Lateralization in the nervous system.* New York: Academic Press, 1977.

Heilman, K. M., Schwartz, H. D., & Watson, R. T. Hypoarousal in patients with neglect and emotional indifference. *Neurology*, 1978, *28*, 229-232.

Heilman, K. M. Neglect and related disorders. In K. M. Heilman & E. Valenstein (Eds.), *Clinical neuropsychology.* New York: Oxford Univ. Press, 1979.

Hilliard, R. D. Hemispheric laterality effects in facial recognition tasks in normal subjects. *Cortex*, 1973, *9*, 246-258.

Hooper, E. *The Hooper Visual Organization Test.* Los Angeles: Western Psychological Services, 1958.

Jones, B. Lateral asymmetry in testing long term memory for faces. *Cortex*, 1979, *15*, 183-186.

Joynt, R., & Goldstein, M. The minor hemisphere. *Advances in Neurology*, 1975, *7*, 147-183.

Kaplan, E., Goodglass, H., & Weintraub, S. *The Boston Naming Test*, experimental edition, 1976.

Kent, R. D., & Rosenbek, J. C. Prosodic disturbance and neurologic site of lesion. *Brain and Language*, in press.

King, F. L., & Kimura, D. Left ear superiority in dichotic perception of vocal non-verbal sounds. *Canadian Journal of Psychology*, 1972, *26*, 111-116.

Klein, D., Muscovitch, J., & Vigna, C. Attentional mechanisms and perceptual asymmetries in recognition of words and faces. *Neuropsychologia,* 1976, *14,* 55-66.

LaPointe, L., & Culton, G. Visual-spatial neglect subsequent to brain injury. *Journal of Speech and Hearing Disorders,* 1969, *34,* 82-86.

LeDoux, J. E. Parietooccipital symptomatology: The split brain perspective. In M. Gazzaniga (Ed.), *Handbook of neuropsychology.* New York: Plenum Press, 1978.

Leehey, S. C., & Cahn, A. Lateral asymmetries in the recognition of words, familiar faces and unfamiliar faces. *Neuropsychologia,* 1979, *17,* 619-635.

Ley, R. G., & Bryden, M. P. Hemispheric differences in processing emotions and faces. *Brain and Language,* 1979, *7,* 127-138.

Marzi, C. A., & Berlucchi, G. Right visual field superiority for accuracy of recognition of famous faces in normals. *Neuropsychologia,* 1977, *15,* 751-756.

Metzler, N., & Jelinek, J. Writing disturbances in patients with right cerebral hemisphere lesions. In R. H. Brookshire (Ed.), *Clinical Aphasiology: Conference Proceedings.* Minneapolis: BRK Publishers, 1976.

McNeil, M. R., & Prescott, T. E. *Revised Token Test.* Baltimore: University Park Press, 1978.

Mills, L., & Rollman, G. Hemispheric asymmetry for auditory perception of temporal order. *Neuropsychologia,* 1980, *18,* 41-47.

Milner, B. Laterality effects in audition. In V. B. Mountcastle (Ed.) *Interhemispheric relations and cerebral dominance.* Baltimore: Johns Hopkins University Press, 1962.

Milner, B. Hemispheric specialiation: Scope and limits. In F. Schmitt & F. Worden (Eds.), *Neurosciences third study program.* Cambridge: MIT Press, 1974.

Morrow, L., Vrtunsk, P. B., Kim, Y., & Boller, F. Arousal responses to emotional stimuli and laterality of lesion. *Neuropsychologia,* 1981, *19,* 65-71.

Myers, P. S. Analysis of right hemisphere communication deficits: Implications for speech pathology. In R. H. Brookshire (Ed.), *Clinical Aphasiology: Conference Proceedings.* Minneapolis: BRK Publishers, 1978.

Myers, P. S. Profiles of communication deficits in patients with right cerebral hemisphere damage. In R. H. Brookshire (Ed.), *Clinical Aphasiology: Conference Proceedings.* Minneapolis: BRK Publishers, 1979.

Myers, P. S. Visual imagery in aphasia treatment: A new look. In R. H. Brookshire (Ed.), *Clinical Aphasiology: Conference Proceedings.* Minneapolis: BRK Publishers, 1980.

Myers, P. S. Right hemisphere communication disorders. In W. H. Perkins (Ed.), *Current therapy in communication disorders.* New York: Thieme-Stratton, in press.

Myers, P. S., & Linebaugh, C. W. The perception of contextually conveyed relationships by right brain damaged patients. Paper presented to the American Speech-Lauguage-Hearing Association Convention, Detroit, 1980.

Myers, P. S., & Linebaugh, C. W. Comprehension of idiomatic expressions by right-hemisphere-damaged adults. In R. H. Brookshire (Ed.), *Clinical Aphasiology: Conference Proceedings.* Minneapolis: BRK Publishers, 1981.

Newcombe, F., & Russell, W. R. Dissociated visual perceptual and spatial deficits in focal lesions of the right hemisphere. *Journal of Neurology, Neurosurgery, and Psychiatry,* 1969, *32,* 78-81.

Ornstein, R. *The psychology of human consciousness.* New York: Harcourt, Brace, Jovanovich, 1977.

Osgood, C. The cross cultural generality of visual-verbal synesthetic tendencies. *Behavioral Science,* 1960, *5,* 146-169.

Paivio, A. Mental imagery in associative learning and memory. *Psychological Review,* 1969, *76,* 241-263.

Paivio, A. *Imagery and verbal processes.* New York: Holt, Rinehart, & Winston, 1971.

Patterson, K., & Bradshaw, J. Differential hemispheric mediation of nonverbal visual stimuli. *Journal of Experimental Psychology*, 1975, *1*, 246-252.

Porch, B. *The Porch Index of Communicative Abilities*. Palo Alto: Consulting Psychologist Press, 1967.

Pylyshn, Z. What the mind's eye tells the mind's brain: A critique of mental imagery. *Psychological Bulletin*, 1973, *80*, 1-24.

Rapaczynski, W., & Ehrlichman, H. Opposite visual hemifield superiorities in face recognition as a function of cognitive style. *Neuropsychologia*, 1979, *17*, 645-652.

Ratcliff, G. Spatial thought, mental rotation, and the right cerebral hemisphere. *Neuropsychologia*, 1979, *17*, 49-53.

Riege, W., Metter, E. J., & Hanson, W. R. Verbal and nonverbal recognition memory in aphasic and non-aphasic stroke patients. *Brain and Language*, 1980, *10*, 60-70.

Rivers, D. L., & Love, R. J. Language performance on visual processing tasks in right hemisphere lesion cases. *Brain and Language*, 1980, *10*, 348-366.

Rizzolatti, C., Umilita, C., & Berlucchi, G. Opposite superiorities of the right and left cerebral hemispheres in a discriminative reaction time to physiognimical and alphabetical materials. *Brain*, 1971, *94*, 431-442.

Ross, E. D. The aprosodias. *Archives of Neurology*, 1981, *38*, 561-569.

Ross, E. D., and Mesulam, M. Dominant language functions of the right hemisphere? *Archives of Neurology*, 1979, *36*, 144-148.

Rowher, W. D. Images and pictures in children's learning: Research results and educational implications. *Psychological Bulletin*, 1970, *72*, 399-403.

Russo, M., & Vignolo, L. A. Visual figure-ground discrimination in patients with unilateral cerebral disease. *Cortex*, *1967*, *3*, 113-127.

Schlanger, B. B., Schlanger, P., & Gerstman, L. J. The perception of emotionally toned sentences by right-hemisphere damaged and aphasic subjects. *Brain and Language*, 1976, *3*, 396-403.

Schuell, H. *The Minnesota Test for Differential Diagnosis of Aphasia*. Minneapolis: University of Minnesota Press, 1957.

Semmes, J. Hemispheric specialization: A possible clue to mechanism. *Neuropsychologia*, 1968, *6*, 11-26.

Shapiro, B., Grossman, M., & Gardner, H. Selective musical processing deficits in brain damaged populations. *Neuropsychologia*, 1981, *19*, 161-168.

Sidtis, J. On the nature of the cortical function underlying right hemisphere auditory perception. *Neuropsychologia*, 1980, *18*, 321-330.

Sparks, R., Helm, N., & Albert, M. Aphasia rehabilitation resulting from melodic intonation therapy. *Cortex*, 1974, *10*, 303-316.

Sperry, R. W. Hemispheric disconnection and unity in conscious awareness. *American Psychologist*, 1968, *23*, 723-733.

Stachowiak, F. F., Huber, W., Poeck, K., & Kerschensteiner, M. Text comprehension in aphasia. *Brain and Language*, 1977, *4*, 177-195.

Stanton, K., Flowers, C., Kuhl, P., Miller, R., & Smith, C. Teaching compensation of left neglect through a language-oriented program. Paper presented to the American Speech-Language-Hearing Association Convention, Atlanta, 1979.

Stanton, K., Yorkston, K. M., Talley-Kenyon, V. T., & Beukelman, D. R. Language utilization in teaching reading to left neglect patients. In R. H. Brookshire (Ed.), *Clinical Aphasiology: Conference Proceedings*. Minneapolis: BRK Publishers, 1981.

Strauss, E., & Muscovitch, M., Perception of facial emotion. *Brain and Language*, 1981, *13*, 308-332.

Suberi, M., & McKeever, W. Differential right hemisphere memory for storage of emotional and non-emotional faces. *Neuropsychologia,* 1977, *15,* 757-768.

Tucker, D. M., Watson, R. T., & Heilman, K. M. Discrimination and evocation of affectively intoned speech in patients with right parietal disease. *Neurology,* 1977, *27,* 947-950.

Wapner, W., & Gardner, H. Profiles of symbol-reading skills in organic patients. *Brian and Language,* 1980, *12,* 303-312.

Wapner, W., Hamby, S., & Gardner, H. The role of the right hemisphere in the appreciation of complex linguistic material. *Brain and Language,* 1981, *14,* 15-33.

Warrington, E. K., & James, M. An experimental investigation of facial recognition in patients with unilateral cerebral lesions. *Cortex,* 1967, *3,* 317-326.

Watson, R. T., Heilman, K. M., Cauthen, J. C., & King, F. A. Neglect after cingulectomy. *Neurology,* 1973, *23,* 1003-1007.

Watson, R. T., Miller, B., & Heilman, K. Nonsensory neglect. *Annals of Neurology,* 1978, *3,* 505-508.

Watson, R. T., Miller, B., & Heilman, K. M. Evoked potentials in neglect. *Archives of Neurology,* 1977, *34,* 224-227.

Weber, R. J., & Bach, M. Visual and speech imagery. *British Journal of Psychology,* 1969, *60,* 199-202.

Weinstein, S. Deficits concomitant with aphasia or lesions of either cerebral hemisphere. *Cortex,* 1964, *1,* 151-169.

Weintraub, S., Mesulam, M., & Kramer, L. Disturbances in prosody: A right-hemisphere contribution to language. *Archives of Neurology,* 1981, *38,* 742-744.

West, J. Imaging and aphasia. In R. H. Brookshire (Ed.), *Clinical Aphasiology: Conference Proceedings.* Minneapolis: BRK Publishers, 1977.

West, J. Heightening the action imagery of materials used in aphasia treatment. In R. H. Brookshire (Ed.), *Clinical Aphasiology: Conference Proceedings.* Minneapolis: BRK Publishers, 1978.

Wilcox, M. J., Davis, G. A., & Leonard, L. B. Aphasic's comprehension of contextually conveyed meaning. *Brain and Language,* 1978, *6,* 362-377.

Winner, E., & Garnder, H. The comprehension of metaphor in brain-damaged patients. *Brain,* 1977, *100,* 719-727.

Yorkston, K. M., & Beukelman, D. R. An analysis of connected speech samples of aphasic and normal speakers. *Journal of Speech and Hearing Disorders,* 1980, *45,* 27-36.

Yorkston, K. M. Treatment of right hemisphere damaged patients: A panel presentation. A. Davis (Moderator), In R. H. Brookshire (Ed.), Clinical Aphasiology: Conference Proceedings. Minneapolis: BRK Publishers, 1981.

Zaidel, E. The elusive right hemisphere of the brain. *Engineering and Science,* 1978, Sept.-Oct., 10-32.

Zurif, E. Auditory lateralization: Prosodic and syntactic features. *Brain and Language,* 1974, *1,* 391-404.

Kathryn A. Bayles

Language and Dementia

Dementia

Dementia is a condition of chronic progressive deterioration of intellect, memory, and communicative function resulting from organic brain disease. In early dementia the behavioral manifestations may be subtle and apparent only to family members and close acquaintances. Eventually intellect, personality, and language become so impaired that the individual is unable to function socially or occupationally.

The term dementia denotes a constellation of behavioral abnormalities. Aretaeus of Cappadocia introduced the term in the second century B.C., to refer to a chronic degenerative mental disease associated with old age. Since then, dementia has been applied to a variety of disorders and often used synonymously with insanity. Emil Kraepelin (1919) redefined dementia in the late 1800s as a mental disorder characterized by memory disturbance and loss of the ability to reason. Kraepelin specified two types, senile and presenile dementia. The presenile form of the disease was described by Alois Alzheimer (1907), a neuropathologist who had observed the progressive deterioration of intellect, memory, and orientation in a 51-year-old woman. After her death, Alzheimer examined the brain and discovered cerebral atrophy and the presence of senile plaques and neurofibrillary tangles in the neocortex.

The disease Dr. Alzheimer described was thought to occur only in the presenium, prior to the age of 65, and a variety of other terms became

---

©College-Hill Press, Inc. All rights, including that of translation, reserved. No part of this publication may be reproduced without the written permission of the publisher.

popular for Alzheimer's disease when it occurred in the senium. The term "chronic brain syndrome" became popular after its use was recommended in the 1952 edition of the *Diagnostic and Statistical Manual on Mental Disorders* (DSM-I). In this edition, a distinction was introduced between the terms "acute" and "chronic" brain syndrome, and dementia became "chronic brain syndrome associated with senile brain disease." The terms "chronic" and "acute" proved confusing because their application involved a clinical judgment about disease onset and progress. Authors of the second edition of the *Diagnostic and Statistical Manual* (DSM-II) (1968), seeking to eliminate confusion, made the use of "acute" or "chronic" optional.

The Committee on Organic Mental Disorders of the American Psychiatry Association reviewed the definition of organic mental disorders preparatory to publishing *DSM-III* (1980). Additional revisions were made in the terminology applied to mental disorders. Dementia was recognized as being caused by several different diseases which were categorized as "primary degenerative" and "secondary degenerative." For the first time, senile, presenile, and circulatory dementias were classified together as "primary degenerative dementias" and senile brain disease was referred to as Alzheimer's disease (AD).

In addition to revising the terminology used to refer to degenerative brain disorders, the Committee on Organic Mental Disorders established a set of diagnostic criteria for differentiating dementia from other disorders. Some of the conditions *must* be present, while others *may* be present. Aphasia, described as a loss of language due to brain dysfunction, is a condition noted to be sometimes present. However, research of the last decade suggests that language impairment is present in all stages of dementia (Bayles, 1982; Irigaray, 1973; Obler & Albert, 1981a). In the early stages, cognitive changes are subtle and it is only with tests of much subtlety that language changes are also detected. Often these language changes are well concealed by patients in everyday interactions. To believe that language is not affected when intellect, memory, attention, and other higher cortical functions are deteriorating is not consistent with what is known about the relationship of thought to language.

Use of the term aphasia to describe language dysfunction associated with dementia is likely to be confusing to speech-language pathologists, because it denotes a loss in the ability to manipulate linguistic symbols as a result of focal brain damage, usually of sudden onset, as a result of cerebral vascular accident. Since none of these conditions apply to dementia, the term "aphasia" seems inappropriate for denoting the language deficits in such patients.

TABLE 7-1.
Types of Dementia. (Foley's taxonomy with modifications noted by *)

Remedial Nonvascular Causes
- Intoxications
- Infections
- Metabolic Disorders
- Nutritional Defects (Korsakoff's Syndrome)*
- Subdural Hematoma
- Benign Intracranial Tumors
- Occult Hydrocephalus (Normal Pressure Hydrocephalus [NPH])
- Sensory Deprivation
- Depression*

Irreversible Nonvascular Dementia with Movement Disorder
- Parkinson's Disease*
- Huntington's Chorea
- Creutzfeldt-Jacob Disease
- Progressive Supranuclear Palsy
- Progressive Subcortical Gliosis

Irreversible Nonvascular Dementia without Movement Disorder
- Alzheimer's Disease
- Pick's Disease
- Senile Brain Atrophy

Vascular Dementia
- Multiple Infarctions

Classification of Dementia-Producing Diseases

Although all dementia-producing diseases are associated with neural degeneration, they can be differentiated from each other in many respects. One classification system that identifies many of the differentiating characteristics is that of Foley's (1972), shown in Table 7-1. Foley distinguishes among the dementing illnesses on the bases of being reversible, associated with movement disorder, or vascular in origin.

Albert (1978) has proposed a classification system in which dementias are designated as cortical or subcortical. This classification appears to the author to be perplexing and premature because it implies that the brain damage causing dementia is solely cortical or subcortical, an implication that remains to be documented. For example, Albert classifies Parkinson's disease as a subcortical dementia, yet degenerative changes, similar to those found in Alzheimer's patients, occur in the neocortex of some Parkinson's disease patients. If intellectual and memory deterioration can be shown to occur in subcortical dementia without observable cortical changes, then Albert's distinction may be useful. While it is true that the majority of neurological changes in Parkinson's disease or Huntington's disease may be subcortical, the changes that result in dementia may not be subcortical.

Prevalence and Incidence of Dementia

One in every 100 persons 65 years or older suffers from severe dementia and 10 from mild dementia (Wang, 1981). In the absence of effective treatment, it has been estimated that the prevalence of dementia should double within the lifetime of our children and triple within the lifetime of our grandchildren (Katzman, 1981). Dementia-producing diseases primarily affect the 65-plus age group, the fastest growing segment of this country's population. There are currently 24.7 million Americans 65 years and older, and by the year 2000 the 65-plus population is expected to rise 32% to 32 million people, or 1 out of every 8 persons. That ratio will change to 1 of every 6 persons by the year 2020.

Because dementia patients are eventually incapable of self-care, many are placed in nursing homes. According to a report of the National Center of Health Statistics (1978), dementia afflicts 58% of the more than 1 million Americans in nursing homes, and is the most common syndrome among nursing home residents. The cost of caring for dementia patients represents 30% of the health care costs of the country (Frederickson, 1981), a figure that will increase with the imminent, dramatic growth of the elderly population.

Incidence

The incidence of dementia diseases, as well as their sex distribution, was studied by Malamud (1972), whose data are presented in Table 7-2.

TABLE 7-2
Distribution of Types of Degenerative Disorders among 1,225 Cases (Malamud, 1972).

	Age range	*# Cases*	*%*	*Male/female ratio*
Senile Brain Disease	65– 98	416	(34)	3:2
Alzheimer's Disease	40– 64	103	(8.4)	2:3
Pick's Disease	35– 72	35	(2.8)	1:1
Creutzfeldt-Jacob Disease	43– 86	32	(2.7)	2:1
Multi-infarct Dementia	42–100	356	(29)	2:1
Mixed: Senile Brain Disease and Multi-infarct Dementia	62– 94	283	(23)	4:3

Senile brain-disease patients comprised the largest category, accounting for 34%. However, Malamud distinguished between senile brain disease and Alzheimer's disease by age of onset. If they are grouped together as they are in many incidence reports, the incidence rate is 42%, only slightly lower than the 50% reported by Tomlinson (1977) in his study of 50 dementia patients. Multi-infarct dementia, a term introduced by Hachinski, Lassen, and Marshall (1974) for dementia resulting from frequent small vascular lesions, is the second most frequently occurring such disease. This finding is consistent with Tomlinson's (1977) report that multi-infarct disease occurs alone in 20% of the cases and with Alzheimer's disease in 18% of the cases.

Incidence figures for dementia do not include dementia patients with Parkinson's disease. Parkinson's disease affects approximately 100 individuals in every 100,000 (Pollock & Hornabrook, 1966) although incidence rises sharply with advancing age as shown in Table 7-3. Presently, in the United States, approximately 375,000 individuals have Parkinson's disease (Reisberg, 1981).

Although dementia is not an inevitable consequence of Parkinson's, it occurs in a significant percentage of cases, a fact that is becoming more widely recognized (Diamond, Markham, & Treciokas, 1976; Martin,

TABLE 7-3
Incidence Rates by Age for Parkinson's disease

Age	Number of affected individuals per 100,000
50–59	239
60–69	758
70–84	1,407

TABLE 7-4
Incidence of Dementia in Parkinson's disease

Year	Author	Percentage
1923	Lewy	77
1949	Mjönes	40
1951	Monroe	33
1966	Pollock & Hornabrook	20
1972	Loranger et al.	36.5 to 57.1
1979	Boller et al.	33
1979	Lieberman et al.	32
1982	Pirozzolo et al.	93

Loewenson, & Resch, 1973; Selby, 1968; Sweet, McDowell, & Feigenson, 1976). The percentage of Parkinson's disease patients who become demented is uncertain, but is probably between 30 and 39%, as can be seen in Table 7-4.

The explanation is still being sought for why some Parkinson's patients develop an associated dementia while others do not. It may be that Alzheimer's disease is co-occurring with Parkinson's disease in patients with dementia because Alzheimer's-like morphological changes have been found in many Parkinson's disease patients with dementia (Hakim & Mathieson, 1979; Selby, 1968). Several investigators suggest there may be two forms of the disease (Boller, Mitzutani, Roessmann, & Gambetti,

1979; Garron, Klawans, & Narin, 1972; Hirano & Zimmerman, 1962; Lieberman, Dziatolowski, Kupersmith, Serby, Goodgold, Korein, & Goldstein, 1979), a motor disorder without dementia in which degenerative changes are limited to subcortical structures, and a second form in which dementia is associated with motor dysfunction and cortical as well as subcortical changes.

Dementia is a certainty in Huntington's disease, a rare autosomal dominant genetic disorder characterized by abnormal involuntary movements, intellectual deterioration, and affective disorders. Four to seven individuals per 100,000 are stricken with Huntington's disease, and at least twice this number are at risk because it is a genetically transmitted disease. Prevalence estimates are scarce because the disease is rare and may often be misdiagnosed or concealed.

Characteristics of Major Dementia-Producing Illness

Alzheimer's Disease (AD): Senile Brain Disease (SBD)

Alzheimer's disease and senile brain disease are neuropathologically indistinguishable and differ only in age of onset. AD occurs in the presenium, and SBD after the age of 65. Because age of onset appears to be the only difference between AD and SBD, there has been an increasing tendency to consider them as a single disease entity. The 1980 edition of the Diagnostic and Statistical Manual eliminated the age of onset as a criterion for AD. AD was defined as a primary degenerative brain disorder which reduces life span and produces dementia.

Morphological changes. The classic neuropathological changes associated with AD are the formation of senile plaques (SP), neurofibrillary tangles (NFT), and granulovacuolar degeneration (GVD) in the neocortex, particularly the temporal lobe and hippocampus. Senile plaques, also called neuritic plaques, consist of an amyloid core surrounded by an outer ring of granular filamentous material (Corsellis, 1962) and are thought to interfere with the transmission of nerve impulses.

Neurofibrillary tangles, the most characteristic change of AD, typically consist of multitudes of twisted intraneuronal fibers, or pairs of helically wound filaments (Kidd, 1963). The fibers making up NFTs have a marked twist unlike normal neurofibers. The nucleus of cells with NFT is essentially normal, except for twisted tubules coursing through the cytoplasm of the cell body, displacing and replacing the organelles normally found in this location (Terry & Wisniewski, 1975). NFT occur throughout the cortical mantle, the hippocampal formation, and the amygdala, but seem to prefer the hippocampus, an area of brain associated with recent memory. When bilateral damage occurs to the hippocampus, recent memory is permanently impaired. The amygdala is a series of nuclei in the temporal lobe that are thought to affect emotion. Degenerative changes in the amygdala may cause the flat affect and passivity characteristic of many dementia patients.

Granulovacuolar degeneration, GVD, the third type of morphological change associated with AD, is a descriptive term for changes occurring inside the cell, namely the accumulation of fluid-filled vacuoles and granular debris. These intracytoplasmic granules are sensitive to silver staining and are seen in the hippocampus (Malamud, 1972).

Particularly intriguing to scientists is the finding that morphological changes characteristic of Alzheimer's disease occur in the brains of the healthy elderly, but to a lesser degree. Tomlinson and Henderson (1976) studied postmortem brain samples and found small numbers of senile plaques in the brains of 15% of people in the 5th decade, in 50% of the people in the 7th decade and 75% of people in the 9th decade. Small concentrations of NFT were found in 10 to 20% of healthy older people, while 40% of dementia patients had numerous, widely scattered tangles. Granulovacuolar degeneration was unusual in 70% of the normal elderly. Tomlinson and Henderson believed the differences between SP, NFT, and GVD in normal and demented were quantitative, not qualitative, and indicated that their presence in the "healthy elderly person" suggests that AD many be an exaggeration of normal aging. Demented individuals had 14 or more plaques per low power field of standard size, and a total volume of 50 ml or more of macroscopically evident softening.

Symptomatology. Memory impairment, mood changes, and personality disturbances are among the first symptoms of AD. Intellectual deterioration is insidious and inexorable. As the disease progresses, impairment in both recent and long-term memory becomes noticeable and the person becomes disoriented for time, place, and self. Eventually, there is global failure of all memory, as well as apathy and incontinence.

Cause(s). Recent research which documents a malfunction in the cholinergic system among Alzheimer's patients may provide a clue to its cause or causes. The cholinergic system is a group of neurons that transmit nerve impulses through acetylcholine. The enzymes CAT (choline acetyltransferase) and ACT (acetylcholinesterase) are necessary for the manufacture of acetylcholine, and the degree to which enzymatic activity is present in the cells reveals the ability of those cells to manufacture acetylcholine. Both CAT and ACT have been found to be reduced by 80% in AD patients (CAT: Davies & Mahoney, 1976; Perry, Perry, Blessed, & Tomlinson, 1977; Reisine, Yamamura, Bird, Spokes, & Enna, 1978; White, Hiley, Goodhardt, Carrasco, Keet, Williams, & Bowen, 1977; ACT: Perry, Perry, Blessed, & Tomlinson, 1978). The brain areas associated with CAT and ACT reduction are the hippocampus, septum, and temporal lobe, precisely those anatomic areas suffering the most extensive degenerative changes in Alzheimer's disease.

Because AD appears to selectively destroy acetylcholine producing neurons, researchers have theorized that raising body levels of acetylcholine might arrest the disease. Because the nervous system is incapable of synthesizing choline (Sparf, 1973; Yavin, 1976), there has been much interest in administering choline derivatives or lecithin, the body's natural source of choline. As yet, results of such treatments are quite nuclear.

Some researches are investigating the possibility that excessive accumulation of environmental toxins and trace metals, most notably aluminum, may cause AD. Crapper, Krishnan, and Quittkat (1976), reported increased levels of aluminum in the brain cells of AD patients. However, McDermott, Smith, Iqbal, and Wisniewski (1977) could not replicate this finding and reported elevated levels of aluminum in both AD patients and age-matched controls. They concluded that intracellular aluminum concentration, particularly in the hippocampus, increases with age. The data of Caster and Wang (1981) suggest that dietary aluminum is neither an essential nutrient nor a toxic element, and tends to accumulate in the membrane tangles in AD. Perl and Brody (1980) examined aluminum levels in hippocampal neurons of three AD patients with scanning electron microscopy and x-ray spectrometry, and found concentrations in the nuclear regions of neurons containing neurofibrillary tangles in both controls and AD patients. Normal-appearing neurons were free of aluminum. Excessive concentrations of aluminum are of concern because their presence is thought to disrupt intracellular protein synthesis (McDermott et al., 1977). As yet, it is unclear whether aluminum concentration may contribute to the neuropathological changes associated with AD or whether it merely increases in the neurons after they have degenerated.

Also under investigation is the possibility that AD results from a slow virus similar to those that result in Creutzfeldt-Jacob disease or Kuru, both of which also are accompanied by dementia. Kuru is a disease once prevalent among the cannibalistic Fore tribe of New Guinea, and is transmitted through ingestion of brain tissue from an affected individual. In 1965, Gajdusek and Gibbs found that when monkeys and chimps were innoculated with brain tissue extracts from Kuru or Creutzfeldt-Jacob disease, they developed degenerative brain disease. Recently, a factor taken from the brains of AD patients was injected into cell cultures of neurons from aborted human fetuses. Neurofilaments with the paired helical pattern typical of AD were produced (Crapper & De Boni, 1979).

Genetics of Alzheimer's Disease. A predisposition to AD may be genetically transmitted; individuals with a first-order relative have a four times greater chance of having the disease than people without such familial relationship (Larsson, Sjörgren, & Jacobson, 1963). This finding has led some researchers to suggest an autosomal dominant mode of inheritance. Others suggest a multifactorial mode (Slater & Cowie, 1970).

Alzheimer's disease is also associated with Down's syndrome (mongolism), a defect characterized by the presence of an extra chromosome, and, like Down's syndrome, may be the consequence of chromosomal abnormality (Reisberg, 1981). The morphological changes characteristic of Alzheimer's disease are found in individuals with Down's syndrome in numbers disproportionate to the normal population. Additionally, there is evidence of an increased incidence of Down's syndrome in families with a history of Alzheimer's disease (Heston & Mastri, 1977; Wisniewski, Howe, Williams, & Wisniewski, 1978).

Malamud (1972) examined the frequency of occurrence of dementia in 347 Down's syndrome cases and 813 cases representing other forms of mental retardation. Of the 347 cases with Down's syndrome, 40 patients (12%), ranging in age from 20 to 69 at the time of death, showed pathologic changes characteristic of senile brain disease, and 60% of these (7% of the total) had severe atrophy. This finding dramatically contrasted with the virtual absence of cortical atrophy among the 813 other retardates. There were no patients with Down's syndrome past the age of 40 in whom such changes were not found. Elam and Blumenthal (1970) suggested the high incidence of cortical atrophy in Down's syndrome cases represented a predisposition toward premature aging, and when associated with signs of delayed maturation, also typical of Down's syndrome, indicated a more rapid aging process. Ball and Nuttal (1980) studied the degree of neurofibrillary tangle formation, granulovacuolar degeneration, and nerve cell loss in serial sections of the hippocampal formation of the brains of five adults with Down's syndrome who were dying. They observed neurofibrillary tangle formation in hippocampal neurons to be more extensive than that occurring in normal elderly subjects. In only one of their subjects were morphological changes within normal limits. Granulovacuolar degeneration, however, fell within the normal range for the three youngest of the five patients, which led Ball and Nuttal to suspect granulovacuolar degeneration may be influenced as much by age as the presence of Down's syndrome. Neuronal density in the hippocampal cortex averaged 60% of that in the control population, and was of the same magnitude as that found in Alzheimer's disease patients. Ball and Nuttal thus hypothesized that a pathogenetic aging mechanism may be the key to understanding Alzheimer's disease.

Multi-infarct Dementia (MID)

Multi-infarct dementia is a term for vascular dementia caused by the accumulation of brain damage resulting from multiple small infarctions. In the majority of cases, one or more large areas of infarction exist and involve the middle and posterior cerebral arteries more often than the anterior. Like stroke, MID is most likely to occur between the ages of 40 and 60 years, and males are more likely to be affected than females. There is usually a history of hypertension or extracerebral vascular disease (Hachinski, et al., 1974), and individuals with MID often also have diabetes, hyperlipidemia, or arteriosclerotic heart disease. Unlike Alzheimer's disease, changes in mental status occur suddenly as a result of stroke and the course is fluctuating due to the occurrence of mild cerebral ischemic episodes. Intellectual functions gradually deteriorate and the exact nature of the person's cognitive and language deficits depends on the site, location, and extent of cerebral infarctions.

Morphological Changes. Diffuse subintimal hyperplasia, a build-up of cells in the inner wall of blood vessels, and multiple small infarctions are common throughout the carotid and vertebrobasilar systems. Often there is evidence of bilateral corticobulbar or corticospinal tract disease manifested as a gait disturbance, or pseudobulbar palsy (Scheinberg, 1978). Focal neurological signs, pathology associated with a specific brain area, appear when more than 50 grams of brain tissue have been destroyed. Destruction of more than 100 grams of tissue throughout the cerebral hemispheres uniformly results in dementia.

Pick's Disease

Pick's disease is a rare primary degenerative dementia usually occurring between the ages of 40 and 60. Its frequent occurrence within a family suggests a dominant autosomal mode of inheritance.

Pick's disease resembles Alzheimer's disease clinically, and many American neurologists do not differentiate them. The hippocampal formation is more preserved in Pick's disease, which may explain why memory is less impaired than in AD. Microscopically, nonspecific degeneration of the cortex particularly in the frontal and temporal lobes, is associated with silver sensitive inclusions called Pick bodies, as well as cell loss, and extensive gliosis (Malamud & Hirano, 1974).

Parkinson's Disease (PD)

There are two basic types of Parkinson's disease, idiopathic (accounting for 85% of the cases), and postencephalitic (accounting for 15%). The idiopathic, or major form, typically occurs in the late 50s (Pollock & Hornabrook, 1966) and has three principal symptoms: rigidity, rest tremor, and bradykinesia. Patients have flexed posture, a slow shuffling gait and are incoordinated. Dementia is often present (Boller et al., 1979) and is manifested as memory impairment, disorientation, impaired concept formation, and expressive-receptive language deficits.

Morphological Changes. Parkinson's disease results from a loss of cells in the substantia nigra, a subcortical structure in the basal ganglia responsible for the production of the neurotransmitter dopamine. The histopathology of the disease is somewhat controversial. Alzheimer-like changes are frequently found in the neurons of the substantia nigra in post-encephalitic PD patients (Wisniewski, Terry, & Hirano, 1970). Whether or not they are a consequence of PD or the result of the co-occurrence of AD and PD is unknown.

Huntington's Disease (HD)

Huntington's disease is a primary degenerative dementia inherited as a Mendelian single-dominant autosomal gene. Autosomal means that it strikes men and women equally, and dominant means that each child of an affected parent has a 50% chance of inheriting the disease. Symptoms usually appear between the ages of 35 and 45, but can occur later; 10% of the cases become apparent before the age of 20. The disease is chronic, progressive, and terminal. Although akinetic forms exist, choreoathetoid involuntary movements are typical and appear first as clumsiness, but eventually involve all body parts. Initial mental changes involve forgetfulness, irritability, depression, and withdrawal. During the disease course there are major reasoning, memory, and linguistic deficits (Fedio, Cox, Neophytides, Canal-Frederick, & Chase, 1979).

Morphological Changes. There is neuronal loss particularly in the striatum, and cerebral atrophy, particularly in the frontal lobes. The constant movements of HD patients are related to the loss of gamma aminobutyric acid and acetylcholine, brain chemicals which inhibit nerve action (Bird, 1980).

Korsakoff's Disease (KD)

In the late 1800s, S. S. Korsakoff, a Russian physician, described a syndrome of polyneuritis and psychological impairment that accompanied alcoholism. The syndrome became known as Korsakoff's psychosis, but, under the new classification system of the DSM-III, was termed Korsakoff's disease (KD). It is a secondary dementia developing after long-term alcohol abuse and vitamin B deficiency (Butters & Cermak, 1976). Vitamin B deficiency is thought to produce atrophy of diencephalic and limbic structures causing the classic symptom of KD amnesia for recent events. Other symptoms include disorientation to time and place, inattentiveness, and misperception.

The most-studied aspect of KD is memory deficit. Research suggests that Korsakoff's patients require more time than normals to process and form durable memories (Butters & Cermak, 1976). Affected individuals do not seem to employ the same memory-encoding strategies, and appear to rely more heavily on phonemic than semantic analysis. Verbal memory is more impaired than nonverbal. With proper diet and thiamine, KD patients may become more alert but memory problems persist.

Morphological Changes. Brain lesions occur in the thalamus (particularly the mammillary bodies which receive strong hippocampal input), hypothalamus, and the frontal and associative areas of the neocortex.

The aforementioned dementia-producing diseases are those most commonly seen by the speech-language pathologist. However, there are several other illnesses associated with dementia, such as progressive supranuclear palsy, progressive subcortical gliosis, Wilson's disease, and Creutzfeldt-Jacob disease.

Literature Review

Language impairment is present in all stages of dementia (Bayles, 1982; Obler & Albert, 1981). Impairment is subtle in the early stages, because cognition is only subtly affected. Speech articulation, or the mechanical production of words, usually is spared in dementing diseases not associated with movement disorders. The mechanics of language production are not reliant on higher-order cognitive processes, but the rules of language are, although our semantic, syntactic, phonologic, and pragmatic competencies are not uniformly affected in dementia. Research has demonstrated that semantic knowledge is more reliant on cognition than phonologic and syntactic knowledge (Bayles, 1982; Irigaray, 1973; Obler, 1977), and clinical observations suggest the same is true of pragmatics, our knowledge of how to use language in social interactions.

The bulk of our information about the effects of dementing illness on language has come from clinical observations of dementia patients, rather than controlled studies of disease effects. Of the studies completed, many have serious methodological limitations, most notably heterogeneous patient samples. Historically, dementia patients have been grouped together with little regard for etiology or severity, which makes interpretation of reported findings difficult.

Naming Research

The most widely studied dementia-associated language deficit is naming. Word finding difficulties and a reduction in functional vocabulary have been reported by Critchley, 1964; Ernst, Dalby, and Dalby, 1970; Stengel, 1964. As dementia worsens, naming errors increase (Bayles & Tomoeda, in press; Overman, 1979).

A popular explanation for the naming errors of dementia patients is impaired perception (Lawson & Barker, 1968; Rochford, 1971). Lawson and Barker compared the performance of 100 dementia patients to that of 40 normal elderly on a 24-item naming task. Dementia patients were found to have longer latencies, particularly for naming less common objects. When object function was demonstrated, naming was facilitated, a finding which motivated the authors to hypothesize that dementia patients are perceptually impaired. Like Lawson and Barker, Rochford (1971) concluded that dementia patients are perceptually deficient. He administered an eight-item naming test to 23 dementia patients, and classified their responses as correct, misrecognized, unclassifiable, or no response. Because the most frequent response was misrecognition, occurring 55% of the time, and because 35% of the responses were visually similar to the stimulus, Rochford concluded dementia patients may be "perceptually off course."

More recent research has failed to substantiate the perceptual impairment hypothesis and has motivated another explanation of the misnamings of dementia patients, that of erosion of referential boundaries in the mental lexicon (Bayles & Tomoeda, in press; Schwartz, Marin, & Saffran, 1979; Warrington, 1975; Wilson, Kaszniak, Fox, Garron, & Ratusnik, 1981). Schwartz, Marin, and Saffran described a woman with senile dementia,

WLP, who was able to name only one object on a 70-item naming test, but who could, nevertheless, demonstrate object recognition through intricate gestures. The authors asked WLP to select the name of stimulus items she could not name from the following five choices: two unrelated object names, a phonologically and orthographically similar name, the name of an item in the same semantic category, and the target name. At the time of initial testing, the patient selected the semantic distractor 85% of the time. Twenty-one months later, the semantic distractor was chosen only 61% of the time, leading the authors to suggest erosion of the associative network that exists between words. A specific example of such semantic erosion was WLP's gradual overextension of the word "dog." Initially "dog" was used to refer to "dogs," then "dogs and cats," and eventually was extended to "squirrels" and "rabbits."

Wilson et al. (1981), who studied the naming ability of 32 dementia patients and 32 age-matched controls, observed a phenomenon similar to that reported by Schwartz and associates. The majority of their subjects' naming errors were words semantically related to the stimulus items or perseverations of previous responses. Bayles and Tomoeda (in press) studied naming errors in four groups of dementia patients for whom dementia etiology and severity were specified, and found the most common response of moderately impaired dementia patients was the name of a semantically associated object (Alzheimer's disease 60%; Huntington's disease 67%; and Parkingson's disease 50%). Bayles and Tomoeda argued that linguistic impairment, rather than perceptual impairment, better accounts for the majority of misnamings of dementia patients. This argument is intuitively appealing because research has shown the semantic aspects of language are most vulnerable to dementia disease effects.

Semantic System More Impaired Than Syntactic and Phonologic

A number of researchers have reported the differential vulnerability of linguistic subsystems to dementia (Bayles & Boone, 1982; de Ajuriaguerra & Tissot, 1975; Irigaray, 1973; Schwartz et al., 1979; H. A. Whitaker, 1976). Irigaray studied the performance of 32 dementia patients on a variety of language tasks and discovered that their semantic and pragmatic subsystems were disturbed, while their morphosyntactic and phonologic subsystems were preserved. Haiganoosh Whitaker described an advanced AD patient who had been silent for years and was incapable of self-care, but who would echo sentences if eye contact was established. An intriguing aspect of her echolalia was her propensity to correct errors of syntax and phonology, but not semantics. Similarly, WLP, the patient of

Schwartz, Marin, and Saffran (1979) described earlier, could disambiguate spoken homophones (i.e., weak/week) with syntactic but not semantic cues. Bayles and Boone (1982) found the inability to perceive semantic errors in sentences to be the most discriminating of five language tasks for identifying senile brain-disease patients. Like Whitaker's patient, the seven severely demented subjects in the Bayles and Boone study frequently made spontaneous corrections of phonologically and syntactically anomalous sentences.

A variety of explanations have been offered for the vulnerabilty of semantic and pragmatic language subsystems in dementia. De Ajuriaguerra suggested that as dementia worsens, affected individuals regress to earlier stages of cognitive development, similar to those specified by Piaget (1923) in his description of the development of higher cognitive functions in children. Dementia patients become less able to perceive that which is illogical, are more likely to talk when performing an action, and become more egocentric.

Whitaker hypothesized the existence of a grammatical filter that operates independently of cognition, and is capable of analyzing syntactic and phonologic features of linguistic stimuli. According to Bayles (1982), intellectually deteriorated individuals retain their ability to analyze phonologic and syntactic features of linguistic stimuli, because the rules of phonology and syntax are finite, learned early, and quite well practiced. Conversely, meaning analysis relies on higher mental operations, because the number of sentences any language can generate is infinite and contextual effects must be analyzed to extract a speaker's communicative intention.

Language Profiles of Etiologically Different Dementia Patients

As we become more knowledgeable about the neurology of dementing illness, it is of clinical and theoretical value to explore the possibility that dementias of different etiologies may be associated with different language performance profiles reflecting their unique patterns of neural degeneration. Halpern, Darley, and Brown (1973) compared patients with aphasia, apraxia, confused language, and general intellectual impairment on ten language tasks. Because the groups were not controlled for severity, intergroup comparisons could not be made. Instead, individual language functions were compared against the group mean, and when a language function retained a fairly constant relation to the mean in all groups, that relation was designated as insignificant for intergroup differentiation. Patients who suffered general intellectual impairment (presumably from dementing disease) were distinguished by impaired reading comprehension, with verbal fluency, writing to dictation, and relevance relatively unaffected. These results are surprising and difficult to interpret because the cause and severity of general intellectual impairment were not specified, and other researchers have reported fluency and relevancy to be impaired in dementia patients (Albert, 1981, Bayles, 1982; Borkowski, Benton, & Spreen, 1967; Irigaray, 1973).

In his previously described dichotomy of dementia, Albert (1978) also argued that, while both cortical and subcortical dementias share some language impairments, each also has a unique profile. The shared deficits of these patients include lack of initiative to speak, perseveration, and naming impairment. Characteristics associated with subcortical dementia patients are slow rate, low volume, disturbances in rhythm, pitch, articulation, decreased output in verbal fluency tests, agraphia, and impaired ability to make verbal abstractions.

Cortical dementia patients, of which AD is the main type, exhibit logorrhea, empty speech, verbal paraphasias, impaired naming, impaired comprehension, preserved repetition, and topic digression. Cortical dementia patients are described as having all the language problems of subcortical patients plus agnosias, apraxias, and aphasias (Obler & Albert, 1981), and were likened to Wernicke's and anomic aphasics. Albert's profiles appear to be based on extensive clinical observation rather than formal studies in which the language behaviors of etiologically different dementia patients controlled for severity were compared.

Mildworf (1978) compared the performance of patients with Huntington's disease, Parkinson's disease, and normals on several language tasks. No significant intergroup differences were found on the confrontation and generative naming tasks for PD and normals. HD patients were, however, significantly more impaired on these tasks. Reading, writing, and oral naming of spelled words were all significantly harder for HD than for PD patients or normal subjects. HD subjects wrote telegrammatic versions of the Cookie Theft picture (Goodglass & Kaplan, 1972) while Parkinsonians used more words than normals to describe the same number of themes. Mildworf was not explicit about whether the PD patients had dementia. Therefore random selection of nondemented PD patients could have accounted for the superior performance of PD patients on some tasks.

Bayles et al. (in progress) compared the performance of patients with AD, HD, PD, and normal elderly on neuropsychological tests and language tasks. The dementia patients, whose average age, IQ, and years of education are presented in Table 7-5, were given a severity rating based on neurological evidence of brain damage and neurobehavioral criteria.

TABLE 7-5
Age, IQ, Years of Education of Dementia Subjects and Normals

Group	Total N	$\overline{X}$ Age	$\overline{X}$ Yrs. Ed.	$\overline{X}$ IQ
AD	22	72	12	113
PD	14	69	14	118
HD	8	45	13	116
Normals	33	70	13	115

Alzheimer's patients were the most impaired of the dementia groups, differing significantly from normals on all 21 variables except the Digit Span subtest of the *Wechsler Adult Intelligence Scale* Wechsler (1955). PD patients ranked second, performing significantly more poorly than normals on 17 tasks. No significant differences were found between PD patients and normals on judgment of syntactic and semantic errors, digit span, and naming. HD patients were least impaired of the disordered groups, a finding which should be interpreted cautiously both because of the small number in the group of subjects and because the HD patients were substantially younger than subjects in other groups. They differed from normals on 7 of the 21 variables: verbal description, *Peabody Picture Vocabulary Test* (PPVT), lexical disambiguation, surface structure disambiguation, selecting speaker intention from context, judging syntax errors, and naming.

When compared to neuropsychological tests, language tasks were found to be of equal or greater sensitivity for detecting dementia. The tasks on which all groups differed from normals were sentence disambiguation (lexical, surface structure, deep structure), verbal description, PPVT, and a pragmatic task of selecting speaker intent given utterance context.

Differences among dementia groups were fewer than those between dementia groups and normals. It must be mentioned that there is great intersubject variability between dementia patients. However, when scores are averaged across a group, AD and PD patients differed significantly only on the confrontation-naming task, although most test scores of AD patients were generally slightly lower. AD patients performed significantly more poorly than HD patients on three tasks: Block Design, *Mental Status Questionnaire*, and naming. HD patients were significantly inferior to PD patients on two sections of the pragmatics test, the ability to select the most appropriate utterance for a particular context from among four choices and the ability to judge the literality of utterances.

Whereas Obler and Albert found naming to be impaired in both subcortical and cortical dementias, a significant naming impairment was not observed in either moderate HD or PD patients (Bayles & Tomoeda, in press). If HD and PD patients are categorized as subcortical dementia patients and AD patients are categorized as cortical, then our data show the groups' common characteristics to include impaired receptive vocabulary, difficulty comprehending the meanings of ambiguous sentences, impaired ability to describe common objects verbally, and impaired ability to identify a speaker's intention in producing a particular utterance.

Language Disturbance During the Progression of Dementing Disease

Longitudinal studies of etiologically specific dementia patients have not been done. Consequently, we cannot specify an order in which language behaviors deteriorate. Nevertheless, numerous researchers have provided descriptions of language impairment at different stages of dementing illness, which enabled us to summarize their common observations (Bayles, 1982; de Ajuriaguerra & Tissot, 1975; Irigaray, 1973; Obler, 1977; H. Whitaker, 1976).

Early Stages

In the early or "forgetful" stage of dementia (Reisberg, 1981), when patients are disoriented for time but generally not for place or person, both short- and long-term memory deficits exist. These deficits are likely to be dismissed as benign forgetfulness. Thus, language impairment is likely to be imperceptible in casual conversation. Affected individuals know that something deleterious is happening to them and may attempt to conceal their shortcomings by avoiding challenging situations, dismissing a task as trivial, or refusing to perform it. In conversation, they are apt to digress from the topic and ramble at length, a behavior that Irigaray (1973) and Obler (1977) called disinhibition. Although the content of such discourse may be somewhat inappropriate due to word boundary erosion, dementia patients adhere to the rules of syntax and phonology. The combined effects of slight cognitive deterioration and semantic-pragmatic impairment may result in an inability to detect humor and sarcasm. As the ability to produce and comprehend language deteriorates, there is greater reliance on clichés.

EXAMPLES

1. Mild

Example 1: Patient was describing a common object.

Examiner: Tell me everything you can about this (a gray button).

Patient: This is a button. This button is grayish in color, and, uh, it is useful. And, uh, I'd say it's grayish in color. (Pause) It's flat. I've already said it's gray. I think. I can't think of anything else.

Example 2: Patient was told an anecdote and had difficulty recognizing contextual effects on speaker intent.

Anecdote: A mother and her son arrive home from shopping with a car full of groceries. The young son rushes from the car empty-handed. The mother says to him: "What's the matter, have you broken your arms?"

Examiner: Why did the mother say, "What's the matter, have you broken your arms?"

Patient: Well, I suppose she's putting over a point that he would understand that he should be careful where he puts his hands and arms.

Middle Stages of Dementia

By now an affected individual is disoriented for time and place, but orientation to self is maintained. Short and long-term memory problems are obvious, and the person is no longer capable of managing personal finances, a job, or his or her medication. Language impairment is apparent, and discourse is vague, empty, and often irrelevant. Terms like "thing" and "this one" are substituted for substantive nouns. Utterances are phonologically wellformed, but syntactic terms affecting meaning are likely to be misused, whereas purely syntactic forms still present little difficulty. Semantic paraphasias are more common than phonemic, and there is an obvious loss of the more specific and abstract semantic features of words. Individuals are no longer able to generate verbal sequences of meaningfully related ideas, and become increasingly apathetic towards other individuals and their environment. Language becomes egocentric, and there is less adherence to the conversational maxims that govern normal conversations. Affected individuals neither ask questions of their conversational partners nor comment on their utterances. Verbal perseverations are frequent, particularly ideational repetition, the repetition of an idea after another idea has been expressed. Self-correction of linguistic errors is rare. The language problems apparent in oral discourse are mirrored in what is written. Just as the mechanics of speech may be spared, so may be the mechanics of reading and writing.

EXAMPLES

2. Moderate

Example 1: Patient was describing a common object.

Examiner: Tell me everything you can about this (a gray button)

Patient: Oh, that's a needle. But...buttonhole scissors. And they go ahead the put buttons or they put, that's how they put buttons on your coat with it. I guess.

Example 2: Patient was asked to explain what it means to describe and guarantee.

Examiner: What does it mean to describe?

Patient: Well, like you're a buttoning your blouse would be an example.

Examiner: What does it mean to guarantee?

Patient: Guarantee you're gonna get it. I guess we're gonna have company or something. That would be a guarantee, wouldn't it?

Late Stages of Dementia

In the late stages of dementing illness, an individual is disoriented for time, place, and person, and frequently does not recognize family members. No longer can the person care for himself, and assistance with dressing, washing, feeding, and toileting is needed. Many severe dementia patients wander aimlessly and require placement in a protective environment. Life may seem to become a continuously fading dream, as one is unable to form new, lasting memories. Persons may be mute, echolalic, palilalic, use only jargon, or produce bizarre nonsensical utterances. Symptom variations probably reflect differences in the distribution of neural lesions. Pragmatic competencies of language may be so devastated that eye contact must be established before these dementia patients recognize that they are being spoken to. Syntax and phonology are grossly disrupted, particularly among jargon and palilalic patients.

EXAMPLES

3. Severe

Example 1: Conversation with a severe dementia patient.

   Examiner: Where did you get these flowers?

   Patient: Just a little bit, this place is always smoky.

   Examiner: Are these flowers yours?

   Patient: It's supposed to be Jesus.

Example 2: Conversation with a severe dementia patient.

   Examiner: Where are we now?

   Patient: Just like, like a n-normal person. And guy, guys, guys, girls in the class. They all pay attention, pay attention. You don't pay attention. Don't say, don't say, don't say...

Example 3: Severe dementia patient was asked to describe a marble.

   Examiner: Tell me about this (marble).

   Patient: Well, that's pretty darn good.

   Examiner: It is. What can you tell me about it?

   Patient: Well, he was standing there looking you know, so I. It's not mine. I didn't have it.

Diagnosing Dementia

Language-speech evaluations have not been conducted routinely as part of the examination of dementia patients. Only recently has there been evidence of language impairment in all stages of dementia (Bayles, 1982; Obler, 1977), a finding that may be important in making differential diagnoses and patient management decisions.

Unfortunately a battery of language tests for evaluating dementia patients with different etiologies does not exist. Further, speech-language pathologists do not have normative data on the performance of dementia patients on individual language tasks. Clinicians must plan evaluations based on literature reports about the nature of such patients' intellectual and linguistic deterioration. Bayles and Boone (1982) studied the efficacy of certain language tasks for diagnosing dementia, and recommended evaluating receptive and expressive skills in patients' phonologic, syntactic, semantic, and pragmatic domains. They used a discriminant-function analysis to analyze the performance of AD, PD, HD, and MID patients on the following tests: For neuropsychological evaluation, Block Design, Digit span, and Similarities subtests of the *Wechsler Adult Intelligence Scale* (Wechsler, 1955), the Nonsense Syllable Learning Task (Alexander, 1973) and the *Mental Status Questionnaire* (MSQ) (Goldfarb & Antin, 1975); for language evaluation, Naming Task, Lexical, Surface and Deep Structure Disambiguation Task, Judgment and Correction of Phonologic, Syntactic, and Semantic Errors, *Peabody Picture Vocabulary Test*, Pragmatics Task (Five parts: P1, P2, P3, P4A, P4B), Verbal Description Task, and Story-retelling Task. Table 7-6 lists the results of the discriminant function analysis, in order of most to least discriminative tests. The discriminant-function equation was found to classify subjects with 75% accuracy. Reliability and validity data are being amassed on these measures and, while they show promise for differentiating among dementia patients and normals, they are unstandardized.

Particularly in its early stages, the diagnosis of a dementia-producing disease frequently requires neurological, physical, and psychological examinations. Of the major dementing illnesses, AD is the most difficult to diagnose and usually becomes diagnosis by exclusion. A thorough case history is needed to identify the associated behavioral and personality changes characteristic of the diagnosis. In addition to the case history, the physician may rely on information from CT Scan, pneumoencephalography, regional cerebral blood flow, and electroencephalography.

CT Scan

The CT scan has become an important tool in the diagnosis of dementia. CT is an acronym for computerized axial tomography, a technique in which a narrow x-ray beam is passed through a succession of axial slices

TABLE 7-6
Measures Included in the Discriminant Function Equation (F ratio significant beyond .01 level).

Measure	Wilk's Lambda	Equivalent r
P3: Choosing best utterance for a particular context	.41	18.2
Block Design (WAIS)	.27	11.8
P2: Selection of speaker intent	.17	10.1
Verbal Description	.12	9.2
Naming	.09	7.8
Peabody Picture Vocabulary Test	.08	6.9
Similarities (WAIS)	.06	6.3
Mental Status Questionnaire	.05	5.8
P4A: Judging literality of utterance	.047	5.3
SCSJ: Ability to make syntactic judgments	.04	4.9
Lexical Disambiguation	.04	4.6
Digit Span (WAIS)	.03	4.3

Measures not included in the Discriminant Function Equation

- P1: Defining illocutionary speech acts
- P4B: Explaining speaker intent
- SCPJ: Ability to judge phonologic errors
- SCPC: Ability to correct phonologic errors
- SCSC: Ability to correct syntactic errors
- SCSEJ: Ability to judge semantic errors
- SCSEC: Ability to correct semantic errors
- Nonsense Syllable Learning Task
- Story Retelling
- Surface Structure Disambiguation
- Deep Structure Disambiguation

of the cranium (Pear, 1977). The resulting image varies with the density of the substance visualized. A CT scan may not distinguish dementia, because it is not uncommon to see dementia in patients showing no evidence of cortical atrophy on the scan; nor is it unusual to see prominent atrophy without clinical manifestations of dementia. Early attempts to correlate intellectual deterioration with brain atrophy were disappointing (Fox, Kaszniak, & Huckman, 1979; Roberts & Laird, 1976), but recent correlational studies using new generation CT scanners have been more encouraging (deLeon, Ferris, George, Reisberg, Kricheff, & Gershon, 1980).

Pneumoencephalography

Before the development of the CT technique, pneumoencephalography was commonly used. In this procedure, air is injected into the ventricles enabling physicians to look at ventricular enlargment.

Regional Cerebral Blood Flow

Another promising diagnostic procedure is regional cerebral blood flow measurement, rCBF. Patients inhale an inert radiolabeled gas, usually xenon 133. Its dispersion is then measured by skull sensors which detect the precise location of the radioactive gas. Information from the skull detectors is sent to a computer which provides a display of the brain regions to which blood is flowing.

In dementia, the parameters of rCBF have shown a flow decrease when there is intellectual degeneration (Freyhan, Woodford, & Kety, 1951; Hagberg & Ingvar, 1976) and the areas of diminished flow correspond to areas in which brain decay is most pronounced in dementia patients at autopsy (Ingvar, Brun, Hagberg, & Gustafson, 1978). Gustafson, Hagberg, and Ingvar (1978) studied flow patterns in presenile dementia patients during speech and found that verbal ability fails only when there is a marked general flow reduction in the dominant hemisphere. Further, a relation was found between the type of language-speech defect and the distribution of rCBF abnormalities in the dominant hemisphere. Receptive language disturbances were associated with marked flow reduction in postcentral regions, particularly in the temporoparietal area, whereas expressive language disturbances were associated with marked frontal and anterior temporal flow reductions. Depending on its ultimate availability, regional cerebral blood flow measurement might be valuable for differentiating between depression and AD, because the general and regional CBF are routinely normal in depressive states (Silfverskiold, Gustafson, Johanson, & Risberg, 1979).

Electroencephalography

Since Berger's report in 1931 of a pathological electroencephalogram (EEG) in an AD patient, there have been many EEG studies of dementia patients. The most commonly reported EEG pattern in AD is a diminution of the alpha rhythm (8-12 Hz in normals) into theta (5-7 Hz) and, eventually, delta ranges (4 or less Hz) (Obrist & Henry, 1958; Short & Wilson, 1971). Slowing of patients' alpha rhythm has been significantly correlated with the number of senile plaques (Deisenhammer & Jellinger, 1974), degree of cognitive deterioration (Mundy-Castle, Hurst, Beerstecker, & Prinsloo, 1954), and vocabulary impairment (Johannesson, Hagberg, Gustafson, & Ingvar, 1979).

Although EEG records provide insufficient evidence for specifying dementia etiology, they are suggestive. For example, diffuse slowing is seen in multi-infarct disease (Muller & Schwartz, 1978), while in Pick's disease, EEG's are often normal (Johannesson et al., 1977). In Huntington's disease a low voltage EEG is not uncommon (Scott, Healthfield, Toone, & Margerison, 1972), and in the advanced stages of Creutzfeldt-Jacob's disease, EEG's are characterized by bilateral rhythmic polyphasic complexes (Burger, Rowan, & Goldensohn, 1972).

Distinguishing the Effects of Normal Aging

In normal aging, changes in the brain and body result in sensory impairments as well as in memory, intelligence, and speed of responding. Familiarity with normal, age-related changes is a prerequisite for evaluating the behavior of mildly demented elderly patients. What follows is a brief review. A more comprehensive description of language in normal aging is provided by Davis's chapter in this volume.

In addition to the relatively well-known changes in the visual and auditory systems, there are age-related changes in the brain. Brain weight and volume decrease with age (Dekaban & Sadowsky, 1978; Pearl, 1922), the ventricles enlarge (Barron, Jacobs, & Kinkel, 1976), and the fissures widen and deepen (Wright, Spink, & Andrew, 1974). Microscopic histological studies of the cortex show the formation of senile plaques, neurofibrillary tangles, and sites of granulovacuolar degeneration (Blessed, Tomlinson, & Roth, 1968).

Age primarily affects long-term memory that requires the synthesis of new information (Craik, 1977). Senescents appear to employ less effective strategies for organizing new information (Craik & Masani, 1967; Mandler, 1967). Short-term memory store, typically 7 ± 2 items (Miller,

1956), is modestly reduced, usually by one item (Botwinick & Storandt, 1974; Freidman, 1974).

Intellectual functions most susceptible to age are those related to physiological abilities such as speed printing, perceptual speed, associative memory, and figural and inductive reasoning (Horn, 1972). Intellectual functions likely to be maintained are those dependent on culturally transmitted information and skills, such as verbal comprehension and general information (Horn, 1972).

Reaction time slows with age (Welford, 1958), and individuals become more cautious in responding (Botwinick, 1971), making many older people reluctant to guess on confusing test items.

Language and Aging

Language skills appear to be more resistant to age effects than some other areas of cognitive functioning. Botwinick (1973) called the maintenance of verbal functions and the decline in performance on adult intelligence tests the "classic aging pattern." This is not to say there are no age effects on languge skills. Comprehension appears to be disturbed in many senescents as a result of loss of hearing acuity (Corso, 1977), the ability to perceive and discriminate speech (Bergman, 1971; Feldman & Roger, 1967; Glorig, 1977), and reduced attention span (Rabbitt, 1965).

Studies of expressive language skills showed discourse patterns of the elderly to be different from younger subjects, but not necessarily inferior. Obler, Mildworf, and Albert (1977) analyzed the written discourse of elderly subjects who wrote descriptions of the Cookie Theft Picture of the Boston Diagnostic Aphasia Examination (Goodglass & Kaplan, 1972). Elderly subjects used more elaborate syntax, more embedded constructions, and more words, but did not express more themes. If fluency is considered, the elderly tend to use more filler words and interjections, and evidence more incomplete phrases (Yairi & Clifton, 1972). This finding may be a consequence of the more cautious demeanor of the elderly, rather than of linguistic impairment (Botwinick, 1971).

Management of Dementia Patients

The first step in patient management should be consultation with the patient's physician to learn the etiology and severity of the dementing illness. When the physician is unsure about the diagnosis, a follow-up medical, psychological, and language-speech evaluation should be rescheduled within

6 to 8 months. In most cases of dementing illness, language functions will have worsened in this period.

The care of an individual with a dementing disease can be an overwhelming experience for an individual or family. In addition to the personal sorrow of watching intellect and personality deteriorate in a loved one, there are usually burgeoning expenses and care-taking responsibilities. Spouses typically become depressed over the loss of their marital partner. As the dementia worsens, the dementia patient requires more and more personal care and eventually needs continuous supervision. It is important to meet with the family members and advise them of what to expect, and discuss how they can cope with the changes they observe in the affected family member. The following list is a modified version of a list of management strategies published in *Family Handbook: A Guide for the Families of Persons with Declining Intellectual Functions, Alzheimer's Disease, and Other Dementias* (Mace & Rabins, 1980).

DO:

Establish a routine

Make the routine simple

Forecast deviations from the routine

Minimize distractions

Keep household objects in the same place

Provide indirect orientation to place and time

Display pictures of family members

Have an identification bracelet made for the affected individual

Dispense the patient's medication

Expect the patient to deny the problem

Expect the patient to blame others for his or her problems

Expect the behavior of the affected individual to worsen with fatigue

Avoid arguing with the dementia patient

Expect to lose your temper

Try not to solve disagreements with the affected individual, but change the subject

Expect a change in the patient's condition when there is a major change in his or her lifestyle

Use more concrete and familiar terms when talking to the patient

Avoid sarcasm

Avoid long complex explanations and anecdotes
Arrange to have frequent relief from care-taking responsibilities
Expect to feel a sense of loss

Therapy

Comparative studies of therapy techniques with dementia patients have not been done. The most widely promoted technique has been "Reality Orientation," in which patients are repeatedly oriented. Reality therapy does not result in lasting change, nor does any other known technique. The outlook for finding a behavioral therapy technique that will arrest the progressive deterioration of language function is poor. More promising may be discovery of techniques by which we can better communicate with persons in the various stages of dementing illness. HD patients for example may live for 15 to 25 years after the onset of the disease. If we know the course of language dissolution and the best way of modifying our verbal input to patients, we may greatly improve their comprehension and ability to function.

More appropriate than therapy for the dementia patient may be therapy for the family. Reisberg and colleagues (1981) have established a therapy program for relatives of dementia patients at New York University. It is reported to be well received, particularly by men. Reisberg (1981) suggested that the reason more men seek counseling is that they have greater difficulty assuming a supportive and care-taking role than women. The frustration they feel in coping with a dementing spouse is manifested most often as anger. Children of dementia patients also have participated in the program. They are primarily concerned over the fate of their sick parent and the possibility they themselves might be affected in their later years. The clinician-counselor should be prepared to answer questions about the cause, treatments, disease course, and current research on dementing illnesses as well as questions about the diagnostic process and its accuracy for a particular individual. If counseling is not available for family members, help can be sought from the following national organizations, which provide information and supportive services:

Alzheimer's disease

Alzheimer's Disease and Related Disorders Association
292 Madison Avenue
8th Floor
New York, NY 10017
(212) 683-2868

Huntington's disease
National Huntington's Disease Association
128A East 74th Street
New York, NY 10021
(212) 744-0302

Parkinson's disease
Parkinson's Disease Foundation
William Black Medical Research Building
Columbia Presbyterian Medical Center
640 West 168th Street
New York, NY 10032
(212) 923-4700

National Parkinson's Foundation
1501 N. W. 9th Avenue
Miami, FL 33136
(305) 324-0156

United Parkinson's Foundation
220 S. State Street
Chicago, IL 60604
(312) 922-9734

Acknowledgment

The author wishes to express her gratitude to Karen K. Eagans and Cheryl K. Tomoeda for their assistance in the preparation of this chapter, and to Richard F. Curlee, PhD, and Daniel R. Boone, PhD, of the University of Arizona for their critical comments in reviewing the manuscript. This work was supported by grant number 5R21 AGO2154-02 CMS from the National Institute of Aging.

References

Albert, M. L. Subcortical dementia. In R. Katzman, R. D. Terry, & K. L. Bick (Eds.), *Alzheimer's disease: Senile dementia and related disorders* (*Aging*, Vol. 7), 173-180. New York: Raven Press, 1978.

Albert, M. L. Changes in language with aging. *Seminars in Neurology*, 1981, *1*, 43-46.

Alexander, D. A. Some tests of intelligence and learning for elderly psychiatric patients: A validation study. *Brit. J. Soc. Clin. Psych.*, 1973, *12*, 188-193.

Alzheimer, A. *Allg. Z. Psychiat.*, 1907, *64*, 146-8.

Aretaeus. In F. Adams (Ed.), *The extant works of Aretaeus, the cappadocian*, 1861, 103.

Ball, M. J., & Nuttall, K. Neurofibrillary tangles, granulovacuolar degeneration and neuron loss in Down's syndrome: Quantitative comparison with Alzheimer dementia. *Annals of Neurology*, 1980, *7*, 462-465.
Barron, S. A., Jacobs, L., & Kinkel, W. R. Changes in the size of normal lateral ventricles during aging determined by computerized tomography. *Neurology*, 1976, *26*, 1011-1013.
Bayles, K. A. Language function in senile dementia. *Brain and Language*, 1982, *16*, 265-280.
Bayles, K. A., & Boone, D. R. The potential of language tasks for identifying senile dementia. *Journal of Speech and Hearing Disorders*, 1982,*47*, 210-217.
Bayles, K. A., & Tomoeda, C. K. Confrontation naming impairment in dementia, *Brain and Language*, 1983, *19*, 98-114.
Berger, H. Uber das Elektrenkephalogramm des Menschen. Dritte Mitteilung. *Archiv Fur Psychiatrie und Nervenkrankheiten*, (Berlin) 1931, *94*, 16-60.
Bergman, M. Hearing and aging. *Audiology*, 1971, *10*, 164-171.
Bird, E. D. Chemical pathology of Huntington's disease. *Annual Review of Pharmacology and Toxicology*, 1980, *20*, 533-551.
Blessed, G., Tomlinson, B. E., & Roth, M. The association between quantitative measures of dementia and of senile change in the cerebral grey matter of elderly subjects. *British Journal of Psychiatry*, 1968, *114*, 797-811.
Boller, F., Mitzutani, T., Roessmann, V., & Gambetti, P. Parkinson disease, dementia and Alzheimer disease: Clinicopathological correlations. *Annals of Neurology*, 1980, *7*, 329-335.
Borkowski, J. G., Benton, A. L., & Spreen, O. Word fluency and brain damage. *Neuropsychologia*, 1967, *5*, 135-140.
Botwinick, J. Sensory-set factors in age difference in reaction time. *Journal of Genetic Psychology*, 1971, *119*, 241-249.
Botwinick, J. *Aging and behavior*. New York: Springer Publishing, 1973.
Botwinick, J., & Storandt, M. *Memory, related function and age*. Springfield, IL: Charles C. Thomas, 1974.
Burger, L. J., Rowan, A. J., & Goldensohn, E. S. Creutzfeldt-Jacob disease, an electroencephalographic study. *Archives of Neurology*, 1972, *26*, 428-433.
Butters, N., & Cermak, L. Neuropsychological studies of alcoholic Korsakoff patients. In G. Goldstein & C. Neuringer (Eds.), *Empirical studies of alcoholism*. Cambridge: Ballinger Publishing, 1976.
Caster, W. O., & Wang, M. Dietary aluminum and Alzheimer's disease—a review. *Science of the Total Environment*, 1981, *17*, 31-36.
Corsellis, J. A. N. *Mental illness and the aging brain*. London: Oxford University Press, 1962.
Corso, J. Presbycusis, hearing aids and aging. *Audiology*, 1977, *16*, 146-163.
Craik, F. I. M. Age differences in human memory. In J. E. Birren & K. W. Schaie (Eds.), *Handbook of the psychology of aging*. New York: Van Nostrand Reinhold, 1977, 384-420.
Craik, F. I. M., & Masani, P. A. Age differences in the temporal integration of language. *British Journal of Psychology*, 1967, *58*, 291-299.
Crapper, D. R., & DeBoni U. Etiological factors in dementia. International Society for Neurochemistry Satellite Meeting on Aging of the Brain and Dementia, Florence, Italy, Aug. 27-29, 1979, *Abstracts*.
Crapper, D. R., Krishnan, S. S., & Quittkat, S. Aluminum, neurofibrillary degeneration and Alzheimer's disease. *Brain*, 1976, *99*, 67-80.
Critchley, M. The neurology of psychotic speech. *British Journal of Psychiatry*, 1964, *110*, 353-364.
Davies, P., & Mahoney, A. J. F. Selective loss of cholinergic neurons in Alzheimer's disease. *Lancet*, 1976, *2*, 1403.

de Ajuriaguerra, J., & Tissot, R. Some aspects of language in various forms of senile dementia. In E. H. Lenneberg & E. Lenneberg (Eds.), *Foundations of Language Development* (Vol. 1). New York: Academic Press, 1975, 323-339.

de Leon, M. J., Ferris, S. H., George, A. E., Reisberg, B., Kricheff, I. I., & Gershon, S. Computed tomography evaluations of brain behavior relationships in senile dementia of the Alzheimer's type. *Neurobiology of Aging, Experimental and Clinical Research*, 1980, *1*, 69-79.

Deisenhammer, E., & Jellinger, K. EEG in senile dementia. *Electroencephalography and Clinical Neurophysiology*, 1974, *36*, 91.

Dekaban, A. S., & Sadowsky, D. Changes in brain weights during the span of human life: Relation of brain weights to body heights and body weights. *Annals of Neurology*, 1978, *4*, 345-356.

Diagnostic & statistical manual of mental disorders. American Psychiatric Association, Washington, DC, 1952.

Diagnostic & statistical manual of mental disorders. American Psychiatric Association. 2nd Edition, 1968.

Diagnostic & statistical manual of mental disorders. American Psychiatric Association, 3rd Edition, 1980.

Diamond, S. G., Markham, C. H., & Treciokas, L. J. Long term experience with L-dopa: Efficacy, progression and mortality. In W. Birkmayer & O. Hornykeiwicz, (Eds.), *Advances in parkinsonism*, Basel: Roche, 1976, 444-455.

Elam, L. H., & Blumenthal, H. T. Aging in the mentally retarded. In H. T. Blumenthal (Ed.), *Interdisciplinary topics in gerontology*. New York: S. Karger, 1970, 7, 87.

Ernst, B., Dalby, M. A., & Dalby, A. Aphasic disturbances in presenile dementia. *Acta Neurologica Scandinavica Supplementum* 1970, *43*, 99-100.

Fedio, P., Cox, C. S., Neophytides, A., Canal-Frederick, G., & Chase, T. N. Neuropsychological profile of Huntington's disease: Patients and those at risk. In T. N. Chase, N. S. Wexler, & A. Barbeau (Eds.), *Advances in neurology, Vol. 23, Huntington's disease*. New York: Raven Press, 1979, 239-255.

Feldman, R. M., & Roger, S. N. Relations among hearing, reaction time and age. *Journal of Speech and Hearing Research*, 1967, *10*, 479-495.

Foley, J. M. Differential diagnosis of the organic mental disorders in elderly patients. In C. M. Gaitz (Ed.) *Aging and the brain*, New York: Plenum Press, 1972, 153-161.

Fox, J. H., Kaszniak, A. W., & Huckman, M. Computerized tomographic scanning not very helpful in dementia—nor in craniopharyngiomia. *New England Journal of Medicine*, 1979, 300.

Frederickson, D. S. Introductory statement: A view from National Institutes of Health. In N. E. Miller & G. D. Cohen (Eds.) *Clinical aspects of Alzheimer's disease and senile dementia (Aging*, Vol. 15). New York: Raven Press, 1981.

Freidman, H. Interrelation of two types of immediate memory in the aged. *Journal of Psychology*, 1974, *87*, 177-181.

Freyhan, F. A., Woodford, R. B., & Kety, S. S. Cerebral blood flow and metabolism in psychosis of senility. *Journal of Nervous and Mental Disease*, 1951, *113*, 449-456.

Gajdusek, D. C., & Gibbs, J. C., Jr. Slow, latent, and temperate virus infections of the central nervous system. *Research Publications-Association for Research in Nervous and Mental Disease*, 1968, *44*, 254-280.

Garron, D. C., Klawans, H. L., & Narin, F. Intellectual functioning of persons with idiopathic Parkinsonism. *Journal of Nervous and Mental Disease*, 1972, *154*, 445-452.

Glorig, A. Auditory processing and age. In H. Shore & M. Ernst (Eds.), *Sensory processes and aging*, 39-60. Denton, TX: University Center for Community Services, 1977.

Goldfarb, A. I., & Antin, S. Unpublished data. In R. Goldman & M. Rockstein (Eds.), *The physiology and pathology of human aging*. New York: Academic Press, 1975.

Goodglass, H., & Kaplan, E. *The assessment of aphasia and related disorders*. Philadelphia: Lea & Febiger, 1972.

Gustafson, L., Hagberg, B., & Ingvar, D. H. Speech disturbance in presenile dementia related to local blood flow abnormalities in the brain. *Brain and Language*, 1978, *5*, 103-118.

Hachinski, V. C., Lassen, N. A., & Marshall, J. Multi-infarct dementia: A cause of mental deterioration in the elderly. *Lancet*, 1974, *2*, 207-210.

Hagberg, B., & Ingvar, D. H. Cognitive reduction in presenile dementia related to regional abnormalities of the cerebral blood flow. *British Journal of Psychiatry*, 1976, *128*, 209-222.

Hakim, A. M., & Mathieson, G. Dementia in Parkinson's disease: A neuropathologic study. *Neurology*, 1979, *29*, 1209-1214.

Halpern, H., Darley, F. L., & Brown, J. R. Differential language and neurological characteristics in cerebral involvement. *Journal of Speech and Hearing Disorders*, 1973, *38*, 162-173.

Heston, L. L. & Mastri, A. R. The genetics of Alzheimer's disease. *Archives of General Psychiatry*, 1977, *34*, 976-981.

Hirano, A., & Zimmerman, H. M. Alzheimer's neurofibrillary changes. *Archives of Neurology*, 1962, *7*, 227-242.

Horn, J. L. Intelligence: Why it grows, why it declines. In J. M. Hunt (Ed.), *Human intelligence*, 53-74. New Brunswick, NJ: Transaction Books, 1972.

Ingvar, D. H., Brun, A., Hagberg, B., & Gustafson, L. Regional cerebral blood flow in the dominant hemisphere in confirmed cases of Alzheimer's disease, Pick's disease, and multi-infarct dementia: Relationship to clinical symptomatology and neuropathological findings. In R. Katzman, R. D. Terry, & K. L. Bick (Eds.), *Alzheimer's disease: Senile dementia and related disorders*, (*Aging*, Vol. 7). New York: Raven Press, 1978.

Irigaray. L. *Le language des dements*. The Hague: Mouton, 1973.

Johannesson, G., Brun, A., Gustafson, L., & Ingvar, D. H. EEG in presenile dementia related to cerebral blood flow and autopsy findings.*Acta Neurologica Scandinavica*, 1977, *56*, 89-103.

Johannesson, G., Hagberg, B., Gustafson, L., & Ingvar, D. H. EEG and cognitive impairment in presenile dementia. *Acta Neurologica Scandinavica*, 1979, *59*, 225-240.

Katzman, R. Early detection of senile dementia. *Hospital Practice*, June, 1981, 61-76.

Kidd, M. Paired helical filaments in electron microscopy in Alzheimer's disease. *Journal of Neuropathology and Experimental Neurology*, 1963, *22*, 629-642.

Kraepelin, E. *Dementia praecox and paraphrenia*. Krieger: Huntington, NY, 1919.

Larsson, T., Sjörgren, T., & Jacobson, G. Senile dementia. *Acta Psychiatrica Scandinavica Supplementum*, 1963, *167*, 39.

Lawson, J. S., & Barker, M. G. The assessment of nominal dysphasia in dementia: The use of reaction time measures. *British Journal of Medical Psychology*, 1968, *41*, 411-414.

Lewy, F. H. *Monographs of Neurological Psychiatry*, 1923, *34*, 32.

Lieberman, A., Dziatolowski, M., Kupersmith, M., Serby, M., Goodgold, A., Korein, J., & Goldstein, M. Dementia in Parkinson disease. *Annals of Neurology*, 1979, *6*, 355-359.

Loranger, A. W., Goodell, H., & McDowell, F. Intellectual impairment in Parkinson's syndrome. *Brain*, 1972, *95*, 402-412.

Mace, L., & Rabins, P. V. *Family handbook: A guide for the families of persons with declining intellectual functions, Alzheimer's disease and other dementias*. Baltimore: Johns Hopkins University, 1980.

Malamud, N. Neuropathology of organic brain syndromes associated with aging. In C. M. Gaitz (Ed.), *Aging and the brain*. New York: Plenum Press, 1972, 63-87.

Malamud, N., & Hirano, A. *Atlas of neuropathology.* Berkeley: University of California Press, 1974.

Mandler, G. Organization and Memory. In K. W. Spence & J. T. Spence (Eds.), *The psychology of learning and motivation: Advances in research and theory* (Vol. 1), 327-372. New York: Academic Press, 1967.

Martin, W. E., Loewenson, R. B., & Resch, J. A. Parkinson's disease: Clinical analysis of 100 patients. *Neurology,* 1973, *23,* 783-790.

McDermott, J. R., Smith, A. J., Iqbal, K., & Wisniewski, H. M. Aluminum and Alzheimer's disease. *Lancet,* 1977, *2,* 710-711.

Mildworf, B. Cognitive function in elderly patients. Unpublished master's thesis, Hebrew University, 1978.

Miller, G. A. The magical number seven, plus or minus two: Some limits on our capacity for processing information. *Psychological Review,* 1956, *63,* 81-97.

Mjönes, H. *Acta Psychiatrica Neurologica, Supplement 54,* 1949.

Monroe, R. T. *Diseases in old age.* Cambridge, MA: Harvard University Press, 1951.

Muller, H. F., & Schwartz, G. Electroencephalograms and autopsy findings in geropsychiatry. *Journal of Gerontology,* 1978, *33,* 504-513.

Mundy-Castel, A. C., Hurst, L. A., Beerstecker, D. M., & Prinsloo, T. The electroencophalogram in the senile psychoses. *Electroencephalography and Clinical Neurophysiology,* 1954, *6,* 245-252.

National Center of Health Statistics, survey conducted 1973-74, reported 1978.

Obler, L. K. Language and brain dysfunction in dementia. In S. Segalowitz (Ed.), *Language functions and brain organization.* New York: Academic Press, 1977.

Obler, L. K., & Albert, M. L. Language in the elderly aphasic and the dementing patient. In M. T. Sarno (Ed.), *Acquired aphasia.* New York: Academic Press, 1981, 385-398. (a)

Obler, L. K., & Albert, M. L. Language and aging: A neurobehavioral analysis. In D. S. Beasley & G. A. Davis (Eds.), *Aging communication processes and disorders,* New York: Grune & Stratton, Inc., 1981, 107-121. (b)

Obler, L. K., Mildworf, B., & Albert, M. L. Writing style in the elderly. Montreal: *Academy of Aphasia Abstracts,* 1977.

Obrist, W. D., & Henry, C. E. Electroencephalographic findings in aged psychiatric patients. *Journal of Nervous and Mental Disorders,* 1958, *126,* 254-267.

Overman, C. A. Naming performance in geriatric patients with chronic brain syndrome. Paper presented at the Annual Convention of the American Speech-Language-Hearing Association, Atlanta, 1979.

Pear, B. L. The radiographic morphology of cerebral atrophy. In W. L. Smith & M. Kinsbourne (Eds.), *Aging and dementia.* New York: Spectrum Publications, 1977, 57-76.

Pearl, R. *The Biology of death.* Philadelphia: J. B. Lippincott, 1922.

Perl, D. P., & Brody, A. R. Alzheimer's disease: X-ray spectometric evidence of aluminum accumulation in neurofibrillary tangle-bearing neurons. *Science,* 1980, *208,* 297-299.

Perry, E. K., Perry, R. H., Blessed, G., & Tomlinson, B. E. Necropsy evidence of central cholinergic deficits in senile dementia. *Lancet,* 1977, *1,* 189.

Perry, E. K., Perry, R. H., Blessed, G., & Tomlinson, B. E. Changes in brain cholinesterases in senile dementia of the Alzheimer type. *Neuropathology and Applied Neurobiology,* 1978, *4,* 273-277.

Piaget, J. *Le language et la pensée chez l'enfant.* Neuchâtel: De la Chaux & Niestlé, 1923.

Pirozzolo, F. J., Hansch, E. C., Mortimer, J. A., Webster, D. D., & Kuskowski, M. A. Dementia in Parkinson disease: A Neuropsychological analysis. *Brain and Cognition,* 1982, *1,* 71-83.

Pollock, M., & Hornabrook, R. W. The prevalence, natural history and dementia of Parkinson's disease. *Brain,* 1966, *89,* 429-448.

Rabbitt, P. An age decrement in the ability to ignore irrelevant information. *Journal of Gerontology*, 1965, *20*, 233-238.

Reisberg, B. *Brain failure*. New York: The Free Press, 1981.

Reisine, T. D., Yamamura, H. I., Bird, E. D., Spokes, E., & Enna, S. J. Pre- and postsynaptic neurochemical alterations in Alzheimer's disease. *Brain Research*, 1978, *159*, 477-480.

Roberts, M. A., & Laird, F. I. Computerized tomography and intellectual impairment in the elderly. *Journal of Neurology, Neurosurgery and Psychiatry*, 1976, *39*, 986-989.

Rochford, G. A study of naming errors in dysphasic and demented patients. *Neuropsychologia*, 1971, *9*, 437-445.

Scheinberg, P. Multi-infarct dementia. In R. Katzman, R. D. Terry, & K. L. Bick (Eds.), *Alzheimer's disease: Senile dementia and related disorders* (Aging, Vol. 7). New York: Raven Press, 1978.

Schwartz, M. F., Marin, O. S. M., & Saffran, E. M. Dissociations of language function in dementia: A case study. *Brain and Language*, 1979, *7*, 277-306.

Scott, D. F., Healthfield, K. G. W., Toone, B., & Margerison, J. H. EEG in Huntington's chorea: A clinical and neuropathological study. *Journal of Neurology, Neurosurgery and Psychiatry*, 1972, *35*, 97-102.

Selby, G. Parkinson's disease. In P. J. Vinken & G. W. Bruyn (Eds.), *Handbook of clinical neurology*. Amsterdam: North Holland, 1968, *6*, 173-211.

Short, M. J., & Wilson, W. P. The electroencephalogram in dementia. In C.E.Wells (Ed.), *Dementia*. Philadelphia: F. A. Davis, 1971, 81-89.

Silfverskiold, P., Gustafson, L., Johanson, M., & Risberg, J. Regional cerebral blood flow related to the effect of electroconvulsive therapy in depression. In Ballus (Ed.), *Proceedings from the Second World Congress of Biological Psychiatry*. Amsterdam: Elsevier/North Holland Biomedical Press, 1979.

Slater, E., & Cowie, V. Senescence, senile and presenile dementias. In *Genetics of mental disorders*. London: Oxford University Press, 1970.

Sparf, B. On the turnover of acetylcholine in the brain. *Acta Physiologica Scandinavica Supplement*, 1973, *397*, 1-47.

Stengel, E. Speech disorders and mental disorders. In A. De Reuch & M. O'Connor (Eds.), *Symposium on disorders of language*. Boston: Little Brown and Co., 1964.

Sweet, R. D., McDowell, H., & Feigenson, J. S. Mental symptoms in Parkinson's disease during treatment with levodopa. *Neurology*, 1976, *26*, 305-310.

Terry, R. D., & Wisniewski, H. M. Structural and chemical changes in the aged human brain. In S. Gershon & A. Raskin (Eds.), *Aging: Genesis and treatment of psychologic disorders in the elderly* (Vol. 2). New York: Raven Press, 1975, 127-142.

Tomlinson, B. E. Morphological changes in dementia in old age. In W. L. Smith & M. Kinsbourne (Eds.), *Aging and dementia*. New York: Spectrum Publications, 1977. 25-56.

Tomlinson, B. E., & Henderson, G. Some quantitative cerebral findings in normal and demented old people. In R. D. Terry & S. Gershon (Eds.), *Neurobiology of aging*. New York: Raven Press, 1976, 183-204.

Wang, H. S. Neuropsychiatric procedures for the assessment of Alzheimer's disease, senile dementia and related disorders. In N. E. Miller & G. D. Cohen (Eds.), *Clinical aspects of Alzheimer's disease and senile dementia*, (Aging, Vol. 15). New York: Raven Press, 1981.

Warrington, E. K. The selective impairment of semantic memory. *Quarterly Journal of Experimental Psychology*, 1975, *27*, 635-657.

Wechsler, D. *Manual for the Wechsler Adult Intelligence Scale*. New York: Psychological Corporation, 1955.

Welford, A. T. *Aging and human skill*. London: Oxford University Press, 1958.

Whitaker, H. A. A case of isolation of the language function. In H. Whitaker & H. A. Whitaker (Eds.), *Studies in neurolinguistics*. (2). New York: Academic Press, 1976.

White, P., Hiley, C. R., Goodhardt, M. J., Carrasco, L. H., Keet, J. P., Williams, I. E. I., & Bowen, D. M. Neocortical cholinergic neurons in elderly people. *Lancet*, 1977, *1*, 668.

Wilson, R. S., Kaszniak, A. W., Fox, J. H., Garron, D. C., & Ratusnik, D. L.Language deterioration in dementia. Paper presented at the 9th Annual Meeting of the International Neuropsychological Society, Atlanta, 1981.

Wisniewski, H. M., Terry, R. D., & Hirano A. Neurofibrillary pathology. *Journal of Neuropathology and Experimental Neurology*, 1970, *29*, 163-176.

Wisniewski, K., Howe, J., Williams, G. D., & Wisniewski, H. M. Precocious aging and dementia in patients with Down's syndrome. *Biological Psychiatry*, 1978, *18*, 619-627.

Wright, E. A., Spink, J. M., & Andrew, W. *Brain structure and aging*. New York: M.S.S. Information, 1974.

Yairi, E., & Clifton, N. Dysfluent speech behavior of preschool children, high school seniors and geriatric persons. *Journal of Speech and Hearing Research*, 1972, *15*, 714-719.

Yavin, E. Regulation of phospholoid metabolism in differentiating cells from rat brain cerebral hemispheres in culture. *Journal of Biological Chemistry*, 1976, *251*, 1392-1397.

Chris Hagen

Language Disorders in Head Trauma

Post-closed-head-injury (CHI) dysfunction presents the speech-language pathologist with a unique and complex diagnostic, prognostic, and treatment challenge. The CHI patient demonstrates a breakdown in communication abilities that is in certain respects similar to, but in many ways quite different from, those language disturbances caused by vascular, penetrating, or space-occupying lesions. While these patients manifest impaired receptive and expressive abilities, they do not seem to be "aphasic" in the same way that a stroke patient is "aphasic." The uniqueness of this population is not only evident in our daily clinical endeavors with them, but also can be seen in the studies that have been conducted with this population.

Language Dysfunction

Early studies (Arseni, Constantinovici, & Iliesca, 1970; Caveness, 1969; Fahy, Irving, & Millac, 1967; Hooper, 1969; Lewin, 1966, Russell, 1932) reported that head-injured patients experienced an initial period of complete dissolution of language abilities, but then gradually and spontaneously recapitulated the ontogeny of language, and eventually attained "normal speech." The most frequent behavioral residuals reported were cognitive problems of impaired concentration and short-term

©College-Hill Press, Inc. All rights, including that of translation, reserved. No part of this publication may be reproduced without the written permission of the publisher.

memory. However, these studies were directed toward the broader issues of charting and identifying the natural course of general recovery from head trauma. Language dysfunction was not a specific area of focus. As a consequence, the evaluation of patients' abilities in this area was quite general and cursory. Heilman, Safron, and Geschwind (1971) also present evidence of specific and isolated post CHI language impairments; they classified their subjects as having anomic disturbances or as having Wernicke's aphasia. Levin, Grossman, Sarwar, and Meyers (1981) found half of their language-impaired subjects to have specific linguistic deficits and half to have generalized receptive and expressive impairments.

The results of several studies suggest that CHI causes multiple language disturbances. Thomsen's (1976) subjects shifted from global to sensory aphasia and eventually stabilized as "amnestic aphasics." Although these subjects demonstrated anomic errors as a predominant feature, the majority of the subjects also had impaired auditory and reading comprehension, verbal paraphasia, and agraphia. This same pattern of deficits has also been reported in other studies. Sarno (1980) found her subjects to have either aphasia, "subclinical" aphasia, or "subclinical" aphasia with dysarthria. For aphasic subjects, Sarno further categorized 39% as fluent aphasics, 38% as nonfluent aphasics, 11% as anomic, and 11% as global aphasics. All groups, those with aphasia, subclinical aphasia, and subclinical aphasia with dysarthria, exhibited a wide range of language impairments. Of significance is the finding that, when compared with the test responses of a normal population, even those with the mildest impairments (subclinical aphasia with and without dysarthria) had significant impairments. Although subjects in the Levin, Grossman, and Kelly study (1976) had predominantly anomic errors and word-finding difficulties, they, too, exhibited a wide range of impairment.

In addition to the types of specific language impairments, other investigators find "confused language" to be a common characteristic of CHI. In general, confused language can be described as receptive/expressive language that may be intact phonologically, semantically, and syntactically, yet is lacking in meaning because the behavioral responses are irrelevant, confabulatory, circumlocutory, or tangential in relation to a given topic, and lacking a logicosequential relationship between thoughts.

Levin, Grossman, Rose, and Teasdale's (1979) subjects had specific aphasic language disorders, as well as conversational language that was frequently fragmented, tangential, and "often drifted to irrelevant topics." Thomsen (1975) found that half of his subjects had symptoms of aphasia and impaired language organization. Groher (1977) found that "confused language" was the primary residual symptom 4 months post onset. All of Groher's subjects initially had anomia as well as other language deficits.

At the end of 4 months, the anomic symptomatology had remitted, but test scores still indicated reduced expressive and receptive language abilities. Many subjects carried on conversations in which their "thought content was confused, seldom relevant to the discussion, and inappropriate in length." Groher concluded that the major post-CHI deficit is the discrepancy between the seemingly normal ability to communicate and impaired organizational and retention skills. Halpern, Darley, and Brown (1973) also found confused language to be characteristic of CHI patients. They investigated the language characteristics of patients with various neurologic etiologies, including head trauma. They measured the subjects' "relevance of responses" as well as more typical language skills. While all patients in the confused-language group manifested some degree of impairment in all areas measured, it was the category of "relevance" that clearly differentiated subjects with head trauma from the other etiologic categories.

Not only is there variability within and between CHI patients, but the literature is not unanimous with respect to the nature and temporal course of post-CHI-language dysfunction. On the basis of the literature, one could respond in at least four different ways to the question: What type of language disorder follows CHI? It could be said that such individuals regain "normal" linguistic abilities. Some may hold that specific and isolated language impairments occur across patients with no single type of disorder common to the population as a whole. Others might contend that such patients are characterized by the presence of multiple language impairments with anomia being a feature common to all. Finally, it might be said that CHI results in either specific or multiple language disorders and a coexisting presence of confused language.

To a certain extent the variability and findings are a reflection of the fact that complete homogeneity does not exist within any of the neurologic etiology categories. However, the variability may also be related, in part, to such factors as the lack of an agreed-upon taxonomy for language disorders, the use of language assessment instruments that do not evaluate the more complex levels of language utilization, or the lack of common agreement as to what constitutes a language disorder. All of these factors influence the manner in which data, either clinical or research, are analyzed and interpreted. For example, it is entirely possible that the separate findings of anomia, word-finding problems, auditory and reading comprehension deficits, and paraphasic responses are all symptoms of an underlying, more common, linguistic dysfunction, rather than five discrete disorders. The majority of language-assessment instruments focus on presence and degrees of absence of specific language abilities. As such, they yield considerable data about language power, but little about process and quality.

In the case of the CHI patient, the critical data are often found in organization of the linguistic data base, rather than in the degree to which the data base is impaired. A CHI patient will often appear to have minimal to no language impairment on the basis of available test instruments, yet manifest significant functional communication difficulties in real-life situations.

The definition of what constitutes a language disorder also heavily influences data interpretation. If one is oriented toward the more classical categorical disturbances such as aphasia and apraxia, Wernicke's and Broca's, or fluent and nonfluent aphasia, then it is entirely possible that patients with confused language, but without these symptoms, would not be considered to have a language disorder. Yet, in my experience, language disorganization is a more frequent cause of impaired ability to communicate than is the presence of a categorical linguistic deficit. For example, when asked to describe what was absurd or wrong about a picture of a man standing in the rain holding a closed umbrella, one patient stated, "First off, he's wearing slippers out in the rain and then, no I guess that's it, ya, he should wear his jacket, he's got his coat off and umbrella off and he's standing in the rain." When asked to describe what was absurd about a picture showing a bride and groom coming out of a barber shop to an awaiting car, with rice being thrown over their heads, another patient stated, "The guy should have gotten his hair cut before he picked up the bride for the wedding. Anyway, that's not the kind of costume to wear into a barber shop." While both patients scored quite well on a frequently used test battery, and while they did not manifest frank symptoms of what is often considered to be aphasia, neither could use language as an effective tool in communication situations above the level of meeting basic needs. Thus, while not aphasic or apraxic, they were nonetheless language-impaired.

The great variability of findings is not solely a reflection of the heterogeneity found within our profession's approach to language disorders. To a considerable extent, it represents the uniqueness and reality of this clinical population. In a sense, variability is their commonality. As such, it is as important to understand the source of variation as it is to identify the areas of similarity. At this time, the most observable sources appear to arise from the cognitive sequelae, as well as the neurological dynamics and pathological consequences of CHI.

Cognitive Dysfunction

Cognitive impairments have been found to be a major residual of CHI. Initially the most frequently reported problems were inability to sustain concentration and impaired memory (Brock, 1960; Hooper, 1969; Jacobsen, 1963; Lewin, 1966; Russell, 1932; Walker, 1969). The primary memory deficits reported were retrograde and anterograde amnesia (Brock, 1960; Lewin, 1966; Russell & Smith, 1961). As early as 1932, Russell (1932) suggested that the memory impairment might be a factor underlying the language dysfunction. The amnesic types of memory loss are not the only memory disturbances caused by CHI. Such patients also experience long-term deficits in immediate and recent memory as well (Brooks, 1972, 1976; Brooks, Aughton, Bond, Jones, & Rizvi, 1980; Jacobsen, 1963; Levin et al., 1979; Schilder, 1934; Smith, 1974). CHI has also been found to produce other cognitive impairments. The Levin et al. (1979) finding that subjects were inefficient in filtering extraneous material suggests possible selective-attention problems. Miller (1970) interpreted his findings of slower reaction time in relation to task complexity as reflecting reduced speed of information processing and decision making. Several investigators (Cronholm, 1972; Miller & Stern, 1965; Thomsen, 1975) have found abstract thought to be impaired. The findings of Schilder (1934), Mandleberg (1976); Mandleberg and Brooks (1975); Dye, Milby and Saxon (1979); Hallgrim and Cleeland (1972) suggest that CHI subjects have particular difficulty with the integration and synthesis of elemental parts of a whole perception. Perhaps these attention impairments of memory, analysis, and synthesis are related to Levin, Grossman, Rose and Teasdale, (1979) finding that their more severe CHI subjects had conceptual disorganization and unusual thought content.

In general, then, the literature indicates that the CHI patient incurs impairments in concentration, attention, memory, nonverbal problem solving, part/whole analysis and synthesis, conceptual organization, abstract thought, and speed of processing. Because these cognitive abilities are inextricably involved in language formulation and processing, it would seem reasonable to assume that post-CHI-language dysfunction is heavily influenced, and in some instances created, by cognitive dysfunction. Consequently, it is conceivable that some of the language variability found within and between CHI patients arises from a dynamic and reciprocal interaction between linguistic and nonlinguistic cognitive dysfunction. It has been my clinical observation that many of the previously noted specific language-disorder symptoms, such as anomia, paraphasia, and impaired auditory comprehension fluctuate considerably in relation to cognitive factors. These fluctuations appear to occur either in relation to the congitive demands inherent in a given linguistic task (test or real-life interactions) or to the intrinsic status of a patient's cognitive functions at any point in time, regardless of task demands. Both of these factors are influenced by the type, nature, and severity of cognitive dysfunction. Depending upon these cognitive factors, a previously observed specific language impairment may become worse, spread, and contaminate more functional language abilities. On the other hand, patients who do not have specific language impairments but do have confused language often demonstrate specific language impairments when their cognitive abilities are challenged.

Neurological Dysfunction

The very nature and dynamics of CHI is another source of the variability of language dysfunction found within this population. CHI is a term used to indicate those cases in which the primary source of brain injury is one of blunt trauma to the skull. There may or may not be a concurrent fracture of the skull and/or discontinuity of neural substance. The use of this term, then, excludes brain injury that is secondary to penetrating head wounds, cerebral vascular insults, and space-occupying lesions.

The force of a blow to the skull is distributed to all parts of the brain. Thus, all parts of the brain suffer to a greater or lesser degree (Brain & Walton, 1969). At the moment of impact, the brain accelerates, rotates, compresses, and expands within the skull. The dynamics of these motions produce pressure waves within the brain substance (Brain & Walton, 1969; Field, 1970). All of these effects function to damage cerebral tissue through the dynamics of compression, tension, and shearing. (Brain & Walton, 1969; Greenfield & Russell, 1963; Tomlinson, 1964; Walker, 1969) Compression forces tissue together; tension pulls it apart; and shearing, which produces contusions and lacerations, develops at the points where the brain impinges upon bony or ligamentous ridges within the cranial vault. Cerebral edema, which produces increased intracranial pressure, occurs shortly after this mechanical displacement and disruption of the brain substance (Meyer & Denny-Brown, 1955). In view of the magnitude and multiplicity of these negative forces, Russell's, (1932) and Adams and Sidman's (1968) descriptions of the effects of CHI as being a "molecular commotion" would appear quite appropriate. The very molecular structure of the brain is disrupted, disorganized, bruised, and/or lacerated. These gross neuropathological effects of CHI have been found to produce permanent microscopic alterations of both white and gray matter. Brain and Walton (1969) report widely scattered punctate hemorrhages throughout the brain associated with CHI. Severe localized demyelination was found by Greenfield (1938), and others (Stritch, 1956; Tomlinson, 1964) have reported wide-spread white-matter degeneration. Nerve cell damage after CHI has been reported both by Courville and Amyes (1952) and Horowitz and Rizzoli (1966). Other permanent neurological impairments result from the contusions, lacerations, and hemorrhages (Brain & Walton, 1969; Courville, 1942) that occur when the brain substance rotates against the bony shelves of the skull, from direct trauma at the site of the blow to the skull, or contra-coup trauma that occurs when the brain strikes the skull on the side opposite the point of trauma. Lesions of the corpus callosum have also been reported (Lindberg, Fisher, & Durlacher, 1955; Rowbotham, 1949; Rubens, Geschwind, Mahowald, & Mastri, 1977; Stritch, 1969).

The variety of the possible neuropathological consequences of CHI suggests that the initial generalized impairment of language/cognitive processes is a manifestation of the massive, yet, to a degree, reversible disruption and disorganization of neurophysiological activity. Conversely, the irreversible neurologic damage could, subsequently, produce a potentially wide variety of cognitive/language impairments that would not be expected to remit spontaneously.

Clinically, there appear to be at least three general phases of post-CHI-neurologic-communicative-cognitive dysfunction. During the initial phase the patient is in a state of "cerebral paralysis" (Russell, 1932). At this time there is a global suppression of all communicative and cognitive functions. In the intermediate phase, a mixture of reversible and irreversible neurologic impairments coexist. Consequently, at this time it is not unusual to observe wide swings in the presence or absence, as well as types of, cognitive/communicative impairment. However, one may also begin to find certain symptoms persisting across time during this phase. The irreversible neurologic impairments and their concomitant communicative and cognitive sequelae become evident during the long-term phase.

Thus, the variability of post-CHI-language dysfunction characterizes the dynamic interactions between the natural course of neurological recovery, the type, extent, and location of residual neurologic impairment, and the degree to which cognitive abilities are disturbed. It has been my experience that three general types of patients ultimately emerge from the diffuse symptomatology of the first two phases: (1) those with disorganized language secondary to cognitive disorganization, who may or may not have a coexisting specific language disorder; (2) those with the predominant feature of a specific language disorder and coexisting minimal cognitive impairment; and (3) those with attentional, retentional, and recent memory impairments, but without language dysfunction. The remainder of this chapter will focus on the assessment and treatment of those patients who fall into the first two categories.

The speech-language pathologist who treats the CHI patient must answer the same critical questions related to clinical management as they do with other disorders, namely to whom, when, what, and how care should be rendered. One cannot reason solely from experience and information related to language disorders secondary to other types of neurological impairments. Head trauma patients cannot be successfully understood, diagnosed, and treated within the framework of our traditional approaches to language disorders. The communicative dysfunction of the CHI patient is quite dynamic. Consequently, our clinical approach must also be dynamic. Ongoing assessment and subsequent modification of the treatment approach is a primary requisite for the appropriate management of this population.

The purpose of this chapter is to present an approach to evaluation and treatment that has been drawn from my clinical experience with more than 2,500 CHI patients over the past 18 years. Other work that broadens the scope in this field may include Adamovich (1981), Adamovich and Brooks (1981), Adamovich and Henderson (1982), Adamovich and Henderson (1983), Ben-Yishay (1978, 1979, 1980), Buschke and Fuld (1974), Butler (1981), Glick and Holyoak (1980), Hedberg-Davis and Bookman (1979), Ledwon-Robinson and Beh-Arendshorst (1980), Lezak (1979), Ligne, Sinatra, and Kimbarow (1979), and Yorkston, Stanton and Beukelman (1981). This approach is based on the premise that the majority of the post-CHI-language dysfunction is a secondary consequence of an underlying impairment, suppression, and/or disorganization of the nonlinguistic cognitive processes that support language processes. This is not to suggest that the CHI patient does not have a language disorder but rather indicates that the observed language disorder is the sum of both linguistic and nonlinguistic cognitive dysfunctions.

Characterictics of Cognitive-Language Disorganization

Typically, our internal and external environment is fluctuating, fluid, and random. Under normal circumstances we bring stability, structure, and organization to this otherwise chaotic world by automatically yet willfully focusing only on those things that we deem necessary and relevant to our needs. At a minimum, this ability to focus our awareness on only certain aspects of our environment is derived from the following seven cognitive processes:

1. Attentional abilities (alertness, awareness, attention, attention span, and selective attention);
2. Discrimination;

3. Sequential ordering of sensory stimuli and internal thoughts;
4. Memory abilities (retention span, immediate, recent, and remote memory);
5. Categorization of sensory stimuli and internal thoughts;
6. Association/integration of sensory stimuli and internal thoughts;
7. Analysis/synthesis of sensory stimuli and internal thoughts.

These seven cognitive processes become disrputed as a result of CHI. The patient is unable to exert the influence of these processes on the internal and external environment. As a result, the patient has difficulty organizing, structuring, and predicting the sequential order of thoughts. This leads to a breakdown in the patient's ability to structure mental processes volitionally to deal differentially with stimuli, to mentally structure ongoing events, to shift cognitive sets, and to modify/dampen emotional reactions. As a result, such individuals become disoriented, disorganized, confused, stimulus bound, and reduced in both initiation and inhibition. As a consequence, the patient's receptive, integrative, and expressive language can also become

1. *Disoriented*—not appropriate to the situation, question, statement or discussion.
2. *Disorganized*—fragmented and incomplete understanding of what has been heard or expressed by the patient.
3. *Confused*—confabulatory, circumlocutory, tangential in relation to the content of the situation, question, statement, or discussion.
4. *Stimulus bound*—relevant to a part, but not the whole idea of a statement, question, or discussion.
5. *Reduced in initiation*—reliant upon others to stimulate the occurence and structure of language responses.
6. *Reduced in inhibition*—Once language response is initiated, it is lacking in specificity and precision in relationship to the original question or statement.

Typically, these six consequences of cognitive disorganization appear in the patient's receptive and expressive language in the form of combinations of the following symptoms:

1. Decreased auditory comprehension;
2. Decreased visual and reading comprehension;
3. Expressive language that does not make sense;
4. Language expressions that are grammatically correct but not relevant to the question, statement, or discussion;

5. Lack of ability to inhibit verbal expressions;
6. Inappropriate ordering of words in sentences and/or inappropriate grammar;
7. Inability to recall specific words.

Many of these symptoms are characteristic of the aphasic disorders found in patients with vascular or space-occupying lesions. A CHI patient may, in fact, have a specific language disorder caused by a focal lesion. However, while many of these receptive and expressive language problems are like aphasia, the majority are symptomatic of the language confusion that results from the underlying disorganization of the seven cognitive processes listed above. Because of this, a major part of the patient's communication rehabilitation program must be directed toward cognitive reorganization. Typically, as cognitive processes become reorganized, there will be a major decrease in the patient's language disorganization.

Assessment

The following variables must be addressed when evaluating the CHI patient: the patient's ability to cooperate with testing, the rapid and random fluctuations in symptoms, clinically apparent language dysfunction with little or no impairment reflected in test scores, and the dynamic interaction between cognitive and language impairments. In the early phases of recovery, patients are confused, disoriented, and unable to deal purposefully with internal and external stimuli. Consequently, assessment should not be completely dependent upon a patient's ability to cooperate volitionally in the more typical stimulus-response test-taking procedures. Structured, systematic, and consistent clinical observation and evaluation of spontaneous behavior will be needed. The rapid and random fluctuations in the type and severity of symptoms necessitate frequent re-evaluation. During the first 4 to 8 weeks of recovery, a patient's communication disorder usually results from the combined effects of the temporary global interruption of neural activity, the language and cognitive disorganization secondary to irreversible diffuse structural damage and, possibly, a specific language disorder secondary to a focal lesion. Fluctuations in symptomatology are reflective of the interplay between the subsidence of reversible neurological dysfunction and the emergence of the long-term neurologic impairments. It is neither practical nor instructive to repeat standardized tests on a daily to weekly basis; however, clinical direction depends upon some form of frequent reassessment. Consequently, during the early phases of recovery the evaluation approach should include a means of describing, categorizing, and scaling the type and nature of language/cognitive behavior at very frequent intervals. Standardized tests should be employed when the more global cognitive disorganization begins to remit.

During the later phases of recovery, it is not unusual to find that patients who demonstrate minimal to no impairment on standard aphasia test instruments will experience difficulty with language in their natural environment. Because of this, one must assess those language abilities that are not evaluated by most aphasia tests, such as the verbal reasoning and thought organization that lie behind the use of language.

The assessment approach that I have found to be the most helpful consists of four evaluation methods: (1) categorizing the patient's spontaneous behavioral responses to randomly occurring environmental stimuli; (2) scaling responses to nontest stimuli that are presented and controlled by someone other than the patient, as in the daily nursing routine; (3) administering a standard aphasia test battery; and (4) administering higher-level cognitive and verbal tests. Depending on the patient's level of functioning, these four assessment approaches may be applied sequentially in steps that parallel the longitudinal course of recovery or, when appropriate, combinations of all four methods may be applied simultaneously.

Categorizing Spontaneous Behavior

Clinical observation is the primary method of identifying and categorizing behavioral manifestations of cognitive/linguistic dysfunction during the early phases of recovery. When present, the symptoms will be readily apparent in the patient's manner of handling daily activities, interacting with others, using familiar objects, and the manner and content of the patient's responses to language tests. Some of the more common behavioral characteristics are the following:

1. *Disorientation*—behavior that is not appropriate to prevailing stimuli; lack of awareness of time, space and place;
2. *Confusion*—behavioral responses that randomly fluctuate between appropriate and inappropriate; difficulty in discriminating between animate and inanimate objects; confabulatory, circumlocutory, tangential, or completely inappropriate language responses;
3. *Distractability and impulsivity*—decreased attention and attention span;

4. *Reduced initiation*—reliant upon external stimuli for the occurrence and structure of responses;
5. *Reduced inhibition*—once responses are initiated, they continue beyond logical point of cessation and usually lack specificity in relation to the stimulus;
6. *Concreteness*—deals with stimuli in their literal sense, responses are relevant to a part of a stimulus, but not the implied whole concept;
7. *Reduced cognitive flexibility*—either does not shift cognitively or carries part of a previous thought/response into a succeeding response, or needs an abnormal length of time to shift from one stimulus condition to another;
8. *Disorganization*—behavioral responses generally appropriate to stimulus, but are organized in an illogical sequential manner and display periodic intrusion of extraneous responses not relevant to stimulus;
9. *Reduction in judgment*—does not grasp cause-effect relationships.

The purpose of categorizing patient's behavior is not simply to generate a diagnostic label. Rather, this information provides a very general statement about the broad area of dysfunction that must be addressed, as well as the general goal of treatment. Categorizing patients is the first step in discerning the differences among patients whose behavior may appear superficially similar. For example, the knowledge that one must decrease confusion in one patient, increase cognitive flexibility in another, and decrease distractibility and impulsiveness in a third will, when combined with other assessment data, assist in the development of a treatment plan that focuses on individual patient needs.

Scaling of Behavioral Responses

Historically, head-trauma patients have been classified according to such categories as coma, stupor, delirium, and confusion (Hooper, 1969; Lewin, 1966). In recent years the Glasgow Coma Scale (Jennett & Teasdale, 1981; Teasdale & Jennett, 1974) has also been extensively used. While the major purpose of the Glasgow Scale is the early prediction of mortality and morbidity, it also provides some very useful general descriptive categories of patient responses which are characteristic of different levels of coma. This scale is particularly useful during the acute phase of treatment. The Levels of Cognitive Functioning (Hagen & Malkmus, 1979) described in abbreviated form in Table 8-1 has been found to be quite helpful in identifying a patient's most intact level of cognitive functioning throughout the entire course of rehabilitation. The Glasgow Coma Scale is used for prognosis.

TABLE 8-1
Levels of Cognitive Functioning.

I. *No Response:* Patient appears to be in a deep sleep and is completely unresponsive to any stimuli.

II. *Generalized Response:* Patient reacts inconsistently and nonpurposefully to stimuli in a nonspecific manner. Responses are limited and often the same, regardless of stimulus presented. Responses may be physiological changes, gross body movements, and/or vocalization.

III. *Localized Response:* Patient reacts specifically, but inconsistently, to stimuli. Responses are directly related to the type of stimulus presented. May follow simple commands such as, "Close your eyes" or "Squeeze my hand" in an inconsistent, delayed manner.

IV. *Confused-Agitated:* Behavior is bizarre and nonpurposeful relative to immediate environment. Does not discriminate among persons or objects, is unable to co-operate directly with treatment efforts, verbalizations are frequently incoherent and/or inappropriate to the environment, confabulation may be present. Gross attention to environment is very short, and selective attention is often nonexistent. Patient lacks short term recall.

V. *Confused, Inappropriate, Non-Agitated:* Patient is able to respond to simple commands fairly consistently. However, with increased complexity of commands, or lack of any external structure, responses are nonpurposeful, random, or fragmented. Has gross attention to the environment, but is highly distractible, and lacks ability to focus attention on a specific task; with structure, may be able to converse on a social-automatic level for short periods of time; verbalization is often inappropriate and confabulatory; memory is severely impaired, often shows inappropriate use of subjects; may perform previously learned tasks with structure, but is unable to learn new information.

VI. *Confused-Appropriate:* Patient shows goal-directed behavior, but is dependent on external input for direction; follows simple directions consistently and shows carry-over for relearned tasks with little or no carry-over for new tasks; responses may be incorrect due to memory problems, but appropriate to the situation; past memories show more depth and detail than recent memory.

VII. *Automatic-Appropriate:* Patient appears appropriate and oriented within hospital and home settings, goes through daily routine automatically, but is frequently robot-like, with minimal-to-absent

TABLE 8-1 (Continued)
Levels of Cognitive Functioning.

---

confusion; has shallow recall of activities; shows carry-over for new learning, but at a decreased rate; with structure, is able to initiate social or recreational activities; judgment remains impaired.

VIII. *Purposeful and Appropriate:* Patient is able to recall and integrate past and recent events, and is aware of and responsive to the environment, shows carry-over for new learning and needs no supervision once activities are learned; may continue to show a decreased ability, relative to premorbid abilities in language, abstract reasoning, tolerance for stress and judgment in emergencies or unusual circumstances.

The Levels of Cognitive Functioning, in contrast, is used to identify a patient's best level of functioning, and, thereby, to indicate the best way to approach the patient during the course of treatment.

The purpose of this type of evaluation is to establish the presence and pattern of change in such basic neurobehavioral dichotomies as:

1. Response to external stimuli versus no responses;
2. Gross undifferentiated response to stimuli versus differentiated response to stimuli;
3. Differentiated response to stimuli, but no continued response after withdrawal of stimuli, versus differentiated and sustained response after withdrawal of stimuli;
4. Sustained response to stimuli only if stimuli brought to patient, versus sustained response on basis of patient's self-directed behavior;
5. Inappropriate versus appropriate responses to stimuli, whether externally presented or self-initiated.

These behavioral responses represent the manner in which the Levels of Cognitive Functioning Scale should be interpreted with respect to levels of information processing. In this regard, Item 1 represents reception of sensory stimuli versus no reception; Item 2 represents reception of stimuli, but with minimal to no relation to specific sensory modalities; Item 3 represents response to specific sensory modalities, but inability to retain the response for purposes of processing; Item 4 represents ability to process information, if information is continually presented, versus ability to process information on a self-initiated basis; and Item 5 represents a qualitative evaluation of the patient's behavioral responses on Items 2 through 4. We have found that, for patients at and between Levels II and VII, the rating scale is most useful when all disciplines interacting with the patient rate him or her.

Such a behavioral-scaling technique is a means for systematically describing and categorizing the patient's level of cognitive/language functioning across time, be it a day, week, or month. In the early phases of recovery, it provides an immediate and sensitive picture of the dynamics of the course of change. This type of assessment has several benefits. Systematic observation and assessment of the type, nature, and quality of a patient's behavioral responses assists in estimating the level at which the patient is functioning in the hierarchy of cognitive processes. Behavioral scaling also allows one, as early as possible, to differentiate between those language-impairment characteristics secondary to temporary interruption of cognitive/language processes, those that reflect potential long-term cognitive/language disorganization, and those that may indicate the presence of a language disorder secondary to a focal lesion. Clear patterns of change emerge through daily-to-weekly charting. Through these patterns, one is able to differentiate between the rapidly resolving, and, therefore, most probably temporary and reversible, symptoms and the more slowly remitting symptoms characteristic of the irreversible diffuse and/or focal damage. By observing the type and nature of the patients' responses to the environment, and, then, to purposefully introduce stimuli that are contextually relevant to the patient's total treatment program, one will find that behavioral responses characteristic of a particular level occur more frequently than others. Most patients have a characteristic range of cognitive function, showing a preponderance of behavior at one level and a scatter of behavioral responses below and above that level. Determining the patient's range of cognitive/communicative behavior provides three types of information important to planning and maintaining an appropriate treatment plan: (1) Knowledge of the patient's most typical cognitive level identifies the highest level of functioning we can expect from a patient at a given point in time. Knowing this, the stimuli we present and the way in which we present them will be consonant with his or her capabilities. A program that presents stimuli in a manner that matches the patient's most stable level of functioning, and that slightly challenges the next highest level simultaneously is optimal. Such treatment decreases the behavioral swings below the most intact level and increases the swings above. In time, the next highest level becomes the patient's most typical level, with a scatter of responses remaining from the previous level, but now the emergence of abilities at the next highest level are observed. (2) Responses below the patient's most consistent level of functioning are extremely important signs. They indicate that the environment should be altered to maintain the patient's highest level of cognitive/communicative organization for the longest period of time.

Responses characteristic of a lower level of function signal regression, and, as such, tell us to alter the way in which we interact with the patient or what we request from the patient. (3) Similarly, the emergence and stabilization of behavioral responses characteristic of the next highest level indicate that it is safe to alter the treatment plan in a manner that challenges the patient to move toward this next level of function. It is on the basis of these three types of information, i.e., the patient's most typical cognitive level, responses below, and above, that level, that one is able to construct the type of treatment plan that will maintain cognitive organization.

Direct Assessment of Cognitive Functioning

Evaluation of language processes should occur concurrently with assessment of the patient's cognitive abilities. Because of the interrelationship and reciprocal interplay between linguistic and cognitive processes, it is necessary to have information regarding type and level of nonlinguistic cognitive dysfunction to interpret the dynamic nature of the linguistic disturbance. The type and nature of cognitive dysfunction will provide information as to why and how the patient is experiencing a breakdown in language organization. At a minimum, one should assess the general cognitive processes of (1) attentional abilities (alertness, awareness, attention, attention span, and selective attention); (2) discrimination; (3) temporal ordering; (4) memory abilities (retention span, immediate, recent, and remote memory); (5) categorization; (6) association/integration; (7) analysis/synthesis; (8) maintenance of sequential goal-directed behavior. At the phonemenological level, language disorganization (i.e., confused language) may appear similar across patients at different points in time. However, the source of the cognitive disorganization that underlies the language disorganization is often different for each patient. Appropriate and effective treatment is heavily dependent on treatment of the specific impaired-cognitive abilities.

All eight cognitive abilities are assessed during the previously described processes of categorizing and scaling spontaneous behavior. But, they cannot be directly assessed until the patient reaches Level VII. Following are examples of tests that can be used to assess these various abilities.

To measure attention, discrimination, temporal sequencing, and retention span abilities, the following tests are used: Visual Sequential Memory subtest of the ITPA (Kirk, McCarthy, & Kirk, 1968); the WAIS Digit Span subtest (Wechsler, 1955); the Auditory Attention Span for Unrelated Words and Related Syllables and the Visual Attention Span for Objects and Letters subtests of the DTLA (Baker & Leland, 1959); the Developmental Test of Visual Perception (Frostig, 1963); the Southern California Figure-Ground Visual

Perception Test (Ayres, 1966); Luria's tests for Perception and Reproduction of Pitch Relationships and Perception and Reproduction of Rhythmic Structures (Christensen, 1975); The G-F-W Sound-Symbol Tests (Goldman, Fristoe, & Woodcock 1974b); and the G-F-W Test of Auditory Discrimination (Goldman, Fristoe, & Woodcock, 1970).

To measure immediate and recent memory abilities, the following tests are used: The Wechsler Memory Scale (Wechsler & Stone, 1945); the Digit Symbol subtest of the WAIS (Wechsler, 1955); The Goldstein-Scheerer Stick Test (Goldstein & Scheerer, 1945); the Benton Revised Visual Retention Test (Benton, 1963); Luria's mnestic tests (Christensen, 1975); and the G-F-W Auditory Memory Tests (Goldman, Fristoe, & Woodcock, 1974a).

To measure categorization, association, integration, and synthesis abilities, we use the Weigle-Goldstein-Scheerer Color Form Sorting Test (1945); the Disarranged Pictures subtest of the DTLA (Baker & Leland, 1959); the Block Design, Object Assembly, and Picture Arrangement subtests of the WAIS (Wechsler, 1955); The Ross Test of Higher Cognitive Processes (Ross & Ross, 1976), and the tests of higher level language organization listed in the section on language, following the section on language assessment. Finally, the Nonverbal Test of Cognitive Skills (Johnson & Boyd, 1981) provides a means of evaluating a number of the various cognitive abilities within the context of a single test battery.

The various tests which have been described do not constitute a "test battery." The list represents tests that can be drawn upon relative-to-specific types and levels of language impairments known to exist in a particular patient. For example, to assess attention, selective attention, or retention span in patients with significant language impairments, one would not use those tests that were dependent upon auditory comprehension or highly intact speech production abilities. Instead, one would select those tests not dependent on these abilities. Because of the need to control for confounding variables such as these, as well as the effect of fatigue, one should use those few tests that focus with the greatest precision on the areas of breakdown.

The various cognitive abilities have been placed in clusters because of the close interaction between them. However, from the standpoint of actual cognitive processing, there is a functional interaction both within and between these clusters of cognitive abilities. Consequently it is not solely the presence or absence of an error that is of significance. It is this *plus* the dynamic nature of the dysfunction. In this regard, the interpretation of the pattern of deficits leads to the determination of cognitive/language dysfunction. This determination is not based on the scores on specific tests. For example, one could not infer the presence of a problem with categorization, association, and synthesis if a patient exhibits severe impairments of attention and memory, even though the patient did very poorly on tests related to those higher level skills. Here, one is undoubtedly observing a cause-effect relationship rather than areas of discrete impairment.

Comparison of behavioral responses under different conditions and analysis of variations in behavioral responses under the same condition provides two means of interpreting the pattern of response errors. For example, a comparison of the type and level of dysfunction that is identified through clinical observation (e.g., categorizing and scaling spontaneous behavior) with the type and level of dysfunction found during direct assessment could lead to one of the following interpretations: Better performance in spontaneous activities requiring cognitive abilities similar to those directly tested would suggest that the patient is able to maintain better cognitive stability and organization when provided with familiarity, contextual cues, and the structure of an actual event. The individual cannot internally evoke and organize these same attributes independently. Conversely, the patient who does better on test tasks than on tasks using environmental stimuli is a person who is more cognitively organized by the structure of tasks, and who has trouble spontaneously and independently organizing the random and fluctuating stimuli of the environment. Table 8-2 presents possible interpretations of variations in the pattern of errors that occur under similar task conditions.

Finally, the interpretation of the quality and pattern of both language and cognitive organization impairments is considerably aided by gathering information relative to factors that are not implicit in the tests themselves. Specifically, it is important to assess and identify the manner in which the patient approaches a given problem. I have found that each patient has an optimal and stable level of performance in relationship to the rate, amount, duration, and complexity of stimulus input. Variations either above or below a patient's optimal level of receiving and processing stimuli act to intensify his or her already impaired ability to remain organized. With respect to the patient's problem-solving approach, I have found it helpful to watch for the following characteristics: immediately recognizes a solution, studies task before attempting solution, is organized and systematic, approaches task in an impulsive or trial-and-error manner, develops alternate strategies when unsuccessful, over-attends to details, must be prompted to start, as well as continue, task, perseverates approach across tasks, benefits from cues and correction, and independently carries cues or corrections over to next task. Knowing the optimal manner for presenting stimuli, as well as the patient's problem-solving approach, is critical diagnostic information. The behavioral-rating scale and the tests yield information that tells us what the level of the problem is, and what should and should not be treated. Knowledge about stimulus presentation and task approach tells how to treat the problem.

TABLE 8-2
Variations in Pattern of Errors Within Similar Task Conditions.

A. Random and fluctuating errors across time—suggests attention span and/or selective attention problems;
B. Errors that occur on the first several stimuli of tasks, but not later in the task, across test tasks—suggestive of attentional/selective attention impairments;
C. Errors that consistently occur during the last several stimuli of tasks, but not earlier—suggestive of attentional, selective attention, or retention span fatigue;
D. Clustering of errors at relatively similar time intervals during a task—suggests problems with amount and duration of stimuli, and gives insight into what would be optimal for a given patient relative to these parameters during treatment;
E. Errors decrease relative to certain types of cues: auditory, visual, visual-motor, contextual, breaking up stimulus into its parts, providing whole idea, etc.—suggestive of problems with categorization, association, and/or analysis/synthesis;
F. Errors increase/decrease with rate, amount, and duration of stimuli—affects all cognitive abilities;
G. Errors increase in relation to complexity—suggestive of impaired memory abilities, including retention span and/or weakened categorization, association, and analysis/synthesis problems;
H. Responds appropriately to parts of stimulus, but not whole or vice versa—suggestive of associative, integrative, analysis/synthesis impairment;
I. Carry-over of responses to previous tasks to succeeding ones—suggestive of cognitive shift problems.

Language Assessment

The previously described approaches to behavioral categorization and scaling also provide a means of on-going language assessment. Charting and describing a patient's behavior across time provides information that is most useful in determining the presence of a specific language disorder, and, if it exists, distinguishing between it and communication impairment secondary to language disorganization. The presence of specific language disorders, such as apraxia or aphasic syndromes, will rapidly become apparent through the persistence of their characteristic symptoms across time, even though their severity levels might vary. Similarly, the presence of language disorganization will also become apparent through the observed persistence of the characteristics noted in Table 8-3.

A high degree of confusion and disorientation decreases the validity of standardized test results prior and up to Level V of cognitive functioning. However, even though validity with respect to isolating specific language disorders is diminished, it is important to present patients with stimuli relative to various communication skills in a categorical and systematic fashion as early as possible. A patient's failure to respond or to give a response that is completely without form and/or meaning is as significant as a response that fits into a more recognizable speech- or language-disturbance category. Tests administered to such severely involved patients will generate very important information regarding language functioning under controlled, identifiable, and systematic conditions; this performance may contrast significantly with performance under spontaneous conditions. The delineation of the difference between responses to structured versus unstructured stimulus conditions generates very important base-line data. For example, the type and quality of responses of a confused and disoriented patient to auditory subtests should be interpreted in relation to the patient's ability to focus attention on a task and remember the instructions, rather than to the auditory tasks themselves. In essence, the purpose of this level of evaluation is to determine the stimulus conditions under which the patient becomes less confused and more oriented, rather than to attempt to determine whether the problem is one of aphasia or apraxia. Diagnosis of specific language impairments become clearer as the patient moves from Level V towards Level VIII.

As patients approach Level VII it is not unusual to find that they have minimal to no deficits in the majority of the categorical language abilities, but, at the same time, observe that they have difficulty using language to understand and convey the meaning of thoughts. This disparity between apparent linguistic competence on tests and poor performance in a natural communication environment is typically the result of two factors. First, the temporary disruption of neural activity that produced the global disturbances of language has, by now, remitted almost completely. Second, since most aphasia tests are oriented primarily toward the assessment of the categorical elements (i.e., phonology, semantic, and syntactic) of language, test results now accurately portray the patient's improvement in these areas of language. This does not necessarily mean that the patient has normal functional language abilities. Our tests do not assess in depth the organizational structure of expressed discursive thought, the use of language as a verbal reasoning tool, or the auditory processing counterpart of these

TABLE 8-3
Language Disorganization.

Language expressions that are
- I. Inappropriate
- II. Irrelevant
- III. Confabulatory
- IV. Fragmented
- V. Have no logical sequential relationship
- VI. Circumlocutious
- VII. Tangential
- VIII. Concrete
- IX. Intermittent and random auditory confusion

expressive functions. Thus, it is entirely possible for a patient to do well on discrete identification, naming, sentence completion/understanding, and short-answer tasks within the structured context of a test, but to be unable to organize these same language processes across time.

In many instances, then, good test performance only reflects the fact that the patient has reached the upper limits of those factors that a particular test was designed to assess. It is the quality of the language behavior that now becomes of diagnostic and therapeutic significance. One must now evaluate to determine whether the language-disorganization characteristics shown in Table 8-3 are present. This usually becomes necessary after a patient has reached Level VI. The following are a number of the tests that can be used to assess the higher levels of language integrity: The Wechsler Adult Intelligence Scale (WAIS)(Wechsler, 1955); subtests of the Detroit Test of Learning Aptitude (DTLA)(Baker & Leland, 1959); the Goldstein-Scheerer Object Sorting Test (Goldstein & Scheerer, 1951); subtests of the Illinois Test of Psycholinguistic Abilities (ITPA)(Kirk, McCarthy, & Kirk, 1968); and Luria's tests of understanding both logical grammatical structures and thematic pictures and texts (Christensen, 1975). Although some of these tests were developed for and standardized on a children's population, the intention in using them is not to derive an age-comparable score, but, rather, to assess the manner in which the patient responds to the tasks.

Treatment

The treatment approach discussed here is based on the following postulates:

1. Treatment should be directed toward the reorganization of the cognitive processes, rather than modification of the abnormal language consequences of the cognitive disorganization.
2. As cognitive processes become reorganized, there will be a commensurate reorganization of phonological, semantic, syntactic, andverbal-reasoning abilities.
3. The reorganization of cognitive abilities follows a predictable and systematic hierarchical sequence, in which the reacquisition and stabilization of lower level processes is necessary for the emergence and stabilization of higher level activities.
4. Cognitive structure is maximized and behavioral responses become more organized when the treatment program progresses sequentially from the patient's highest level of cognitive abilities through all of the necessary steps following that level.
5. Treatment stimuli should be presented through the patient's single-most intact sensory modality, and generalized to other modalities only as increasing cognitive abilities support the ability to deal with multiple stimuli.
6. Regardless of the level of cognitive abilities toward which treatment is directed, the manner of stimulus input is critical to the elicitation of structured and appropriate behavioral responses. Consequently, one must manipulate the rate, amount, duration, and complexity of stimulus input in a manner consistent with the patient's cognitive abilities at any given time.

The goal of treatment is to promote the conscious processing of language stimuli in an orderly, sequential manner. This is accomplished through the appropriate manipulation of the patient's environment, as well as through direct treatment of cognitive-linguistic disorganization.

Environmental Manipulation

The rate, quality, and ultimate level of recovery is critically dependent upon the degree to which the patient's environment allows him or her to function at the threshold of his most intact level of cognitive abilities. Maintaining a balance between the type and manner of stimulus input and the patient's most intact level of cognitive functioning is the single-most critical factor in the successful reorganization of cognitive/communicative abilities. A patient is able to process internal and/or external stimuli in the most organized manner, and, consequently, to function at his or her optimum level when the demands of the environment match existing cognitive abilities. Environmental stimulation that is below the patient's most functional level will not challenge recovery in a structured, controlled, and predictable manner. Stimulation above a patient's optimum level of functioning will be overwhelming, and, as a result, will suppress and impede recovery. The speech-language pathologist can provide guidance to other members of the rehabilitation team regarding the manner in which a patient's environment can be optimally structured. In addition to the usual recommendations relative to increasing awareness of a patient's most functional receptive and expressive modes of communication, the recommendations that follow are pertinent.

LEVELS I, II, AND III: NO, GENERALIZED, AND LOCALIZED RESPONSE

The goal of treatment for Levels I and II is to activate a behavioral response and, thereby, initiate the patient's movement toward the early phases of awareness of his or her environment.

Activation of behavioral responses will occur within the context of routine patient care. Special efforts outside this routine are unnecessary. Stimulating the patient toward Level III will, however, be enhanced by giving special consideration to the manner in which the nursing routine is carried out. The following ways of interacting with patients have good potential for stimulating awareness of the environment:

1. Be calm and soothing in manner of speech and physical manipulation of the patient;
2. Do not talk to others when working with the patient;
3. Assume that the patient can understand all that is said. While the degree to which patients can actually understand will be unknown at this time, it is wiser not to risk his or her hearing comments about themselves or other patients. Hearing and understanding such conversations can be traumatizing and create emotions that potentially affect the course of future recovery. Consequently, all comments or discussions of medical status, behavior, prognosis, and family concerns, as well as discussions about other patients, should be avoided in the patient's presence.
4. Talk to the patient. It is quite difficult to carry on a conversation with an unresponsive patient; however, one should try to avoid

concluding that since the patient cannot answer, there is not much point in talking to him or her. Talking is a natural form of stimulation. Use appropriate greetings such as, "Good morning Mr. or Mrs. Smith." Describe what you are going to do with the patient before you do it, describe such occurrences as family visits, upcoming occupational therapy treatment, etc., talk about the weather conditions, or even things or events that are of personal interest to you. Try to learn about the patient's family and/or friends so that you can talk about them by name and describe some of the things they are doing. However, it is important not to overwhelm the patient with talking. Talk slowly and calmly. Describe what you are about to do with the patient; then, without talking, do it and then describe the next event. It will be important to leave moments of silence between verbal stimuli.

5. Manage environmental stimuli. While activation of the patient's behavioral responses at these lower levels is dependent on the presence of external stimulation, too much stimulation can suppress an increasing awareness of environment. A TV or radio is a very useful source of stimulation. However, it is important to use them sporadically and for short durations. The patient will rapidly get habituated and fail to respond to such stimuli when they are on continuously. Only one source of stimulation should occur in the environment at a time. For example, if talking is occurring, then the radio or TV should be off.

6. Determine which type of stimuli seems to cause the patient to respond. Certain topics, statements, TV programs, music, etc. may elicit a response. Often family voices or the voice of a particular staff member seem to stimulate a response. In the case of these latter two, tape recordings can be made of those to whom the patient reacts, and these can be played intermittenty. Identify key stimuli and present them to the patient on a routine basis. The patient, however, will become fatigued and overwhelmed if such stimuli are allowed to continue for long periods of time. To a large extent, arousal and awareness depend on the novelty of the stimulus. In this regard, all activities should be kept very brief. Present several different types of stimuli rather than a single lengthy stimulus.

7. Encourage the family to follow the above pattern of interaction. Special caution should be taken to describe the problems of presenting simultaneous multiple stimuli and stimulating the patient for too long a period of time. If family members do not understand the problems, they can unknowingly overwhelm the patient.

LEVEL IV:
CONFUSED-AGITATED

The goals for this level are to increase the patient's awareness of, and attention to, the environment, to minimize the frequency of occurrence of agitated behavior, and to decrease the duration of agitated behavior when it occurs.

One's physical handling and moving of patients, as well as one's manner of interacting with them, is most important at this stage. Patients are beginning to be aware of, and alert to, the environment and are trying to process information. Their neurological status at this time, however, is such that they often make exaggerated responses to internal and external stimuli. Thus, patients at this level are susceptible to the triggering of defensive motor reflexes and emotional reactions, such as acute fear, anxiety, and anger. Many of these behavioral responses occur spontaneously and are unavoidable, but the nurse can take steps to minimize the degree and duration of such responses. However, the degree to which one is able to keep from triggering the patient's defensive responses relates to the degree to which the patient is neurologically ready to move towards the environment rather than away from it. The following approaches can be taken with patients at this level:

1. Be calm and soothing in manner when handling the patient;
2. Move slowly around the patient and move the patient slowly when it is necessary to change his or her position or range, to bathe, or to transfer the patient;
3. Talk slowly and softly. Talking loudly may trigger a startle reflex, and speaking rapidly will be overwhelming;
4. Do not talk to others while working with the patient. Multiple stimuli—such as physical manipulation and an ongoing conversation with others—will be more than a patient can handle;
5. Always describe what you are going to do with the patient before you do it. Even if what you say is not totally understood by the patient, the patient will have time during the explanation to adjust to your presence in the room and to become aware that something is going to happen;
6. Before physically handling patients in accordance with the desired task, take time first to simply touch them, gently rub one of the extremities, head, or back, and/or gradually move an extremity. Such activities will decrease the occurrence of defensive motor reflexes and emotional reflexes—that is, the activities allow time to adjust;

7. If the patient becomes upset, allow time for self-adjustment. Do not try to talk a patient out of his or her reaction. At this time, talking will be an additional external stimulus that will only act to intensify the reactions;
8. If the patient remains upset, either remove him or her from the situation or remove the situation from him or her;
9. Watch for early signs that the patient is becoming agitated (e.g., more-than-usual motor movement activity, increase in vocal loudness, resistance to activity) and modify the environment immediately. It is far better to cease all of your activity than to launch the patient into a prolonged state of agitation. It will take far less time to wait then it will to calm the patient down.

LEVELS V AND VI: CONFUSED, INAPPROPRIATE, NON-AGITATED, AND CONFUSED-APPROPRIATE

The goal of this phase of rehabilitation is to create the environmental conditions whereby the patient can produce purposeful and appropriate responses to external and internal stimuli with greater frequency and duration. There are two approaches to creating the appropriate conditions. One involves the use of the more automatic behavioral responses found in some of the activities of daily living. Such activities can be used as a means of eliciting purposeful behavior and to provide environmental structure. Activities of daily living, such as dressing, eating, toilet and leisure time tasks provide numerous opportunities to gently challenge a patient to move toward purposeful and appropriate responses. For example, putting a pant leg or shirt sleeve partially over one extremity, but not over the other, encourages the patient to complete the task. Rather than allowing the patient to randomly attempt to organize the act of tooth brushing, someone should stay with him or her, lay out the various components of the task in the appropriate order, and help the patient to move stepwise through each component of the task sequence. Eating meals can be structured in the same way. In essence, any and all routine tasks that a patient carries out can be turned into cognitive reorganization tasks. All that is needed is to see the tasks as such, then assist the patient by breaking the tasks into subcomponents, initiate the first step or two, and maintain the patient's structure as he or she proceeds through the task. If the patient begins to become confused, the staff can intervene and assist in initiating the next appropriate behavioral response in the sequence, then withdraw, and allow the patient to continue.

The following are suggestions that will assist in turning routine unit tasks into a medium to help patients at this level of functioning to become cognitively organized:

1. Be calm and soothing in manner; move slowly, talk slowly and softly;
2. Present patients with only one task at a time, and allow them to complete the entire task or a subpart of it before presenting the next task. Multiple tasks and instructions will only confuse patients further;
3. Tell the patient what you want done several minutes before you actually start the task. Then tell the patient again just before you ask him or her to attempt it. This gives the patient time to become aware of you and the task and to begin to think about how to complete it. Having sufficient time to process and organize the request and response is essential to helping the patient remain cognitively organized;
4. If the patient becomes confused and resists you and your request, do not continue the activity or begin talking. Wait until the patient appears relaxed and is attending to you and then explain the activity again and continue with it;
5. Give instructions at a time or in a place that is the most quiet and least distracting;
6. Before giving an instruction, place yourself in a postion where you can be seen. Be sure the patient is paying attention to you and then touch the patient before you begin talking;
7. First, tell the patient what you want done and why it should be done, then demonstrate what you want done, and give the instruction;
8. When giving instructions, use gestures, demonstrations, and only a few of the most necessary and important words;
9. Once the sequence of routine unit activities has been established, do not change it, and, whenever possible, do not change the staff person who carries it out. Any such changes produce a completely new task. Enhancing the predictability of a routine is a major means of assisting the patient to remain cognitively organized.

Maintaining a structured environment is critical to patients at Levels V and VI. The environment includes the physical setting, the particular activity at hand, and the verbal and nonverbal interactions between the patient and others. The purpose of providing environmental structure is to keep the patient's environment as unconfusing as possible. If the activities are random, chaotic, and confusing, they will match—thereby indirectly reinforce—the patient's own inner confusion.

Because patients at Levels V and VI are experiencing internal confusion, one of the best ways to treat the confusion is to make the environment less confusing. It is easier to modify the external confusion than to request patients to modify their internal confusion. An orderly, predictable, and structured environment will help patients remain at their highest level of functioning. The following are ways in which the environment can be modified so as to engender congitive organization rather than to precipitate disorganization:

1. Continue to employ suggestions 1 through 9 from the approaches to the previous level.

2. Describe the unit routine on a daily basis. This will help patients to understand why certain things are being done to, and around, them. Relate the description of the various unit routines to the different points in time in which they occur. In this way patients can gradually be helped to predict what is most likely to occur next in their environment. The nurse can describe schedules for meals, medication, OT and PT, time to get up, time to go to bed, bathroom activities, visiting hours, etc., in relation to past and future events. For example: "It is 12:00, and you have finished lunch, next you will go to O.T." Activities which do not occur on a predictable basis should be described to the patient several times before the patient engages in them. These might be such things as special appointments, rounds and conferences, special tests, any changes in schedule, etc.;

3. Provide a constant verbal description of what the patient was doing, is now doing, and will be doing. While it might be somewhat boring to the staff, verbal description of what has occurred, is occurring, and will occur will help the patient to structure his or her behavior and relate the activity to things occuring in the environment;

4. Present all requests or instructions slowly and concisely. The patient should be given a few moments to think about what has been said before responding. Do not talk during these few moments because the added speech will be confusing. If the patient does not respond appropriately, the request should be repeated. When it is repeated, attempt to use the same vocabulary and word order you originally used. Any slight change in either of these often causes the patient to think that you are asking something entirely different;

5. Keep the patient mentally challenged. Since CHI patients have difficulty structuring their environment, it will help if they are purposefully

presented with structured tasks. Often, if patients are allowed to remain alone, they attend only to their fleeting and disjointed perceptions and thoughts. It is quite possible that this is one of the factors that eventually causes a patient to become agitated, combative, and even further confused.

Some of the following things might be done to challenge patients mentally during their free time:

1. Encourage them to watch television;
2. Ask another patient to either talk with them or go with them around the unit area and talk with people they meet;
3. Ask another patient or volunteer to read to the CHI patient, or play checkers, or some similar game, that will focus his thoughts on a task.

LEVELS VII AND VIII: AUTOMATIC-APPROPRIATE, AND PURPOSEFUL-APPROPRIATE

The goal for this level is to assist patients to carry out daily unit routines with minimal-to-no supervision. One must be careful not to withdraw structured assistance too early from Level VII patients. A this point, they seem to look and act "normal," and, as a result, one may assume they can carry out their daily tasks in an appropriate manner. However, the appearance of normal functioning is only superficial. Underneath, the patient is still somewhat disorganized cognitively, and retention span and short memory impairments are beginning to surface as significant problems. While it may not be apparent, the major reason a patient is able to function with the appearance of normalcy is because of the structure provided by the environment. If the structure is removed prematurely, the patient will begin to fluctuate between Levels VI and VII. Consequently, the approach should be to continue with the suggestions for Level VI but to alternate the way in which they are used. Specifically, one should continue to supply the type of structure implicit in all of the suggestions given for Levels V and VI, but now only assist the patient to initiate the activity and help the patient with each task component. Now, verbal instructions need not be given several moments before a task, nor must they be repeated when it is initiated. However, it will still be important to present only one task and one instruction at a time. Providing structure and predictability of behavior through verbal descriptions can be substantially decreased at this point, but not eliminated. Verbal structure should be used only for those activities or times when the patient is becoming confused.

At this time, reduced retention span and short-term memory are beginning to emerge as the patient's more significant cognitive/communicative impairments. The staff should find the following suggestions helpful in assisting the patient:

1. Have the patient's schedule located where he or she can easily read it. Be sure it is clearly marked with respect to morning and afternoon, as well as the individual hours of the day. Be sure that it is up to date. The patient should be requested to refer to the schedule before and after each activity. If a staff member is with the patient, the patient should be encouraged to discuss the activity just completed and the one that is to be done next;

2. Have a clock and large calendar located in a place to which the patient has easy visual access. Have the date of the given day indicated on the calendar. When a patient is away from the schedule, he or she should be asked to use the calendar and clock to determine what is next in the routine. If difficulty occurs he should be asked to review the schedule. You should not give the information. However, if the patient becomes confused, then go together to the schedule board and review it until the patient is reoriented to what is to be done next;

3. Patients in this phase of recovery are prone to becoming lost. This is a manifestation of the short-term memory problem. Because of this, it can be helpful to review with the patient how to go to and return from activities. The patient should be the one to supply most of the information, with the staff intervening only to supply correct information. It will be helpful to have a floor-plan drawing available with key areas, such as the patient's room, the nursing station and other treatment areas clearly marked, for use if there is difficulty with verbally describing the route. The patient should trace and simultaneously describe where he or she is expected to go;

4. Have the patient keep a written daily log of activities. Depending on length of the patient's short-term memory, he or she may need to fill out the log after each activity, at the end of a small block of time, or at the end of the day.

Direct Treatment of Cognitive-Linguistic Disorganization

Treatment is the process of causing the patient to re-establish an equilibrium between the linguistic, cognitive, and psychosocial spheres of communicative behavior. Typically, the patients's nonlinguistic cognitive abilities provide the greatest residuals for achieving this balance. Maximizing cognitive abilities increases the patient's conscious ability to:

1. Deal differentially with impinging internal and external stimuli;
2. Structure inner mental processes;
3. Mentally structure ongoing environmental events;
4. Predict most probable and appropriate responses on the basis of previous information; and
5. Shift cognitive sets fluidly and appropriately in relation to an ever fluctuating and random environment.

Regardless of the level of dysfunction, these five cognitive abilities are central to a patient's ability to deal with and benefit from treatment. In addition they form the basic structure within which the patient can continue to maintain the necessary equilibrium independent of the structured treatment setting.

Treatment serves to challenge and channel spontaneous recovery, maximize residual function, and compensate for lost abilities. The critical therapeutic factor in all three of these phases of language rehabilitation is the creation of the critical balance between the patient's most appropriate level of cognitive functioning and type and manner of stimulus input. When the balance is maintained, the patient is able to process internal and/or external stimuli in the most organized manner and, consequently, utilize language processes at a more organized level. To this end the speech-language pathologist uses treatment tasks specifically designed to cause the patient to (1) attend to the stimulus (attention); (2) attend for a sufficient length of time to grasp its form and quality (attention span); (3) suppress irrelevant stimuli (selective attention); (4) recognize the differences between stimuli (discrimination); (5) analyze groups of stimuli and determine the whole on the basis of the parts (temporal ordering, retention span, categorization); (6) relate this information to similar past learned information (association/memory); (7) associate and integrate this information with information from other areas of stimulus analysis (association/integration/memory); (8) determine the most appropriate sequence of behavioral events by analyzing and synthesizing information derived from steps (6) and (7) (analysis/synthesis/memory); (9) transmit the sequence; (10) attend to the output; (11) compare the actual with the intended output; (12) determine whether change is necessary; and (13), if necessary, produce a modified response.

Depending upon level of severity, some patients must begin at the level of first stabilizing attending abilities, and sequentially work their way through each subsequent cognitive skill. Others may already possess a number of the lower level abilities. Consequently, their treatment begins at a higher level and progresses sequentially from that point. Still others may exhibit marginally functional abilities at all of these levels, but the abilities rapidly disintegrate under stress. Thus, for some, this treatment process is carried out as a series of separate goals over a period of months. For others, the progression through these thirteen steps occurs within a given treatment session, while, for others, the goal may be to cause the patient to apply the steps consciously as a strategy for dealing with and solving a treatment task, or, possibly, identifying a discrete stimulus with a task. However, we have found that for patients whose lower level cognitive skills (e.g., attention, discrimination, temporal ordering, categorization) are functional, we must still use treatment tasks that cause them to consciously begin with attending abilities and progress to the level that is the focus of treatment. If treatment commences only at the level of deficit, the patient often experiences a weakening of the lower level skills because of the increased cognitive demands. Under such conditions, the patient then must rapidly solve two cognitive tasks. Simultaneously, he or she must try to deal with the original stimulus and attempt to maintain the weakening subskills. By beginning with the lower level skills, the patient is provided with the external structure that will be necessary to deal with the tasks that are at the level of dysfunction.

The therapeutic value of this approach does not lie in proceeding repetitively through these steps (though mass practice is extremely necessary) or in the stimuli that are used to elicit a response, or in the response itself. These three factors are simply the media through which the patient is taught cognitive strategies for processing language information. The general strategy is that he or she now must do something consciously that the brain previously did automatically. The secondary strategies arise because the patient must learn to evaluate his or her cognitive/language behavior in any given situation, consciously to determine at what point in this hierarchy of thirteen steps the breakdown is experienced and then to focus attention on consciously manipulating the information through that particular stage. Within this context, treatment tasks are oriented towards both strengthening weakened abilities and learning compensatory mechanisms. Treatment for any of these cognitive abilities must first be directed toward increasing the power of the ability, and, then, once power is established, moved toward increasing the quality of the skill. Power is improved by increasing the rate, amount, and duration of stimulus input that a patient can handle while holding complexity constant. Quality of ability is enhanced by increasing complexity while holding rate, amount, and duration constant.

Manipulation of Treatment Stimuli

Several parameters are critical to the success of treatment, regardless of cognitive/linguistic level. One should present stimuli at the rate, amount, duration, and complexity that is optimal for the patient. The task solutions should not require a level of problem solving above the patient's ability. Treatment tasks should initially require nonverbal congitive skills, and move toward their linguistic counterparts when proficiency at the nonverbal level is demonstrated. For example, the ability to selectively attend to nonlinguistic stimuli should be fairly stable prior to presenting tasks such as identifying embedded target words. Tasks that require nonlinguistic analysis and synthesis, such as block designs, should be presented prior to tasks that require the patient to synthesize part-whole language concepts, such as those that occur in story-telling.

I have found the following sequence of tasks to be quite helpful: visual-visual (e.g., pointing to pictures that are similar to stimulus pictures), visual-motor (e.g., tracing, copying, or supplying the missing parts of a visual stimulus), visual-auditory (e.g., identifying the visual response to an auditory stimulus); auditory-motor (e.g., producing a motor response to an auditory stimulus); and auditory-verbal (e.g., producing a verbal response to an auditory stimulus).

A given patient's movement from nonlinguistic to linguistic tasks and visual-visual to auditory-verbal analysis and response modalities will be dependent on the severity of the dysfunction. For some, these treatment parameters will represent the various sequential steps they will take over a period of months, whereas others will progress through them within a given treatment session or treatment task. The treatment value does not exist in the stimulus per se but rather in the increase in the patient's ability to handle higher and higher levels of rate, amount, duration, and complexity of stimulus processing. A treatment program that requires a higher level of cognitive functioning than the patient is capable of producing, that appeals to all sense modalities simultaneously, and that attempts to elicit and modify language before the lower level cognitive abilities necessary to support it have been stabilized will impede progress. Initially, the speech-language pathologist creates the balance between the patient's most functional level of cognitive functioning and the type and manner of presenting stimuli. The goal of treatment should be to transfer the responsibility for maintaining this critical balance to the patient.

References

Adamovich, B. B. Language vs. cognition: The speech-language pathologist's role. *Clinical Aphasiology Conference Proceedings, 1981*. Minneapolis: BRK Publishers, 1981.

Adamovich, B. B., & Brooks, R. A diagnostic protocol to assess the communication deficit of patients with hemispheric damage. *Clinical Aphasiology Conference Proceedings, 1981*. Minneapolis: BRK Publishers, 1981.

Adamovich, B. B., & Henderson, J. Cognitive changes in head trauma patients following a treatment period. Presented at the American Speech-Language-Hearing Association convention, Toronto, 1982.

Adamovich, B. B., & Henderson, J. Treatment of communication deficits resulting from traumatic head injury. In W. H. Perkins (Ed.), *Current therapy of communication disorders*. New York: Thieme-Stratton, 1983.

Adams, R., & Sidman, R. L. *Introduction to neuropathology*. New York: McGraw-Hill, 1968.

Arseni, C., Constantinovici, A., & Iliesca, D. Considerations of post traumatic aphasia in peacetime. *Psychiatrica, Neurologica, Neurochirurgica*, 1970, *73*, 105-112.

Ayres, A. J. *Southern California Figure-Ground Visual Perception Test*. Los Angeles: Western Psychological Services, 1966.

Baker, H. J., & Leland, B. *Detroit Test of Learning Aptitude*. Indianapolis: Bobbs-Merrill, 1959.

Benton, A. L. *The Revised Visual Retention Test*. New York: Psychological Corp., 1963.

Ben-Yishay Working approaches to remediation of cognitive deficits in brain damaged patients. Institute of Rehabilitation Medicine, New York University Medical Center, Department of Behavioral Sciences. Supplements for June 1978, May 1979, May 1980. (Studies for grant 13-P-556 23 and RT-93.)

Brain, L., & Walton, J. N. *Brain's diseases of the nervous system* (7th ed.). New York: Oxford University Press, 1969.

Brock, S. *Injuries of the brain and spinal cord* (4th ed.). New York: Springer, 1960.

Brooks, D. N. Memory and head injury. *Journal of Nervous and Mental Disease*, 1972, *155*, 350-355.

Brooks, D. N. Wechsler memory scale performance and its relationship to brain damage after severe closed head injury. *Journal of Neurology, Neurosurgery and Psychiatry*, 1976, *39*, 593-601.

Brooks, D. D., Aughton, M. E., Bond, M. R., Jones, P., & Rizvi, S. Cognitive sequelae in relationship to early indicies of severity of brain damage after severe blunt head injury. *Journal of Neurology, Neurosurgery and Psychiatry*, 1980, *43*, 529-534.

Buscke, H., & Fuld, P. Evaluation, storage, retention and retrieval in disordered memory and learning. *Neurology*, 1974, *24*, 1019-1025.

Butler, K.G. Mnemonic and retrieval strategies for language disordered adolescents. Paper presented at American Speech-Language-Hearing Association convention, Los Angeles, 1981.

Caveness, W. F. Introduction to head injuries. In E. Walker, W. Caveness, & M. Cutchley (Eds.), *The late effects of head injury*. Springfield, IL: Charles C. Thomas, 1969.

Christensen, A. L. *Luria's neuropsychological investigation*. New York: Spectrum, 1975.

Courville, C. B. Coup, contre-coup mechanisms of craniocerebral injuries: some observations. *Archives of Surgery*, 1942, *45*, 19-43.

Courville, C. B., & Amyes, E. W. Late residual lesions of the brain consequent to dural hemorrhage. *Bulletin of the Los Angeles Neurology Society*, 1952, *17*, 163.

Cronholm, B. Evaluation of mental disturbances after acute head injury. *Scandinavian Journal of Rehabilitation Medicine*, 1972, *4*, 35-38.

Dye, O. A., Milby, J. B., & Saxon, S. A. Effects of early neurological problems following head trauma on subsequent neuropsychological performance. *Acta Neurologica Scandinavia*, 1979, *59*, 10-14.

Fahy, T. J., Irving, M. H., & Millac, P. Severe head injuries. *Lancet*, 1967, 7514.

Field, J. R. Head injuries pathophysiology. *Journal of the Arkansas Medical Association*, 1970, *66*, 340-347.

Frostig, M. *Developmental Test of Visual Perception*. Chicago: Follett, 1963.

Glick, M. L., & Holyoak, K. J. Analogical problem solving. *Cognitive Psychology*, 1980, *12*, 306-355.

Goldman, R., Fristoe, M., & Woodcock, R. W. *G-F-W Test of Auditory Discrimination*. Circle Pines, MN: American Guidance Service, 1970.

Goldman, R., Fristoe, M., & Woodcock, R. W. *G-F-W Auditory Memory Tests*. Circle Pines, MN: American Guidance Service, 1974. (a)

Goldman, R., Fristoe, M., & Woodcock, R. W. *G-F-W Sound-Symbol Tests*. Circle Pines, MN: American Guidance Service, 1974. (b)

Goldstein, K., & Scheerer, M. *Goldstein-Scheerer Stick Test*. New York: Psychological Corp., 1945.

Greenfield, J. G. Some observations on cerebral injuries. *Proceedings of the Royal Society of Medicine*, 1938-1939, *32*, 45.

Greenfield, J. G., & Russell, D. S. Traumatic lesions of the central and peripheral nervous systems. In W. Blackwood (Ed.), *Greenfield's neuropathology*. Chicago: Year Book Medical Publishers, 1963.

Groher, M. Language and memory disorders following closed head trauma. *Journal of Speech and Hearing Research*, 1977, *20*, 212-223.

Hagen, C., & Malkmus, D. Intervention strategies for language disorders secondary to head trauma. American Speech-Language-Hearing Association Convention Short Course, Atlanta, 1979.

Hallgrim, K. & Cleeland, C. S. The relationship of neuropsychological impairment to other indicies of severity of head injury. *Scandinavian Journal of Rehabilitation Medicine*, 1972, *4*, 55-60.

Halpern, H., Darley, F. L., & Brown, J. R. Differential language and neurologic characteristics in cerebral involvement. *Journal of Speech and Hearing Disorders*, 1973, *38*, 162-173.

Hedberg-Davis, N., & Bookman, M. An information processing approach to language and learning disabilities appraisal. Presented at the American Speech-Language-Hearing Association convention, Atlanta, 1979.

Heilman, K. M., Safron, A., & Geschwind, N. Closed head trauma and aphasia. *Journal of Neurology, Neurosurgery, and Psychiatry*, 1971, *34*, 265-269.

Hooper, R. *Patterns of acute head injury*. Baltimore: Williams & Wilkins, 1969.

Horowitz, N., & Rizzoli, H. V. Complications following the surgical treatment of head injuries: Clinical neurosurgery. *Proceedings of the Congress of Neurological Surgeons*, 1966, 277-287.

Jacobsen, S. A. Disturbances of mental function: Effects of head trauma on mental function. In S. A. Jacobsen (Ed.), *The post-traumatic syndrome following head injuries: Mechanisms and techniques*. Springfield, IL: Charles C. Thomas, 1963.

Jennett, B., & Teasdale, G. Management of head injuries. Philadelphia: F. A. Davis, 1981.

Johnson, G. O., & Boyd, H. F. *Nonverbal Test of Cognitive Skills*. Columbus: Charles E. Merrill, 1981.

Kirk, S. A., McCarthy, J., & Kirk, W. D. *Illinois Test of Psycholinguistic Abilities*. Champaign: University of Illinois, 1968.

Ledwon-Robinson, E., & Beh-Arendshorst, M. University of Michigan Cognitive protocol: Pragmatically assessing verbal-nonverbal communication. Presented at the American Speech-Language-Hearing Association Convention, Houston, 1980.

Levin, H. S., Grossman, R. G., & Kelly, P. J. Aphasic disorder in patients with closed head injury. *Journal of Neurology, Neurosurgery, and Psychiatry*, 1976, *39*, 1062–1070.

Levin, H. S., Grossman, R. G., Rose, J. E., & Teasdale, J. Long term neuropsychological outcome of closed head injury. *Journal of Neurosurgery*, 1979, *50*, 412–422.

Levin, H. S., Grossman, R. G., Sarwar, M., & Meyers, C. A. Linguistic recovery after closed head injury. *Brain and Language*, 1981, *12*, 360–374.

Lewin, W. *The management of head injuries*. Baltimore: Williams & Wilkins, 1966.

Lezak, M. D. Recovery of memory and learning functions following traumatic brain injury, *Cortex*, 1979, *15*, (1), 63–72.

Ligne, M. E., Sinatra, K. S., & Kimbarow, M. L. Language assessment battery for evaluation of closed head trauma patients. Paper presented at the American Speech-Language-Hearing Association convention, Atlanta, 1979.

Lindberg, R., Fisher, R. S., & Durlacher, S. H. Lesions of the corpus callosum following blunt mechanical trauma to the head. *American Journal of Pathology*, 1955, *31*, 297–317.

Mandleberg, I. A. Cognitive recovery after severe head injury. *Journal of Neurology, Neurosurgery and Psychiatry*, 1976, *39*, 1001–1007.

Mandleberg, I. A., & Brooks, D. N. Cognitive recovery after severe head injury. *Journal of Neurology, Neurosurgery, and Psychiatry*, 1975, *38*, 1121–1126.

Meyer, J. S., & Denny-Brown, D. Studies of cerebral circulation in brain injury: II. Cerebral concussion. *Neurophysiology*, 1955, *7*, 529–544.

Miller, E. Simple and choice reaction time following severe head injury. *Cortex*, 1970, *6*, 121–127.

Miller, H., & Stern, G. The long term prognosis of severe head injury. *Lancet*, 1965, 225–229.

Ross, J. D., & Ross, C. M. *Ross Test of Higher Cognitive Processes*. Novato, CA: Academic Therapy Publications, 1976.

Rowbotham, G. F. *Acute injuries of the head*. Baltimore: Williams & Wilkins, 1949.

Rubens, A. B., Geschwind, N., Mahowald, M. W., & Mastri, A. Post traumatic cerebral hemispheric disconnection syndrome. *Archives of Neurology*, 1977, *34*, 750–755.

Russell, R. W. Cerebral involvement in head injury. *Brain*, 1932, *55*, 549–603.

Russell, W. R., & Smith, A. Post-traumatic amnesia in closed head injury. *Archives of Neurology*, 1961, *5*, 4–17.

Sarno, M. T. The nature of verbal impairment after closed head injury. *The Journal of Nervous and Mental Disease*, 1980, *168* 11, 685–692.

Schilder, P. Psychic disturbance after head injuries. *American Journal of Psychiatry*, 1934, *91*, 155–188.

Smith, E. Influence of site of impact on cognitive impairment persisting long after severe closed head injury. *Journal of Neurology, Neurosurgery, and Psychiatry*, 1974, *37*, 719–726.

Stritch, S. J. Diffuse degeneration of the cerebral white matter in severe dementia following head injury. *Journal of Neurology and Psychiatry*, 1956, *19*, 163.

Stritch, S. J. The pathology of brain damage due to blunt head injuries. In A. E. Walker, W. F. Caveness, & M. Critchley (Eds.), *The late effects of head injury*. Springfield, IL: Charles C. Thomas, 1969.

Teasdale, G., & Jennett, B. Assessment of coma and impaired consciousness. *Lancet*, 1974, 2.

Thomsen, I. V. Evaluation and outcome of aphasia in patients with severe closed head trauma. *Journal of Neurology, Neurosurgery, and Psychiatry*, 1975, *38*, 713-718.

Thomsen, I. V. Evaluation and outcome of traumatic aphasia in patients with severe verified focal lesions. *Folia Phoniatrica*, 1976, *28*, 362-377.

Tomlinson, B. E. Pathology. In G. F. Rowbotham (Ed.), *Acute injuries of the head* (4th ed.). Edinburgh: Livingstone, 1964.

Walker, E., Caveness, W., & Critchley, M. (Eds.). *The late effects of head injury*. Springfield, IL: Charles C. Thomas, 1969.

Wechsler, D. *Wechsler Adult Intelligence Scale*. New York: Psychological Corp., 1955.

Wechsler, D., & Stone, C. P. *Wechsler Memory Scale*. New York: Psychological Corp., 1945.

Weigle, E., Goldstein, K., & Scheerer, M. *Color Form Sorting Test*. New York: Psychological Corp., 1945.

Yorkston, K. M., Stanton, K. M., & Beukelman, D. R. Language-based compensatory for closed head injured patients. *Clinical Aphasiology Conference Proceedings, 1981*. Minneapolis: BRK Publishers, 1981.

Kathryn M. Yorkston
Patricia A. Dowden

Nonspeech Language and Communication Systems

Normal speech is an extremely rapid, efficient and concise means of communication. It requires so little physical effort and preplanning that it comes almost automatically for the normal speaker. Often the complexity of speech is not fully appreciated until one is confronted with the task of developing a functional alternative communication system for an adult who has lost the ability to communicate verbally, as a result of a brain injury or a degenerative neurological disorder. Watching these individuals interact in natural communicative situations confirms an observation made by Holland (1977) that severely speech-impaired adults "communicate better than they talk." (p. 173) Wertz (1978) states the same idea in an eloquent way when he writes:

> Somewhere behind the insolvable ejaculations of neurologically impaired patients is a music awaiting lyrics. Putting words to the music is the primary task in patient management, and the variety of songs eventually sung is the primary test of its effectiveness. (p. 17)

The "words" which we are able to provide adults who are not independent verbal communicators may take a number of forms. The systems may be divided into two broad categories (ASHA Ad Hoc Committee on Communication Processes and Nonspeaking Persons, 1980). "Unaided" communication augmentation systems are those that do not require physical aids, for example, gestural techniques. "Aided" communication systems are those that require a physical board or chart, or a mechanical

©College-Hill Press, Inc. All rights, including that of translation, reserved. No part of this publication may be reproduced without the written permission of the publisher.

or electronic device. These systems may serve three functions: (1) as a replacement when no verbal communication is possible, (2) as a supplement when verbal communication is not sufficiently understandable, or inefficient in certain situations, or (3) as a facilitator when speech flows more easily when accompanied by gestures. In some cases, the nonspeech communication systems described here are permanent in that they provide a long-term alternative to verbal communication. With progressive neurological deterioration, however, the communication systems change in order to meet the increasing demands of the nonspeaking individual. In other cases, the systems are used temporarily to provide a means of communication during the early stages of recovery and are eliminated when speech becomes functional once again.

The task of selecting and training an individual to use an appropriate nonspeech communication system, whether aided or unaided, is a challenging one. It requires the clinician's thorough familiarity with systems available and the demands each system would place on a user. It also requires that, in serving a nonspeaking individual, a clinician make at least three decisions in parallel. One, the clinician must decide if an individual is a candidate for a communication augmentation system. This requires a thorough knowledge of the nonspeaking individual's capabilities in such diverse areas as speech, language, cognition, and motor control. Two, the clinician must identify the communication needs of the individual so that an appropriate match can be made between the abilities and needs of the patient, and the communication system. Three, the clinician must decide which of the many alternative communication systems are appropriate for the individual, and consider making modifications based on performance trial results.

The nonvocal adults described in this chapter are individuals who are not independent verbal communicators, and may be labelled as nonvocal, nonoral, nonspeaking, or anathric (Harris & Vanderheiden, 1980). This population is diverse in the etiology and the nature of their communication disorders, as well as in their needs as communicators. The course of the disorder may vary depending on the etiology. Some disorders, such as amyotrophic lateral sclerosis, are degenerative. Others, such as brain stem stroke or traumatic head injury, are characterized by sudden onset followed by a period of recovery and later stabilization. Nonspeaking adults may be diagnosed as having aphasia, apraxia of speech, and dysarthria, or a combination of these disorders. For our purposes, *aphasia* is defined as a disorder of the central language process which underlies the various language modalities, including listening, speaking, reading, and writing (Darley, 1964). It is an impairment in the ability to interpret and formulate language symbols as a result of brain damage. Most typically, the etiology of aphasia is left-cerebral vascular accident, but other common etiologies include arteriovenous malformations, tumor, and focal head injury. *Apraxia of speech* is a sensory motor disorder of articulation and prosody. Although apraxia may exist as an entity, it frequently accompanies aphasia, and may also coexist with dysarthria (Rosenbek, 1978). The apraxic individual does not exhibit significant weakness or incoordination when performing reflexive or automatic movements. There is, instead, an impaired ability to program the positioning of the speech mechanism and to sequence the movements for volitional speech. In its most severe form, apraxia can render expressive verbal communication impossible, while leaving the patient's auditory comprehension relatively intact. *Dysarthria* refers to a disorder of motor control of the speech mechanism resulting from damage to the central or peripheral nervous system, and is characterized by weakness, slowness, and incoordination of the speech mechanism musculature (Darley, Aronson, & Brown, 1975). Dysarthric speakers usually have normal auditory comprehension, can select words correctly, and order them into grammatical strings without difficulty. They usually possess intact reading and spelling skills. The damage to the nervous system may be a consequence of a number of adult onset disorders, including closed head injury, anoxia, brain stem stroke, amyotrophic lateral sclerosis, multiple sclerosis, or Parkinson's disease. The speech disorder may or may not be part of more general motor control disorder, which may limit ambulation and restrict use of the extremities.

Although initially a group consisting of aphasic, apraxic, and dysarthric speaker may seem quite diverse, there are a number of reason for considering the group as a whole. First, a clinical case load in an adult rehabilitation center typically includes patients from each of these diagnostic categories. Second, these disorders often coexist in a single patient. The overlap in communication diagnosis is especially characteristic of the closed head-injured population, where the cerebral damage is diffuse rather than focal. Third, these individuals share one overriding characteristic—the severity of their impairment. Nonspeech systems, whether aided or unaided, should be considered only when an individual cannot communicate independently via speech. Even marginally functional speakers with poor speech intelligibility and speaking rates of 15 to 20 words per minute often find it quicker to communicate verbally with those who are familiar with them than to use a communication augmentation system. However, when interacting with unfamiliar partners, communication may break down more often and a communication augmentation system may be more effective and less frustrating than verbal communication. Fourth, this population is similar in that their language skills developed in a normal manner prior to the onset of the communication disorder. This implies that they have internalized many "rules" of normal communicative interaction such as turn taking, attention getting, or leave taking.

The focus of this chapter will be a clinical one. The authors hope to provide the readers with information that will help them make certain clinical management decisions. First, we will focus on the aided and unaided systems available, analyzing each system in terms of its components and the demands placed on the user. We will also discuss the implications of research and case study literature regarding these systems. For the aided systems, we will touch on the structure of service delivery and future trends. The end of the chapter will be devoted to the needs assessment, which must be completed prior to any system selection, whether aided or unaided systems are under consideration.

Gestural Systems

Gestural communication systems have long been appealing to clinicians working with nonspeaking adults. Indeed, there are a number of clinical case reports which suggest that gestural communication can serve as an acceptable alternative to speech for some individuals. However, there is a growing body of research literature which indicates that gestures should not be considered a panacea for the nonspeaking individual. This literature documents the nearly universal presence of gestural deficits in nonspeaking adults with language-based or motor speech impairments. This discussion will focus on the clinical implications of the theoretical studies and the clinical case reports. First, however, it is necessary to analyze the demands that the different gestural systems place on the user.

Components of Gestural Systems

A number of gestural systems are available and are reviewed in detail by Silverman (1980). Appropriate selection of these systems is dependent upon the clinician's understanding of the characteristics of each system, specifically the symbolic load, motoric complexity, and communicative function of the system. Before electing to teach any gestural system, the clinician must decide if the patient's skills are commensurate with the requirements of that system, and if the system has the potential for meeting the patient's communication needs.

Symbolic Load

Each system of gestural communication carries a different symbolic load, that is, the systems vary in the extent to which a gesture is an arbitrary symbol for the concept it conveys. According to Peterson and Kirshner (1981), the most symbolic gestures "bear a codified or arbitrary relationship to their referent" (p. 335). Listeners must be familiar with the particular code, as in American Sign Language, in order to understand the letter, word, morpheme, or phoneme intended.

Gestures that do not have an arbitrary or symbolic relationship with a referent are typically placed in three other categories: iconic, referential, or coverbal. Iconic gestures are those in which the meaning is expressed in the form of the movement, or where there is a widely accepted interpretation. American Indian Sign Language (Amerind) comprises both types of iconic gestures. For example, "baby" is conveyed by crossed arms swaying cradle-style, and "bad" is conveyed by the widely understood movement, "thumbs down." Amerind is not a language, but a signal system with simple, but vivid concrete representation of the dominant characteristics of objects, actions, or persons. (Skelly, 1979) There is theoretically nothing arbitrary in the gesture-referent relationship and there is no true syntactic structure. Amerind is considered by Skelly to be highly intelligible to the untrained viewer.

Referential, or indicative, gestures are less symbolic than iconic gestures in that meaning is conveyed in the presence of the object itself, for example, pointing to or showing the function of an object in its presence. Perhaps the least symbolic types of gestures are the paraverbal or coverbal movement. According to Katz, LaPointe, and Markel (1978), these nonverbal behaviors "communicate information such as emotional states, attitudes, relative status, turn taking during conversations and other affective and regulatory information fundamental to dyadic interaction" (p. 164–165). These more or less universal gestures, including eye contact, eyebrow raising, smiles, and head movements carry no specific proportional content, but play a significant role in conversational interactions.

It is important to assess the symbolic load of a gestural system for a number of reasons. First, the symbolic load has an impact on the language-impaired patient's ability to learn the gestural system (Griffith, Robinson, & Panagos, 1981). One could predict that a severely language-impaired individual is not likely to learn the large number of symbolic gestures necessary for functional communication. If, for this reason, a less symbolic system is selected for a patient, the potential messages that can be conveyed are limited. For example, referential gestures can only be used in relationship to an object, and coverbal gestures are only meaningful when accompanied by speech. Second, highly symbolic gestural systems are limited in their usefulness for individuals who need to communicate with listeners unfamiliar with the system. The less symbolic systems may be understood without training, as in the case of iconic gestures, or do not need to be understood by the communication partner, as in the case of the gestures used for facilitation of speech.

Motoric Complexity

The second dimension along which gestures vary is motoric complexity. A single gesture may involve only a fairly simple movement, or entail a highly complex sequence of movements. Similarly, some gestural systems consist of simple repetitive movements, such as the "finger tapping" suggested by Simmons (1978). Other systems comprise a large number of unique gestures, such as the 250 concept labels included in Amerind (Skelly, 1979). Furthermore, some gestures are more or less automatic and are paired with other activities, for example, coverbal behaviors associated with speech. Other gestures are clearly volitional movements requiring complex planning and execution of sequential movements.

Motoric complexity is an important consideration in system selection because successful use of some gestural systems may be precluded by problems in motor learning or motor control. Individuals with apraxia of speech often have motor sequencing problems, with movements of their hands similar to the motor-planning problems seen in the speech mechanism. Individuals with severe dysarthria are often unable to make rapid or precise movements with their hands. Several authors are systematically assessing the motor control requirements of signing and its impact in learning (Kohl, 1981; Shane & Wilbur, 1980).

Communicative Function

Gestures may serve a number of communicative functions. At times, they are a replacement for speech when verbal expression is not functional. A number of authors (Eagleson, Vaughn, & Knudson, 1970; Simmons & Zorthian, 1979; Skelly, Schinsky, Smith, Donaldson, & Griffin, 1975) reported favorable results in training adults with aphasia and/or apraxia to use gestures to express basic self-care needs. Others use gestures to facilitate or "deblock" verbal expression. Rosenbek, Collins, and Wertz (1976), for example, suggested that gestures can be used as a form of "intersystemic organization," in which gestures accompany the speech act in a unique form with unique regularity. These gestures are then faded as verbal communication improves. Rao and Horner (1978) described the use of gesture to deblock receptive and expressive skills in an adult aphasic. Skelly, Schinsky, Smith, and Fust (1974) reported increased verbal performance for patients trained in Amerind gestural code.

Davis and Wilcox (1981) suggested that gestures can supplement speech as one of the multiple channels of communication. In their treatment approach, Promoting Aphasics Communicative Effectiveness (PACE), they proposed that gestures be used to supplement verbal expression, writing, communication aids, and other possible means of expression. Selection of a communication mode is based on its effectiveness, and the aphasic individual is encouraged to use any modality or combination of modalities, as long as the message is conveyed successfully. Coverbal behaviors can be described as serving a supplementary function, since they convey certain information necessary for conversational interaction, but do not carry the primary content of the communication.

It is obvious that the three components of gestural systems—symbolic load, motoric complexity, and function—are interrelated. Typically, the most symbolic gestures are relatively independent of speech, and are capable of expressing a large repertoire of unique ideas. These symbolic gestures also require complex sequences of movements. On the other hand, the less symbolic gestures, i.e. referential or coverbal behaviors, require less complex movements, but are more limited in terms of the concepts which can be expressed. An understanding of each of these components is critical in making appropriate decisions about the selection of a gestural system. Figure 9-1 is a schematic representation of the components of gestural communication systems and illustrates the characteristics of two gestural systems. A simple deblocking gesture uses nonmeaningful, repetitive movements to facilitate speech, while Amerind uses the moderately symbolic, iconic gestures and simple unilateral movements to replace speech.

Studies in the Nature of Gestural Deficits

The observation that nonspeaking individuals often do not attempt to communicate gesturally has spurred research into the nature of gestural deficits and the consequences of damage to the left hemisphere. Although much of the research addresses theoretical issues, the results have implications for the clinical management of aphasic or apraxic individuals and must be taken into account in attempting to select a gestural communication system for a nonspeaking individual. Peterson and Kirshner (1981), in their review of gestural impairment, suggested that there are two broad schools of thought regarding the basis of gestural deficits. The first holds that the deficits are related to motor apraxic impairments; the second maintains that the deficits are a manifestation of underlying linguistic deficits.

FIGURE 9-1
A Schematic Representation of the Components of a Gestural Communication System. Illustrated are the components of "deblocking" gestural system and Amerind sign.

Components of Gestural Communication Systems

Symbolic Load	*Motoric Complexity*	*Function*
Arbitrary	Bilateral, complex motor sequences	Replacement to Speech
Iconic	**Simple, unilateral movements**	Facilitative to speech
Referential		
Nonmeaningful	**Simple repetitive movements**	
	Automatic gestures, e.g., facial expressions	Supplementary to speech

Amerind ---→ Iconic
Deblocking gestures ---→ Nonmeaningful

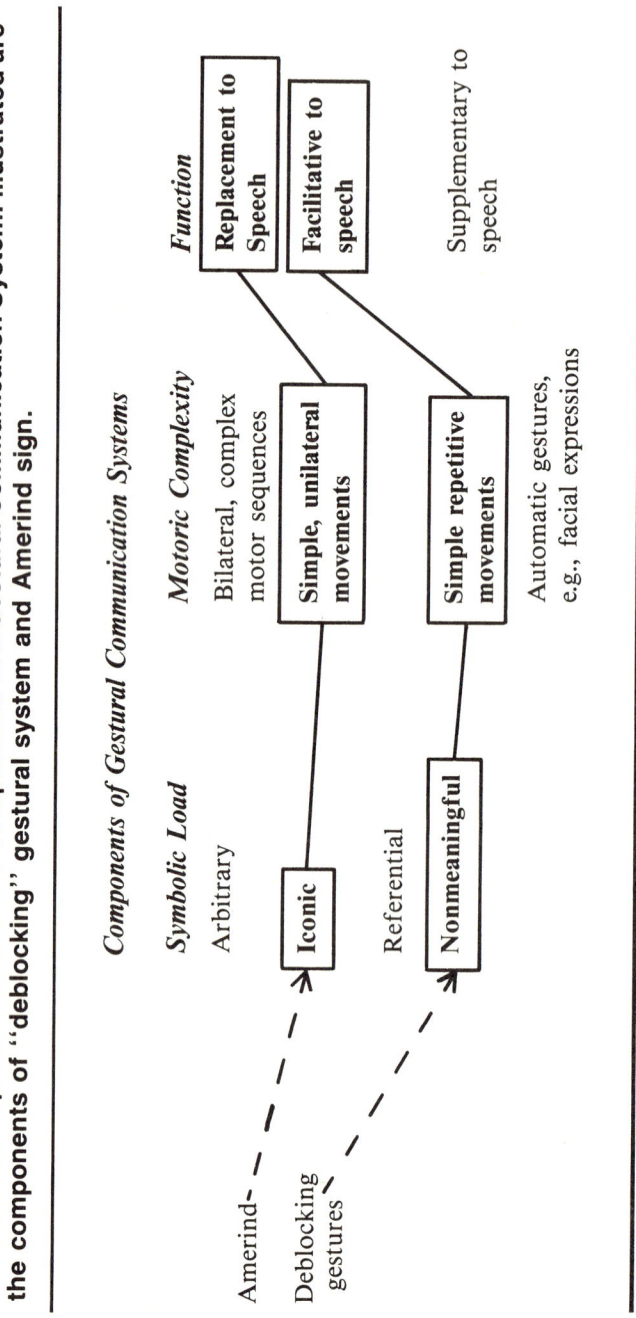

Apraxic Motor Theory

Goodglass and Kaplan, in their 1963 study, proposed that gestural deficits in aphasia are correlated with deficits in motor programming. Their subjects included 20 "mixed, predominantly expressive" aphasic patients ranging from mild to moderately severe, matched for age and "intellectual efficiency" to a group of nonaphasic controls from the neurological ward. The subjects were asked to perform a series of gestural tasks including the following: naturally expressive gestures, conventional gestures, simple pantomime, action with objects, and object description. The results led the authors to conclude that aphasics have a gestural deficiency which is best understood as an apraxic disorder. Goodglass and Kaplan concluded, further, that gestural deficits could not be considered a "central communication disorder" for two primary reasons. First, there was no strong correlation in their study between the severity of the aphasia and gestural deficit. There was, in fact, a "relative independence of severity of aphasia and gestural deficiency" (p. 715), making it difficult to maintain a common underlying cause. Second, their results suggested that the gestural disturbance was related specifically to deficits in the execution of movements, since the aphasic group was disproportionately poor in the ability to imitate gestures.

Kimura and her colleagues (Kimura, 1976; Kimura & Archibald, 1974; Kimura, Battison, & Lubert, 1976) provided additional evidence that the gestural deficits which appear in aphasia may be related to certain motor dysfunctions. In her 1976 review, Kimura stated that the cortical areas important in symbolic language processing may also play an important role in the production of motor sequences. She provided four lines of evidence for this theory:

1. The association between hand preference and speech lateralization;
2. The frequent association of hand movements with speaking in normals, and of vocal utterances with hand signing in the deaf;
3. The frequent association of ideomotor or ideational limb apraxia with aphasia in left hemisphere lesions; and
4. The fact that disorders of manual communication in the deaf occur from left hemisphere lesions, as do disorders of vocal communication. (p. 146)

Kimura suggested an overlap in the neural control of symbolic motor sequences in both the gestural and vocal modalities.

DeRenzi, Motti, and Nichelli (1980) examined gestural imitation ability in an interesting extension of Kimura's theory. Specifically, they studied three dimensions: (1) independent finger movement versus whole hand movement, (2) holding of position versus carrying out motor sequences, and (3) symbolic versus nonsymbolic gestures. Their experimental groups included 80 patients with history of right hemisphere damage, 100 patients with left hemisphere damage, and 100 patients with no evidence of brain damage. Their finding that the left hemisphere-damaged group performed more poorly on nonsymbolic than symbolic gestures led them to conclude that the gestural deficits are not directly related to the "symbolic value" of the gesture. Furthermore, there were no critical differences in whether the movements involved fingers or whole-hand movements, or entailed holding a position or carrying out sequences of movement. Their conclusion was, "what seems to be critical was whether the patient has to organize a sequentially ordered motor program on verbal or visual command, in the absence of contextual or inner motivation, or if the gesture meets a real need" (p. 10). It appears, then, that the motor patterns still exist in these patients, but they are somehow inaccessible without a particularly strong flow of stimulation.

Language-Based Theory

A number of researchers have suggested that gestural deficits are not due to apraxia, but are a consequence of underlying language-based deficits. Several of the authors have come to this conclusion after studying aphasic subjects' productions of propositional and subpropositional gestures. Duffy and Buck (1979) studied both pantomime and facial expression abilities in groups of aphasic, right hemisphere-damaged patients and control subjects. Their results indicated that the aphasic subjects performed poorly, compared to the patients with right hemisphere damage and controls, on tasks including pantomime expression and recognition. However, there were no differences among the groups in the performance of facial expressions, their measure of subpropositional behavior. It was concluded that aphasic patients are impaired in their ability to produce propositional gestures, but not in their ability to make subpropositional, coverbal movements appropriately. Similar results were reported by Katz et al. (1978) who found that coverbal behaviors of a group of 10 mild and moderate aphasic subjects did not differ from normal. No significant differences were found in the mean rate, duration, and average length of these nonpropositional behaviors of the control and aphasic groups. It was concluded that mild and moderate aphasic subjects are not impaired in their use of coverbal behaviors.

Other studies examined the relationship between receptive and expressive language deficits and gestural ability. Gainotti and Lemmo (1976), in their study of 128 patients with unilateral hemisphere damage, found that "within the aphasic group, the inability to understand the meaning of symbolic gestures is highly related to verbal semantic impairment" (p. 457). The authors stressed the link between semantic disintegration in the verbal and nonverbal modalities. Pickett (1978) studied gestural deficits in 28 brain-injured adults and 25 control subjects on eight experimental verbal and gestural tasks, as well as on the *Porch Index of Communicative Ability* (PICA), (Porch, 1967). Of interest in his results is the conclusion that gestural deficits appeared to be "part of the total communicative involvement of the aphasic patient and not a function of apraxia. (p. 102)

Cicone, Wapner, Foldi, Zurif, and Gardner (1979) studied two anterior and two posterior aphasic subjects and their use of gestures in spontaneous speech. Results indicated that gestures closely paralleled speech; that is, the Broca's aphasic subject used simple unelaborated units, whereas the Wernicke's subject produced elaborate and complex gestures which were often vague and unfocused. These findings led the authors to suggest that speech and gestures are either dependent upon language or that there may be a central organizer directing both. Similar results were reported by Duffy, Duffy, and Mercaitis (1979). These investigators studied pantomime performance of two chronic aphasic subjects who showed equivalent overall severity, but distinctive subtypes of aphasia. The subjects' gestures were analyzed in terms of the number of pauses, the numbers of total arm movements and different arm movements, ratings of effort and smoothness, and the average number of seconds per response. All measures were analogous to those used to describe motor speech performance. Results indicated that both subjects exhibited deficits in their ability to convey information through gestures, but their gestural patterns were quite distinctive and paralleled their speech pattern. Specifically, the gestural performance of the Broca's patient was characterized as "constricted," with brief, sparse and unelaborated movements of the hand; the gestures of the Wernicke's patient was termed "excessive," with elaborate arm, head, and torso movements which seemed irrelevant and tangential.

Duffy and Duffy (1981) took a statistical approach in examining the causal relationship between language and gestural deficits. In the first of the three studies cited, these authors examined pantomime recognition in groups of aphasic patients, right hemisphere-damaged patients ($N = 27$), and a control group. Significant deficits in pantomime recognition were found in the aphasic group. Further, a strong relationship existed between deficits in verbal and nonverbal behavior. In their second study, they examined the relationship among deficits in pantomime expression, pantomime recognition, and three verbal measures. Duffy and Duffy concluded that: (1) there was a strong relationship between pantomime recognition and expression, and (2) expressive and receptive pantomime deficits correlated highly with verbal deficits. In the third study, the causal theories of pantomime deficits were examined. From the results of zero order correlations, partial correlations, and multiple regression analyses, the authors concluded that neither limb apraxia nor intellectual deficits were the cause of pantomimic deficits in the aphasic population. Instead, the results supported two possible theories: (1) that deficits in pantomime are due to central symbolic deficits which are also responsible for the language deficit, or (2) that the pantomime impairments are due to the verbal deficits, because nonverbal behaviors may be dependent on verbal modality. According to Duffy and Duffy, aphasia is not primarily, or solely, a verbal impairment, but a communication deficit in the verbal and nonverbal modalities. They maintain that to understand the nature of aphasia, one must also understand the nature of the nonverbal deficits, which are a fundamental component of the communication deficit.

Clinical Implications

Regardless of the differences among these theoretical studies in terms of the conclusions and the models postulated, all the findings are similar in one respect. All researchers agree that individuals with left hemisphere damage and communication impairment exhibit some deficits in the expression of propositional gestures. This finding is not surprising in light of the fundamental similarities between verbal and gestural communication. Both modes of expression have a symbolic component, relying on some arbitrary relationship between words or gestures and the meaning expressed. Both rely on complex sequences of movement which require a combination of volitional and automatic movements, possibly governed by a single neuromechanism. The existence of gestural deficits in the aphasic population comes as no surprise to the experienced clinician who has seen severely apraxic patients who cannot imitate gestures, or severely aphasic patients who do not use either iconic or referential gestures spontaneously.

This review of theoretical literature has been presented here not as part of a critical review of the related models of aphasia, but in order to draw the clinician's attention to the wide range of possible deficits which may limit a patient's use of gestures. It is clear that there is a need for more precise diagnostic protocols that would assess both motor control/motor learning abilities and symbolic/language ability as they relate to gestures. Research has been based on widely varying sampling techniques (Daniloff, Noll, Fristoe, & Lloyd, 1982; Duffy & Duffy, 1981; Koller & Schlanger, 1975; Pickett, 1974). Some tasks sample understanding of gestural communications; others sample gestural expression. Some of the tasks provide instructions verbally; while others base their instructions solely on gestural input. Some of the tasks use pictorial depictions of gestures; some use examiner-presented gestures; still others use video-taped presentations. Some tasks are based on recall and others are based on recognition. In short, the tasks which sample gestural performance are a mixed bag of instruction modes, task types, and levels of difficulty. With the possible exception of Pickett (1974), none appears to provide the broad representation needed to sample gestural performance in the clinical settings.

The "ideal" diagnostic tool would sample gestural performance along several dimensions, including symbolic load and motoric complexity. This diagnostic protocol would also sample the use of gestures in a variety of functions, including the replacement, supplementation, and facilitation of speech. Further, a complete diagnostic protocol would allow the clinician to compare the relative effectiveness of gestural and verbal communication. Some research has suggested such differential effectiveness. For example, Davis, Artes, and Hoops, (1979) found that some aphasic patients used expressive pantomime more effectively than verbal expression. Beukelman, Yorkston, and Waugh (1980) found that severely involved individuals followed single-stage directions given in a combined verbal and pantomime mode as accurately, or more accurately, than when given in either the verbal or pantomime mode alone. It would seem that whether or not gestures are useful for a given patient needs to be assessed empirically with standard clinical protocols. However, complete understanding of a nonspeaking individual's gestural ability is probably not possible solely from an "in-clinic" stimulus-response task format—no matter how complete the task sampling. Clearly, there is a need to supplement this direct testing with observational data obtained in natural communication settings (Holland, 1982). The observation of spontaneous expression and understanding of gestures is especially important in the assessment of severely impaired individuals who may not accurately demonstrate their potential in direct-testing situations.

Clinical Reports

Despite these words of caution found throughout the literature relating to gestural deficits, it would be misleading to conclude that all tasks and approaches in the nonverbal modality should be abandoned for patients with gestural deficits. It is no more appropriate to abandon the gestural mode on the basis of gestural deficits than it is to abandon the verbal modality because of speech or language deficits. According to Duffy (in press), the presence of a deficit does not mean "the absence of a communication skill" in the area of the deficit. Duffy suggested that the best approach is to determine which communication system, or combination of systems, is most functional for a given patient for short or long term communication needs, and then to direct treatment accordingly. Duffy suggested further that gestures have a place in the clinical setting because they may be more "primitive" than verbal communication and, therefore, may require less of the patients' symbolic abilities than speech. This would apply, of course, to the less symbolic gestures as defined above, such as coverbal, referential, or some iconic gestures. From his point of view, gestures may also circumvent some "non-aphasic" communication problems. There are some apraxic or dysarthric patients for whom gestures may be the most appropriate means of communication.

Successful application of gestural systems for nonspeaking individuals has been reported and reviewed in the clinical literature (Peterson & Kirshner, 1981; Silverman, 1980). This literature has important implications for the clinical management of these patients. The selection of an appropriate communication mode requires that the clinician be familiar with factors that have contributed to a successful match between systems and users for other clinicians.

The clinical and research literature contains reports describing the training of a number of gestural systems which differ in symbolic load. Glass, Gazzaniga, and Premack (1973) used a highly symbolic system to study the ability of global aphasic patients to learn symbols. They trained seven global aphasic patients to use an "artificial language," in which paper symbols of various colors, sizes, and shapes were associated with words. Although learning varied from patient to patient, some learned to express simple action statements using symbols.

A number of authors have described the use of iconic systems, such as Amerind gestural code, for training aphasic and/or apraxic individuals (Dowden, Marshall, & Tompkins, 1981; Rao & Horner, 1978; Skelly, 1979; Skelly, Schinsky, Smith, Donaldson, & Griffin, 1975; Skelly, Schinsky, Smith & Fust, 1974). Amerind signs in combination with signs derived from Ameslan (Kirshner & Webb, 1981) or modified Amerind signs (Simmons & Zorthian, 1979) have also been employed. Schlanger (1976) and her colleagues (Schlanger & Freiman, 1979; Schlanger, Geffner, & DiCarrado, 1974; Schlanger & Schlanger, 1970) have written extensively on the application of pantomime training for aphasic individuals.

Iconic signs or nonpropositional limb movements have been used as facilitators of verbal output. Rosenbek, Collins, and Wertz (1976) suggested the use of emblems, a form of iconic gestures, in an intersystemic reorganization program. Simmons (1978) used a finger-counting system to facilitate verbal output for an aphasic/apraxic patient. The author attributed an increased verbal score on the PICA to the "systematic and exaggerated use of this simple and nonmeaningful gesture in a facilitory task hierarchy" (p. 177). Sparks and Holland (1976) used finger-tapping and melody to facilitate speech in their Melodic Intonation Therapy program.

The literature does not provide any clearly defined rules that allow the clinician to predict which patients will benefit from training in gestural communication. However, some trends emerge when one reviews case reports of success with gestural communication. The pattern of these cases suggests that the usefulness of gestural systems, or the extent of the training required, can be predicted by the nature and pattern of the patient's communication deficits. Gestural training has been most successful with patients with predominantly "expressive" disorders, such as nonfluent aphasia, apraxia of speech, and dysarthria. For example, the patient in Eagleson et al. (1970) was described as "right hemiplegic and predominantly expressive" in aphasia type. Schlanger's group of patients (1976) included the following: one patient with hemiparesis, one with apraxia, one with dysarthria, one with "halting, inarticulate" speech and one with "perserverative jargon and good auditory comprehension." Skelly et al.'s patients in 1974 included six apraxic patients, one glossectomee, one dysphonic, one laryngectomee, and one dysarthric patient. Reports of success with patients who exhibit auditory comprehension impairment also appear, although it seems that the training programs must be prolonged. Simmons and Zorthian (1979) report that a fluent aphasic began using trained gestures spontaneously after the seventh month of training, and self-generated signs after the ninth month.

Rao and Horner (1978) listed some possible prerequisite abilities for the use of gestures as verbal facilitators. According to these authors, six skills are positive prognostically for the use of subpropositional gestures to facilitate speech. These include (1) gestural recognition ability, (2) gesture production, including object use, imitation of gestures and spontaneous use of pantomime, (3) facilitation of auditory and visual comprehension when paired with gesture, (4) verbal imitation of single words, (5) good scores on the Raven's Progressive Matrices Test, and (6) motivation to communicate.

Aided Systems

The term *aided communication* refers to a broad group of communication augmentation systems including boards, books, and mechanical or electronic devices, which serve functions similar to those described above for the gestural systems. These aids are designed to replace, supplement, or facilitate the verbal communication of individuals who are not independent verbal communicators in all situations. In contrast to the gestural communication, the area of aided communication is a relatively new one characterized by an ever-changing computer-based technology. During the past several years, an increasing number of systems have become commercially available. These systems, ranging from a modified electric typewriter to computer-based systems with synthesis and rapid printing output, have joined the simple communication boards and books in the clinical management of some patients. Undeniably, communication augmentation devices have enhanced the communication speed, flexibility, and independence of the nonvocal adult for whom appropriate aids have been selected. It has become possible to serve many individuals who had been unable to communicate due to severe physical, linguistic, and cognitive limitations.

Users of Communication Devices

The extent to which communication aids are being used clinically is well beyond the number of reports which have become published literature. Perhaps the best source of personal accounts of devices by their users and descriptions of one-of-a-kind systems is *Communication Outlook*, a newsletter which focuses on communication aids and techniques. (*Communication Outlook* is edited and published jointly by the Artificial Language Laboratory, Michigan State University, and the TRACE Center for the Severely Communicatively Handicapped, University of Wisconsin.) Preliminary descriptions of successful users of communication aids are beginning to appear in the literature. Beukelman, Yorkston, Gorhoff, Mitsuda, and Kenyon (1981) described a series of 13 adults for whom Canon Communicators (distributed by Telesensory Systems, Inc., 3408 Hillview Ave., P. O. Box 10099, Palo Alto, CA 94304) were recommended. This group varied in many respects including age, etiology, funding source, and communication environments. The decision-making process which led to a recommendation of a communication augmentation system also varied from patient to patient. On the basis of this preliminary work, the population appears to be diverse. Disorders may be either degenerative, stable, or improving; they may be adult onset or congenital. The use of devices may be temporary or long term.

Communication aids may serve a variety of functions. They most typically serve as a replacement for speech for chronic severely impaired patients, (Beukelman et al. 1981), for patients who are respirator-dependent, or for patients with acute neurological disease (Henry, 1981).

Some aids also serve to supplement speech. Picture and alphabet boards may be used as a means to re-establish early communication for the recovering brain stem-injured patient (Beukelman & Yorkston, 1978). Alphabet boards have also been used as a means of making the transition from dependence upon a communication aid to independent speech. Beukelman and Yorkston (1977) describe a system in which the individual is taught to point to the first letter of words on an alphabet board as each word is spoken. By providing the listener with additional information, this system permits the patient to attempt functional speech at a point earlier in the treatment program than the level of intelligibility would permit without assistance. Although this system is clearly serving a supplementary function, it may also be facilitating the recovery of speech, since the severely dysarthric patient is able to practice speaking in a functional context. Warren and Datta (1981) reported a case in which a communication aid may have facilitated the recovery of speech. Their patient was a severely head-injured individual with a diagnosis of severe nonfluent aphasia, who was trained to use a communication device with speech synthesized output (Handivoice 110, distributed by H C Electronics, 250 Camino Alto, Mill Valley, CA 94941). Although the patient was considered stable when the aid was introduced, verbal communication began to appear after only a short period of system use.

Despite the diversity existing in the population of nonspeaking adults, these users of communication aids share a number of characteristics that distinguish them from severely physically handicapped nonspeaking children. Often in the adult, severe physical deficits are combined with intact language skills. Unlike nonvocal children, many adults who use communication aids exhibit good reading comprehension, spelling proficiency, and extensive vocabularies. Together, these skills provide the language base which may allow the use of complex communication devices. Further, nonvocal adults, especially those who have a history of normal language development prior to onset, are able to use devices functionally because they do not need to be taught the underlying principles of communication interaction, such as turn taking, attention getting, leave taking, etc. The communication interaction patterns of nonvocal adults are discussed by Beukelman and Yorkston (1982).

Nonvocal adults who use communication aids may also be distinguished from nonvocal children in terms of their communication needs. Because of their intact language skills, nonvocal adults often prefer to communicate subtle differences in meaning with unique vocabulary selection and grammatical constructions. Often these adults are not satisfied with the relatively restricted vocabulary that may be appropriate for use with children who are acquiring language skills, as well as learning to operate the communication augmentation device. In addition to their need to produce unique messages, adults often need to be independent communicators, and may require multiple communication systems, each of which meet specific needs. For example, nonspeaking adults may use one system for preparation of printed output and another for face-to-face conversational interactions. In short, the communication needs of the adult are dictated by a number of social, residential, educational and vocational requirements.

Device Components

It is beyond the scope of this chapter to present a detailed discussion of all possible communication aids. Vanderheiden's *Nonvocal Communication Resource Book* (1978) provides a yearly update of systems and devices. The 1978 version contained over 60 commercial, precommercial, and experimental communication aids. The variety of systems available may initially be somewhat confusing for the clinician who is attempting to select a communication aid. However, like the gestural systems, aided systems may be evaluated in terms of their basic components. For aided systems, these components are control, process, and output.

Control

The control component of a communication aid is the means by which the user operates the system, involving a display and an interface. The *display* refers to the means by which selections are presented to the user. For example, the display for a conventional typewriter is the keyboard containing the complete alphabet and digits. A second type of display consists of a panel or grid containing a number of locations which may be illuminated to offer selections to the user. Some systems contain no control display. For example, in some systems the selections are presented auditorily, and in others, the user memorizes codes, such as Morse Code, in order to operate the system.

The *interface* refers to the means by which the user actually operates the device. Interfaces may involve single or multiple control switches activated by displacement, touch, light intensity, temperature, moisture, or EMG control (Preston, 1980). The selection of an interface for a communication aid depends primarily upon the physical control ability of the user. Minimal physical control may require a single-switch interface in which the user is presented with a series of options that can be either accepted or rejected by means of that switch. Such a system is typically described as a "scanning system." Users with greater motor control can make selections by directly activating a large number of switches. A conventional typewriter is a familiar example of a multiple-switch, direct-selection interface.

The choice of the control option is perhaps the most critical step in the selection of a communication aid for a severely physically handicapped adult. Without an appropriate display and interface, even the most elaborate of aids cannot be used effectively. The display or presentation mode is selected on the basis of the user's visual abilities, cognitive, and language skills. For example, an individual with reduced visual acuity may need an enlarged display in order to make reliable selections, or an individual with poor reading skills, either pre-or postmorbidly, may be unable to use systems with extensive written messages in their display.

The selection of the interface requires the greatest team effort. For adults with severe motor control deficits, the team must develop proper seating and head control before interface selection can be considered. The selection of the most appropriate interface must be made on the basis of specific motor capacity. Specifically, it is necessary to assess the nature of the most reliable voluntary movement, the speed and accuracy of that response, and the effects of fatigue, positioning, and communicative pressure upon the reliability of those movements. The selection of an interface has important implications for the ultimate efficiency that can be expected from a given communication aid. The selection of single switches, although it may be appealing from the perspective of motor control, may be undesirable when one considers the severely slow communication rate which is a characteristic of single-switch scanning systems. On the other hand, the selection of a direct-selection interface, which is relatively rapid but quite fatiguing, may be less appropriate than the selection of a slower, but more reliable single-switch scanning system. In short, a number of important factors must be weighed in making any decision about the most appropriate interface for a severely impaired nonspeaking individual. For adults with less severe motor control deficits, several interface options may be available. In such cases, selection of an interface may be secondary to other considerations, such as the processes or output potential of the aid.

Systems Processes

The processes that can be performed by a communication aid vary considerably in sophistication, from those systems which only transmit messages without enhancing, storing, or decoding them (for example, a conventional typewriter) to systems with complex microprocessing computer-based processes. The general goal of any of these processes is to improve the user's communication efficiency. For the language-intact, but severely physically impaired adult, this is typically an attempt to increase the communication rate beyond the extremely slow rate produced in letter-by-letter selection.

Memory storage and retrieval is a process available in a number of commercial systems. This process allows the user to prepare a message, store it, and retrieve the message by activating a single "memory read" or "recall" switch. For example, the Handivoice 110 contains two memory storage units which can be programmed by the user. The chief benefit of this process is the reduction of the communication partners' time commitment. Using such a system, nonspeaking individuals take as much time as they need to prepare a message correctly; the message can then be delivered to the partner at a relatively rapid rate.

Encoding is a process by which words, phrases, and sentences may be stored in specific locations on a device and called up by the selection of a relatively short code. Communication aids which have encoding capability differ in flexibility. Some are programmed at the factory and cannot be changed without modifying the hardware of the system. Others can be programmed by the manufacturer to meet specific vocabulary needs of the users. Other units are programmable in the field by the user, an attendent, or any adult who has knowledge of the particular system. The field-programmable units offer the most flexibility because their vocabulary or selection options can be altered or enhanced at any time when new communication demands are placed on the user. The Express I (distributed by Prentke Romich Co., Shreve, OH) is an example of a field-programmable unit in which a number of locations can be programmed, and messages called up with the selection of a single entry.

Another process available in some microprocessor-based systems is prediction. Here, the computer predicts the completion of the message on the basis of the first units entered. A language-based prediction system which is currently operating is a Morse Code-based communication device (Wilson, 1981). After the first letter of a word is selected, the device offers the user (on a control display) the most probable completion of the word. If the computer has "guessed" correctly, the user selects a space and the complete word is selected. If the prediction is incorrect, the user simply selects the next letter of the word, and with this additional information, another prediction is made. This continues until the prediction is accepted or until the word is spelled correctly, letter by letter. Linguistic information, as well as the user's most frequently occurring vocabulary, have been programmed into the system to assist the accuracy of the computer guessing. Still another process available in most microprocessor-based systems is that of text editing. Here, the user is able to make corrections in the text, insert or delete portions, or shift the order of elements before the text is printed in its final form.

Selection of the most appropriate process depends to a great extent on the communication needs, along with the user's ability to learn to operate the system correctly. Some individuals require a system to express only basic needs, concerns, and self-care requests to persons who are familiar with them. Others require a system that can be used to express complex messages in educational, vocational settings to strangers. Individuals who must use single switches with scanning displays, or who are extremely slow as they press keys on the keyboard, need communication aids which are capable of speeding up communication. A system with code retrieval, encoding, or predictive capability has this potential.

System Output

Output choices available in communication aids can be divided into these three broad categories—visual, auditory, and electronic. Some visual, and all auditory, output are transient in nature. For example, the output of a communication board is visually transient; the communication partner observes as letters or words are indicated by the user, and no permanent record is left. Visual output systems such as television screens and marquee-type displays are semitransient in that the output is displayed only temporarily. Many communication aids such as a typewriter, strip printer, or computer-driven printer produce permanent visual output. The output of some communication aids is electronic in that the output controls the operation of another system or device. For example, the Prentke-Romich Lapboard Strip Printer (distributed by Prentke Romich Co., Shreve, OH) may operate a TTY computer.

As in the case of the selection of the system processes, output selection depends heavily on the communication needs of the individual. For example, when the communication environment demands that the nonvocal individual interact either with people out of visual contact or several partners at a time, as in a classroom, synthesized speech might be a useful output option. On the other hand, for patients in nursing homes, systems are selected so that messages can be prepared in advance and transmitted rapidly. This requires the selection of systems with either hard copy output or systems which have memory or storage capacities.

Figure 9-2 is a schematic representation of the components of communication aids. The components of some communication aids are simple. For example, the Canon Communicator is a portable tape typewriter, in which the control display contains the letters of the alphabet, and the interface consists of multiple switches or keys which the user depresses as selections are made. The Canon is capable of one-system process, that of direct conversion of the keys selected to letters, and the output is printed

FIGURE 9-2
A Schematic Representation of Communication Augmentation Devices, Including Control, Process, and Output. The Components for Canon Communicator are illustrated.

Components of Communication Augmentation Devices

Control	*Process*	*Output*
Display	**Direct Conversion**	**Visual** — — → Canon Communicator
-letters	Memory storage & retrieval	-letters & -words
-word		Auditory
-control characters	Encoding	-synthesized speech
-no display	Prediction	
	Test Editing	Electronic signals to control other systems
Interface		
-single switch		
-multiple switch		
-direct selection		

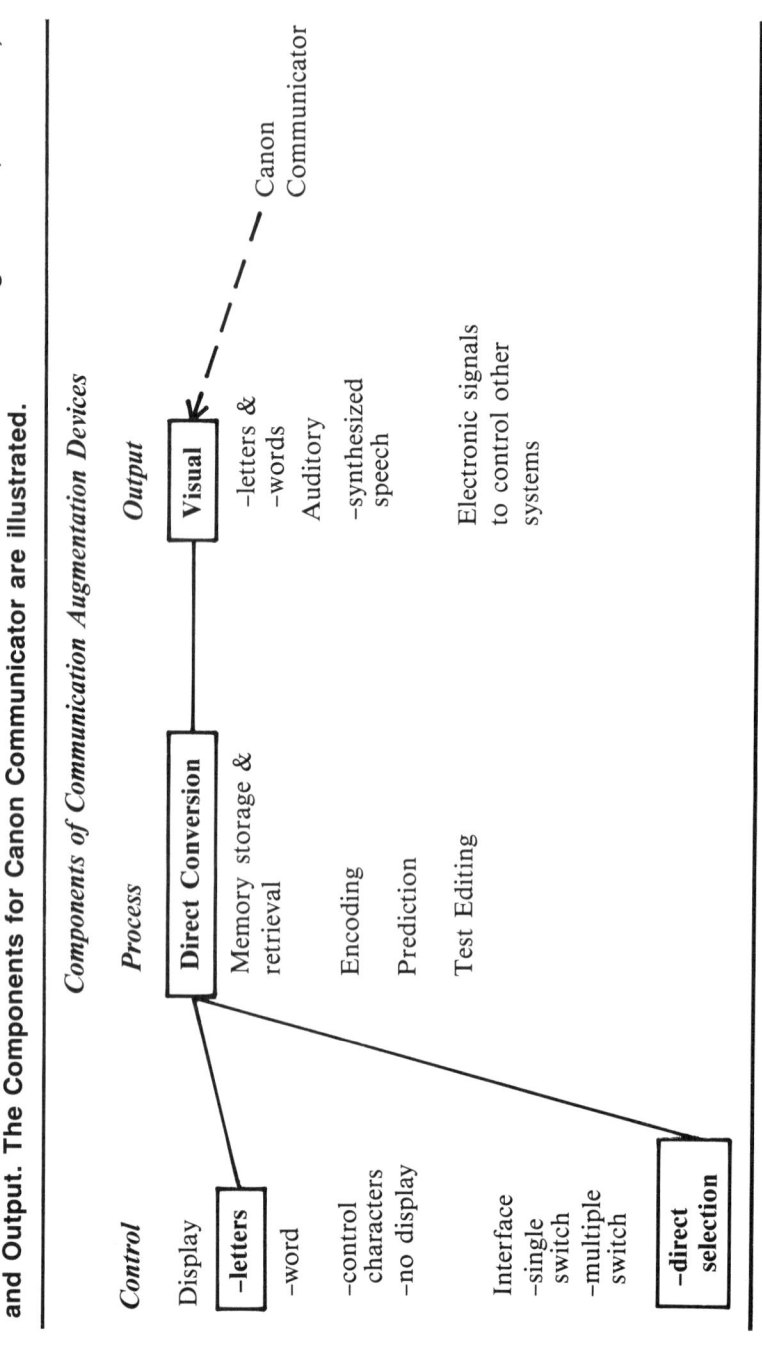

letters on a strip of thermal-sensitive tape. Other communication aids have multiple component options. For example, the Express III system (Prentke Romich) uses a display that contains letters, words, and control characters. A number of single- and multiple-switch interfaces may be used to control the system. The processes include direct conversion of letters into print, memory, and encoding to call up entire preprogrammed messages. The output of such a system may be the printed word, synthesized speech, or electronic output to control other devices.

Service Delivery Systems

An interdisciplinary approach to the selection process is now required in light of the extensive skills and knowledge necessary as part of the service delivery process. Often the selection and customization of communication aids is carried out in large centers where family members together with professionals in communication, engineering, physical control, and adaptation of devices can cooperate. Their efforts are supplemented by the expertise of individuals in the area of medicine, psychology, social services, and vision. Shane and Bashir (1980) suggested that the evaluation process involves two phases—election and selection. The election phase leads to a decision about whether or not a nonvocal individual is a candidate for a communication aid. This process requires both formal and informal assessment of intelligence, language, memory, motor control, reflex pattern, vision, and hearing. Once the election process has been completed and the decision about candidacy made, selection may begin. Selection involves the careful review of the capabilities and communication needs of the nonspeaking individual. Components of the communication aid are then matched to these capabilities and needs.

A third phase of the evaluation process, called performance evaluation, may also be added. The performance evaluation typically involves a period of training followed by a period of trial use of the aid. These trials can be carried out in the clinical setting by obtaining information about the rate and accuracy with which the individual is able to perform a series of message-preparation tasks. Performance evaluation may also be carried out in natural communication settings (Beukelman & Yorkston, 1980). Assessment of performance in natural settings is especially useful in addressing such issues as the frequency of communication exchanges, patterns of communicator initiation, patterns and frequency of communication breakdown and message types.

Future Trends

Communicative efficiency is clearly one of the greatest limitations in the use of communication aids by adults in natural interactions. Even the most optimistic rate of 20 words per minute is nearly 10 times slower than a normal verbal communication rate. Beukelman and Yorkston (1982) reviewed a number of approaches being developed to increase the efficiency of communication aids. Some of these enhancement approaches have been described earlier, including encoding, memory storage, retrieval systems, and prediction.

Other systems designed to maximize communication efficiency use the retrieval of phoneme or letter sequences rather than individual sounds or letters. Goodenough-Trepagnier (1980) and Goodenough-Trepagnier and Prather (1981) have suggested two such approaches for increasing the message preparation. SPEEC, or Sequence of Phonemes for an Efficient English Communication, contains frequently occurring sequences of sounds; WRITE contains frequently occurring sequences of letters. These sound or letter sequences can be combined by the user to form a message.

Another approach to enhancing efficiency is through the optimization of entry locations. Goodenough-Trepagnier and Rosen (1981) have suggested a computer-based model for retrieving the "best key set" for a nonspeaking individual. Three factors included in this model are the number of language units per word, the average number of acts required to encode each unit, and the average time for each act. Beukelman and Poblette (1981) have developed a computer simulation of a row-column scanning system in an effort to identify the optimum location of entries in a scanning system. The relative time to communicate a message can be computed for a variety of display arrangements in a 10 x 10 matrix. The most efficient systems were found to be those in which the most frequently occuring letters were located in the upper left quadrant of the display.

Speculations about future trends in the field of communication augmentation often revolve around the application of computer technology to aid the handicapped. Clearly there has been a trend toward customization in the recent past. This has often taken the form of interface customization. Commercially available devices are often adapted to unique motor needs by customizing switches to allow the user to control the device. As low-cost microprocessing computers become widely available, there is also a trend toward customization of the processes available in communication aids. For example, specific vocabulary and messages can be entered and stored, or any number of output options—including printed output and synthesized speech—may be selected by the user. Microprocessing computers may also function in areas other than communication

(Vanderheiden, 1981). These applications may include recreation and educational activities, as well as systems for management of information, or for control systems for work or home environments.

Needs Assessment

To say that needs assessment is important in the selection of communication augmentation systems seems at first to be a statement of the obvious. However, a thorough understanding of the communication needs of the individual is not a trivial matter. Clinicians often do a better job of assessing the capabilities of their patients, and matching these capabilities with the demands of the systems, than they do in identifying specific communication needs of their patients. Failure to understand and account for these needs often results in selection of a system which is inappropriate, not because it is too demanding, either linguistically or motorically, but because it does not allow the user to perform needed communication functions.

Inappropriate system selection may be avoided by making a needs assessment an integral part of every phase of the selection and customization process. Although no formal evaluation format is available, a needs assessment may be thought of as a listing of a series of specific "needs statements." Many of these needs statements revolve around the messages which the patient needs to communicate. For example, a partial list of needs statements for a patient who is confined to bed may include:

> This man needs to call the nurse.
> This man needs to ask for his glasses.
> This man needs to ask for the bedpan.
> etc.

Other needs statements specify listener requirements. For example, a list of needs statements for a handicapped individual who lives in a residential center might include:

> This woman needs to communicate with nonreaders.
> This woman needs to communicate with people who are not familiar with her.
> This woman needs to deliver her message to listeners rapidly.
> This woman needs to communicate with people who are not sufficiently mobile to come to her.

Finally, needs statements may reflect environmental requirements:

> This woman needs to communicate when she is in her wheelchair.
> This woman needs to communicate when she is in her bed.
> This woman needs to communicate when she is outdoors.

Once a complete list of needs statements is made, it will have a bearing on both the selection and the customization process. There are patients for whom the selection of a device is made on the basis of their specific communication needs rather than on their capabilities. Consider the patient who is able to use an alphabet board, an electric typewriter, and a Canon Communication with equal proficiency, but who resides in a nursing home where staff time is limited and portability is necessary. The needs statements would dictate the selection of the Canon Communicator because it clearly would meet more communication needs than the other systems.

Needs assessment is also an important part of the customization process, in which systems are individualized for specific motor control requirements and vocabulary needs. Severely aphasic/apraxic individuals may not need to communicate many of the "standard" messages that are easily picturable in communication books, or easily understood with simple iconic gestures. For example, most commercially available picture communication boards contain a picture representing the notion "drink." Patients who have independent mobility would be more likely simply to get the drink than to ask for it. Some sampling of the patient communication needs in a natural environment may be required in order to select messages appropriately. Often the patient's spouse or nurse will be able to supply this type of information by keeping a diary for several consecutive days. This diary would contain all messages that the patient is expressing—either independently via spontaneous gestures, or with the assistance of a communication partner who leads the patient through a series of questions and answers. From this raw material a relatively small corpus of messages can be developed. Some of these messages are more easily pictured through a communication book. For example, a calender may be used for communication of time-related messages. Other messages may be more easily gestured. An example of such a message is the universally understood signal for "come here." Working from a relatively small corpus of "needed messages" allows the clinician to train specific messages, as well as to select the most appropriate communication vehicle to transmit those messages. Often, for severely impaired adults, multiple communication systems are appropriate. Perhaps the patient may use highly codified gestures with familiar partners and a communication book with others.

In closing, we will reiterate that nonspeech language and communication systems cannot be as efficient or as flexible as speech. However, they may be the only alternative for individuals who are severely limited verbally as the result of motor-control, motor-planning, or language deficits. There are no hard and fast rules dictating system selection. Of course, the capabilities of the patient and the demands of the system must be taken into account. It is clear that communication needs must also be considered in order to select the most effective system possible. Systematic observation of nonspeaking individuals in natural communication situations would appear to be essential for understanding their needs. This in turn would help us to select appropriate systems, as well as to develop new systems to better meet the needs of our patients.

References

ASHA Ad hoc Committee on Communication Processes in Nonspeaking Persons. "Nonspeech Communication: A position paper." *Asha*, 1980, *22*: (4). 267-272.

Beukelman, D. R., & Poblette, M. Maximizing communication rates of row-column scanning communication systems. A paper presented at the annual convention of the American Speech-Language-Hearing Association, Los Angeles, November, 1981.

Beukelman, D. R., & Yorkston, K. M. A communication system for the severely dysarthric speaker with an intact language system. *Journal of Speech and Hearing Disorders*, 1977, *42*, 265-270.

Beukelman, D. R., & Yorkston, K. M. A series of communication options for individuals with brain stem lesions. *Archives of Physical Medicine and Rehabilitation*, 1978, *59*, 337-342.

Beukelman, D. R., & Yorkston, K. M. Non-vocal communication: Performance evaluation. *Archives of Physical Medicine and Rehabilitation*, 1980, *61*, 272-275.

Beukelman, D. R., & Yorkston, K. M. Communication interaction strategies for severely speech impaired adults. *Topics in Language Disorders*, 1982, *2*(2), 39-54.

Beukelman, D. R., Yorkston, K. M., Gorhoff, S. C., Mitsuda, P. M., & Kenyon, V. T. Canon Communicator use by adults: A retrospective study. *Journal of Speech and Hearing Disorders*, 1981, *46*, 374-378.

Beukelman, D. R., Yorkston, K. M., & Waugh, P. F. Communication in severe aphasia: Effectiveness of three instruction modalities. *Archives of Physical Medicine and Rehabilitation*, 1980, *61*, 248-252.

Cicone, M., Wapner, W., Foldi, N., Zurif, E., & Gardner, H. The relationship between gesture and language in aphasic communication. *Brain and Language*, 1979, *8*, 324-349.

Daniloff, J. K., Noll, J. D., Fristoe, M., & Lloyd, L. L. Gesture recognition in patients with aphasia. *Journal of Speech and Hearing Disorders*, 1982, *47*, 43-47.

Darley, F. L. *Diagnosis and appraisal of communication disorders*. Englewood Cliffs, NJ: Prentice-Hall, 1964.

Darley, F. L., Aronson, A. E., & Brown, J. R. *Motor speech disorders*. Philadelphia: W. B. Saunders, 1975.

Davis, G. A., & Wilcox, M. J. Incorporating parameters of natural conversation in aphasia treatment: PACE therapy. In R. Chapey (Ed.), *Language intervention strategies in adult aphasia*. Baltimore: Williams & Wilkins, 1981.

Davis, S., Artes, R., & Hoops, R. Verbal expression and expressive pantomime in aphasic patients. In Lebrun & Hoope (Eds.), Problems of Aphasia, a volume in Series *Neurolinguistics*. Swets & Zeitliyer B. V., Lisse: 1979.

DeRenzi, E., Motti, F., & Nichelli, P. Imitating gestures: A quantitative approach to ideomotor apraxia. *Archives of Neurology*, 1980, *37*, 6-10.

Dowden, P. A., Marshall, R. C., & Tompkins, C. A. Amer-Ind sign as a communicative facilitator for aphasic and apraxic patients. *Proceeding of the Clinical Aphasiology Conference*, Minneapolis: BRK Publishers, 1981, 133-140.

Duffy, J. F. Comment on Baratz's Case study. *Aphasia, Apraxia and Agnosia* (in press).

Duffy, R. J., & Buck, R. A. A study of the relationship between propositional (pantomime) and subpropositional (facial expression) extraverbal behaviors in aphasics. *Folio Phoniatrica*, 1979, *31*, 129-136.

Duffy, R. J., & Duffy, J. R. Three studies of deficits in pantomimic expression and pantomimic recognition in aphasia. *Journal of Speech and Hearing Research*, 1981, *24* (1), 70-34.

Duffy, R. J., Duffy, J. R., & Mercaitis, P. A. Pantomimic Motor Behaviors of a Broca's and a Wernicke's Aphasic. A paper presented at the Annual Convention of the American Speech-Language-Hearing Association, Atlanta, GA, November 1979.

Eagleson, H. M., Vaughn, G. R., & Knudson, A. B. C. Hand signals for dysphasia. *Archives of Physical Medicine and Rehabilitation*, 1970, *51*, 111-113.

Gainotti, G., & Lemmo, M. A. Comprehension of symbolic gestures in aphasia. *Brain and Language*, 1976, *3*, 451-460.

Glass, A. V., Gazzaniga, M. S., & Premack, D. Artificial language training in global aphasics. *Neuropsychologia*, 1973, *11*, 95-103.

Goodenough-Trepagnier, C. Rate of Language Production with SPEEC Nonvocal Communication System. *Proceedings of International Conference on Rehabilitation Engineering*. Ottawa: Canadian Medical Biological Engineering Society, 1980.

Goodenough-Trepagnier, C., & Prather, P. Communication systems for the nonvocal based on frequent phoneme sequences. *Journal of Speech and Hearing Research*, 1981, *24*, 322-330.

Goodenough-Trepagnier, C., & Rosen, M. J. Model for computer based procedure to prescribe optimal "keyboard." Paper presented at the 4th Annual Conference in Rehabilitation Engineering, Washington, DC, September, 1981.

Goodglass, H., & Kaplan, E. Disturbances of Gesture and Pantomime in Aphasia. *Brain*, 1963, *86*, 703-720.

Griffith, P. L., Robinson, J. H., & Panagos, J. M., Perception of iconicity in American Sign Language by hearing and deaf subjects. *Journal of Speech and Hearing Disorders*, 1981, *46*, 388-397.

Harris, D., & Vanderheiden, G. C. Enhancing the development of communication interaction. In R. L. Schiefelbusch (Ed.), *Nonspeech language and communication: Analysis and intervention*. Baltimore: University Park Press, 1980, 227-259.

Henry, C. Communication for hospital patients acutely deprived of speech. Paper presented at the annual convention of the American Speech-Language-Hearing Association, Los Angeles, 1981.

Holland, A. L. Some practical considerations in aphasia rehabilitation. In M. Sullivan & M. S. Kansmers (Eds.), *Rationale for adult aphasia therapy.* Lincoln: University of Nebraska Medical Center, 1977.

Holland, A. L. Observing functional communication of aphasic adults. *Journal of Speech and Hearing Disorders*, 1982, *47*, 50-56.

Katz, R., LaPointe, L., & Markel, N. Coverbal behavior and aphasic speakers. *Clinical Aphasiology Conference Proceedings*. Minneapolis: BRK Publishers, 1978, 164-173.

Kimura, D. The neurological basis of language qua gesture. In H. Whitaker & H. A. Whitaker (Eds.), *Studies in neurolinguistics* (Vol. 2). New York: Academic Press, 1976.

Kimura, D., & Archibald, Y. Motor functions of the left hemisphere. *Brain*, 1974, *97*, 337-350.

Kimura, D., Battison, R., & Lubert, B. Impairment of nonlinguistic hand movements in a deaf aphasic. *Brain and Language*, 1976, *3*, 566-571.

Kirshner, H., & Webb, W. Selective involvement of the auditory - verbal modality in an acquired communication disorder: Benefit from sign language therapy. *Brain and Language*, 1981, *13*, 161-170.

Kohl, F. Effects of motoric requirements on the acquisition of manual sign responses by severely handicapped students. *American Journal of Mental Deficiency*, 1981, *85* (4), 396-403.

Koller, J., & Sclanger, P. Identification of action words and activity pantomimes by aphasics. Paper presented at the annual convention of the American Speech and Hearing Association, Washington, DC, 1975.

Pickett, L. An assessment of gestural and pantomime deficits in aphasic populations. *Acta Symbolica*, 1974, *5* (3), 69-86.

Pickett, L. Assessment of gestural and pantomimic deficit in aphasia patients. In R. Brookshire (Ed.), *Clinical Aphasiology: Collected Proceedings, 1972-1976*. Minneapolis: BRK Publishers, 1978, 86-103.

Peterson, L., & Kirshner, H. Gestural impairment and gestural ability in aphasia: A review. *Brain and Language*, 1981, *14*, 333-348.

Porch, P. E. *Porch Index of Communicative Ability*. Palo Alto, CA: Consulting Psychologists Press, 1967.

Preston, J. *Controls: Reference catalog to aid physically limited people in operation of assistive devices*. Palo Alto, CA: Rehabilitiation Engineering Center, Children's Hospital at Stanford, 1980.

Rao, P. R. & Horner, J. Gesture as a deblocking modality in a severe aphasic patient. In R. Brookshire (Ed.), *Proceedings of Clinical Aphasiology Conference*. Minneapolis: BRK Publishers, 1978, 180-187.

Rosenbek, J. C. Treating apraxia of speech. In D. F. Johns, (Ed.), *Clinical management of neurogenic communication disorders*. Boston: Little, Brown & Company, 1978.

Rosenbek, J. C., Collins, M. J., & Wertz, R. T. Intersystemic reorganization for apraxia of speech. In R. Brookshire (Ed.), *Proceedings of the Clinical Aphasiology Conference*. Minneapolis: BRK Publishers, 1976, 255-260.

Schlanger, P. H. Training the adult aphasic to pantomime. Paper presented at the annual convention of the American Speech-Language-Hearing Association, Houston, November, 1976.

Schlanger, P., & Frieman, R. Pantomime therapy with aphasics. *Aphasia-Apraxia-Agnosia*, 1979, *1* (2), 34-39.

Schlanger, P., Geffner, D., & DiCarrado, C. A comparison of gestural communication with aphasics: Pre- and post-therapy. Paper presented at the annual convention of the American Speech and Hearing Association, Las Vegas, 1974.

Schlanger, P., & Schlanger, B. Adapting role-playing activities with aphasic patients. *Journal of Speech and Hearing Disorders*, 1970, *35*, 229-235.

Shane, H. C., & Bashir, A. S. Election criteria for the adaption of an augmentative communication system: Preliminary considerations. *Journal of Speech and Hearing Disorders*, 1980, *45*, 408.

Shane, H. D., & Wilbur, R. B. Prediction of experience sign potential based on motor control. *Sign Language Studies*, 1980, Winter, 331-348.

Silverman, F. H. *Communication for the speechless.* Englewood Cliffs, NJ: Prentice-Hall, Inc., 1980.

Simmons, N. Finger counting as an intersystemic reorganizer in apraxia of speech. In R. Brookshire (Ed.), *The Proceedings of the Clinical Aphasiology Conference*, Minneapolis: BRK Publishers, 1978, 174-179.

Simmons, N., & Zorthian, A. Use of symbolic gestures in a case of fluent aphasia. In R. Brookshire (Ed.), *The Proceedings of the Clinical Aphasiology Conference*, Minneapolis: BRK Publishers, 1979, 278-285.

Skelly, M. *Amerind gestural code based on universal American Indian hand talk.* New York: Elsevier North Holland, 1979.

Skelly, M., Schinsky, L., Smith, R. W., Donaldson, R. C., & Griffin, J. M. American Indian sign: A gestural communication system for the speechless. *Archives of Physical Medicine and Rehabilitation*, 1975, *56*, 156-160.

Skelly, M., Schinsky, L., Smith, R. W., & Fust, R. S. American Indian sign (Amerind) as a facilitator of verbalization for the oral verbal apraxic. *Journal of Speech and Hearing Disorders*, 1974, *39* (4), 445-455.

Sparks, R., & Holland, A. Method: Melodic intonation therapy for aphasia. *Journal of Speech and Hearing Disorders*, 1976, *41*, 287-297.

Vanderhieden, G. *Nonvocal communication resource book.* Baltimore: University Park Press, 1978.

Vanderheiden, G. C. Practical application of microcomputers to aid the handicapped. *Computer*, 1981, 54-61.

Warren, R. L., & Datta, K. D. The return of speech 4½ years post head injury: A case report. In R. Brookshire (Ed.), *Proceedings of the Clinical Aphasiology Conference*, Minneapolis: BRK Publishers, 1981, 301-308.

Wertz, R. T. Neuropathologies of speech and language: An introduction to patient management. In D. F. Johns (Ed.), *Clinical management of neurogenic communication disorders.* Boston: Little, Brown & Company, 1978.

Wilson, W. R. A alternative communication system for the severely physically handicapped. Grant to Handicapped Media Services and Captioned Films Program. Department of Education, 1981.

AUTHOR INDEX

Abrams, R., 17
Ackerman, N., 137
Adams, R., 252
Adams, R. D., 85
Adamovich, B. B., 56, 194
Adamovich, B. L., 20, 192, 194, 195, 200, 252
Adelson, R., 51, 52
Ahern, M. B., 133
Aitchison, J., 135
Alajouanine, T., 46
Albert, M., 59, 171, 190
Albert, M. L., 3, 33, 35, 37, 53, 84, 92, 133, 136, 159, 167, 210, 212, 221, 225, 235
Alexander, D. A., 231
Alexander, M. P., 9, 133, 136, 159, 167
Alzheimer, A., 209
Amyes, E. W., 250
Anders, T. R., 87
Anderson, T., 46
Andrew, W., 234
Andrews-Kulis, M. S., 105
Antin, S., 231
Appell, J., 10, 21, 35, 37
Archibald, Y. M., 6, 33, 291
Aretaeus, 209
Aronson, A. E., 5, 17, 18, 29, 30, 35, 40, 41, 43, 285
Arseni, C., 245
Artes, R., 295
Aten, J., 59
Atlas, L., 58
Aughton, M. E., 249
Ayres, A. J., 261

Bach, M., 183
Baker, E., 92, 137, 138, 141
Baker, H., 20
Baker, H. J., 260, 261, 265

Baker, W. D., 135, 152
Baldwin, M., 90, 96
Ball, M. J., 218
Baltes, M. M., 51
Baltes, P. B., 51
Barker, M. G., 222
Barresi, B., 59, 145, 164, 165, 168, 174
Barron, S. A., 234
Barton, M., 182
Barton, M. I., 137
Bashir, A. S., 305
Basili, A. G., 116
Basso, A., 47, 60
Bates, E., 149
Battig, W. F., 104
Battison, R., 291
Bayles, K. A., 7, 12, 21, 22, 24, 27, 34, 58, 64, 210, 221, 222, 223, 224, 225, 227, 231
Beasley, D. S., 2, 13, 84
Becher, B., 142
Beerstecker, D. M., 234
Beh-Arendshorst, M., 252
Belmore, S. M., 98, 99, 100
Benson, D., 147
Benson, D. F., 5, 8, 9, 16, 17, 18, 30, 59, 60, 92, 136, 137, 138
Benton, A. L., 11, 18, 20, 23, 121, 182, 184, 193, 225, 261
Ben-Yishay, Y., 57, 252
Berg, L., 21
Berger, H., 234
Bergman, M., 84, 235
Berlucchi, G., 187
Berndt, R. S., 135, 143
Bernholtz, N. A., 138, 145
Berry, W. R., 123
Beukelman, D. R., 19, 57, 105, 124, 125, 126, 127, 180, 181, 185, 197, 252, 295, 298, 299, 305, 306

Bierwisch, M., 133, 136, 139
Bird, E. D., 217, 221
Birren, J. E., 83
Bisiach, E., 179, 180, 182
Bisiacchi, P., 92
Blazer, D., 27
Blessed, G., 217, 234
Bloom, L. M., 59
Blumenthal, F. S., 56
Blumenthal, H. T., 218
Blumstein, S., 138, 166
Blumstein, S. E., 135, 138, 147
Bogen, J., 184, 202
Boller, F., 188, 214, 220
Bollinger, R. R., 34
Bond, M. R., 249
Bookman, M., 252
Boone, D. R., 21, 22, 223, 224, 231
Borkowski, J. G., 11, 18, 20, 121, 193, 225
Borod, J. C., 81, 94, 103, 106
Botwinick, J., 81, 83, 87, 235
Bourestom, N., 46
Bowen, D. M., 217
Bower, J. H., 182
Bowers, J. K., 82, 188
Boyd, H. F., 261
Bradshaw, J., 202
Bradshaw, J. L., 187, 194
Brain, L., 251
Brain, W. R., 180
Branch, C., 33
Brandt, S. D., 14, 52
Brassell, E. G., 10, 23, 47
Brock, S., 249
Brody, A. R., 217
Brooks, D. D., 249
Brooks, D. N., 249
Brooks, R., 252
Brooks, R. L., 20, 192, 194
Brookshire, R. H., 96, 115, 121, 134, 135
Brosin, H., 42
Brown, C. S., 116
Brown, J., 4, 12, 15, 18, 20, 29, 34, 35, 36, 40, 43, 92, 138
Brown, J. R., 224, 246, 285
Brown, R., 16
Brun, A., 233, 234
Bryden, M. P., 188
Buck, R., 189, 292
Buckingham, H. W., 105, 135, 139, 141, 147
Buckley, C. E., 141

Bugeleski, B. R., 182
Burger, L. J., 234
Burke, D. M., 88, 90
Burns, M. S., 147
Buschke, H., 24, 25, 252
Butler, K. G., 252
Butters, N., 182, 221

Cahn, A., 187
Caltagirone, C., 194
Calvin, J., 139, 141
Camp, C. J., 95
Campanella, D., 172
Canal-Frederick, G., 220
Canero, P., 44
Canter, G. J., 122, 139, 147
Capitani, E., 47, 60, 180
Cappa, S., 148
Caramazza, A., 135, 139, 141, 143, 144
Carpenter, P. A., 96
Carmon, A., 186, 194
Carrasco, L. H., 217
Carroll, J. B., 8
Castaigne, P., 46
Caster, W. O., 217
Caton, C. L. M., 43
Cauthern, J. C., 180
Cavallotti, G., 148
Caveness, W. F., 41, 245, 249, 250
Cermak, L., 221
Chaika, E., 16
Chapey, R., 59, 103, 127, 149, 150
Chapman, J., 5, 16
Chase, T. N., 220
Chedru, F., 15, 42, 43, 54
Christensen, A. L., 261, 265
Cicirelli, V. G., 91, 98, 100
Cicone, M., 173, 188, 293
Citrin, R., 52
Clark, L., 82
Cleeland, C. S., 249
Clifton, N., 235
Coben, L. A., 21
Cohen, G., 55, 79, 81, 84, 87, 97, 98, 105, 202
Cohen, R., 17
Cole, R. E., 82
Collins, M., 142, 180
Collins, M. J., 48, 57, 288, 296
Constantinovici, A., 245
Cooper, L. D., 128

Author Index

Cooper, W., 166
Corsellis, J. A. N., 215
Corso, J., 235
Costa, L., 178, 187, 202
Court, J. H., 82
Courville, C. B., 250, 251
Cowie, V., 218
Cox, C. S., 220
Craik, F. I. M., 86, 87, 88, 90, 234
Crapper, D. R., 217, 218
Critchley, M., 6, 179, 180, 222, 249, 250
Cronholm, B., 249
Crook, T. H., 83
Crosson, B., 11
Cullinan, W. L., 116
Culton, G., 180, 185
Culton, G. L., 56
Cutler, A., 144

Dalby, A., 35, 222
Dalby, M. A., 35, 222
Damasio, A., 8
Daniloff, J. K., 294
Danziger, W. L., 21
Darby, J. K., 15
Darley, F. L., 4, 5, 7, 8, 10, 12, 14, 15, 17, 18, 20, 24, 29, 30, 34, 35, 36, 40, 41, 43, 60, 115, 127, 128, 139, 224, 246, 284, 285
Datta, K. D., 299
Davies, P., 217
Davis, G. A., 2, 13, 59, 82, 84, 96, 107, 114, 135, 142, 149, 150, 200, 289
Davis, S., 295
Dawson, J. M., 80, 85
de Ajuriaguerra, J., 223, 227
Deal, J. L., 12, 19, 21, 33, 35, 37, 47, 48, 192
Deal, L. A., 8, 12, 19, 20, 33, 47, 48, 60, 192
DeBoni, U., 218
Deisenhammer, E., 234
Dekaban, A. S., 234
Dekosky, S., 188
DeLeon, M. J., 233
Delis, D. C., 11, 196
Deloche, G., 145
Denes, G., 92, 198
Denny-Brown, D., 6, 180, 250
DeRenzi, E., 11, 17, 18, 97, 116, 121, 124, 164, 184, 291
De Wolfe, A. S., 17
Diamond, S. G., 213
Diamond, S. J., 187

Di Carrado, C., 296
Diggs, C. C., 116
Diller, L., 56, 57, 181
Di Simoni, F. G., 5, 17, 18, 29, 30, 35, 40, 41, 43
Dixon, D., 53
Dixon, M. M., 127
Donaldson, R. C., 288, 296
Dowden, P. A., 296
Drenth, V., 44
Dresser, A. C., 41
Drummond, S. S., 15, 139
Duffy, J. F., 295
Duffy, J. R., 14, 38, 83, 94, 133, 293, 294
Duffy, R. J., 189, 292, 293, 294
Durlacher, S. H., 251
Dwyer, C., 12, 19, 33, 48, 192
Dye, O. A., 249
Dziatolowski, M., 215

Eagleson, H. M., 288, 297
Ehrlichman, H., 187
Eisenson, J., 6, 11, 46, 47, 63
Elam, L. H., 218
Elmore, C. M., 5
Elmore-Nicholas, L., 115
Emerick, L., 11
Enders, M., 190
Enna, S. J., 217
Ernst, B., 35, 222
Escourolle, R., 46
Esibill, N., 44
Ewanowski, S. J., 139
Eysenck, M. W., 102

Faglioni, P., 116, 184
Fahy, T. J., 245
Fairbanks, H., 16
Farber, R., 17
Farmer, A., 147
Fedio, P., 220
Fedor, K. H., 140, 141, 142, 146
Feier, C., 81, 87, 96
Feigenson, J. S., 214
Feinsilver, D., 64
Feldman, R. M., 235
Feldstein, S., 16, 55
Ferrari, C., 124
Ferris, S. H., 233
Fibiger, C. H., 43
Field, J. R., 250

Author Index

Finkel, S. I., 55
Finlayson, R. E., 13, 27, 28, 34, 53
Fisher, R. S., 251
Fishman, M., 10, 21, 35, 37
Fitch-West, J., 59
Fitzpatrick, P. M., 145, 164, 168, 174
Flamm, L., 200
Flowers, C., 126, 127, 180
Flynn, M., 142
Fogel, M. L., 18
Foiles, S. V., 82
Foldi, N., 173, 293
Foley, J. M., 7, 211
Folsom, J., 14
Fordyce, W., 57
Forer, S., 44
Fox, J. H., 222, 223, 233
Fozard, J. L., 87, 102, 103
Fradis, A., 136
Frazier, S. H., 17
Fredericks, J. A. M., 179
Frederickson, D. S., 212
Freeman, F. R., 45
Freidman, H., 235
Freyhan, F. A., 233
Friden, T., 19, 37, 48
Friederici, A. D., 145
Friedland, R., 45
Frieman, R., 296
Fristoe, M., 261, 294
Fromkin, V. A., 16
Frostig, M., 260
Fuld, P., 252
Fullerton, A. M., 86, 87, 88, 89, 90
Fust, R. S., 288, 296, 297

Gainotti, G., 292
Gajdusek, D. C., 217
Galin, D., 184
Gallagher, A. J., 144
Gallagher, T. M., 139
Galper, R. F., 187
Gambetti, P., 214, 220
Gardner, H., 6, 138, 173, 188, 194, 196, 198, 199, 200, 293
Garron, D. C., 215, 222, 223
Gates, A., 194
Gazzaniga, M., 202, 296
Geffin, G., 187
Geffner, D., 296

George, A. E., 233
Gershon, S., 233
Gerson, S. N., 17
Gerstman, J., 180
Gerstman, L., 57, 81, 87, 96
Gerstman, L. J., 89, 189
Geschwind, N., 15, 26, 42, 43, 54, 55, 135, 137, 164, 167, 246, 251
Gianotti, G., 186, 194
Gibbs, J. C., 217
Glass, A. V., 296
Gleason, J. B., 138
Glick, M. L., 252
Glorig, A., 235
Goldberg, E., 178, 202
Golden, C. J., 11
Goldensohn, E. S., 234
Goldfarb, A., 13
Goldfarb, A. I., 231
Goldiamond, I., 55
Goldman, R., 261
Goldstein, K., 261, 265
Goldstein, M., 179, 215
Goldstein, M. N., 5
Golper, L. A., 44, 123, 126
Goodenough-Trepagnier, C., 306
Goodglass, H., 9, 11, 17, 19, 20, 23, 81, 92, 94, 101, 103, 106, 113, 118, 133, 134, 135, 136, 137, 138, 139, 141, 144, 145, 147, 159, 167, 169, 192, 193, 225, 235, 291
Goodgold, A., 215
Goodhart, M. J., 217
Goodkin, R., 57
Gordon, E., 44
Gordon, H., 194
Gordon, S. K., 97
Gordon, W., 57
Gorham, D. R., 5
Gorhoff, S. C., 298
Gorman, B., 52
Graves, R., 169
Green, E., 142, 145
Greenberg, R., 47
Greenfield, J. G., 250
Greenspan, B., 17
Grembowski, C., 164
Griffin, J. M., 288, 296
Griffith, P. L., 287
Grissel, J. L., 56
Grober, E., 92, 138

Groher, M., 246
Grossman, M., 196
Grossman, R. G., 246, 249
Gustafson, L., 233

Hachinski, V. C., 213, 219
Hagberg, B., 233, 234
Hagen, C., 256
Haggard, P., 186
Haire, A., 59
Hakim, A. M., 214
Hallgrim, K., 249
Halper, A., 92
Halperin, Y., 194
Halpern, H., 4, 12, 15, 18, 20, 29, 34, 35, 36, 40, 43, 55, 224, 246
Halstead, W. C., 11
Hamby, S., 198, 200
Hammeke, T. A., 11
Hand, C. R., 135
Hannay, J., 182
Hansch, E. C., 187
Hanson, W. R., 193
Harasymiw, S. J., 92
Harris, C., 58
Harris, D., 284
Harris, E. H., 133
Harrison, R. J., 10
Hartman, J., 47
Harvey, R. F., 41
Haynes, S. M., 118, 149
Head, H., 180
Healthfield, K. G. W., 234
Hecaen, H., 6, 33, 35, 37, 186
Hedberg-Davis, N., 252
Heilman, K. M., 35, 144, 172, 179, 180, 181, 186, 188, 189, 190, 246
Heimburger, R. F., 11
Helm, N., 59, 66, 127, 128, 133, 136, 159, 165, 166, 167, 171, 190
Helm-Estabrooks, N., 145, 164, 166, 167, 168, 169, 171, 174
Henderson, G., 216
Henderson, J., 252
Henoch, M. A., 84
Henry, C., 298
Henry, C. E., 234
Herbon, M., 58
Heston, L. L., 218

Heyman, A., 21, 35
Hier, D. B., 142
Hildebrand, B. H., 118, 149
Hiley, C. R. 217
Hilliard, R. D., 187
Hirano, A., 215, 220
Holland, A. L., 3, 9, 11, 13, 23, 24, 27, 51, 82, 92, 105, 106, 107, 113, 119, 127, 128, 133, 135, 149, 150, 151, 163, 169, 283, 295, 297
Holmes, R. L., 10
Holyoak, K. J., 252
Hooper, E., 19, 20, 184, 192
Hooper, R., 245, 249, 256
Hoops, R., 295
Horel, J. A., 166
Horenstein, S., 6, 180
Horn, J. L., 235
Hornabrook, R. W., 213, 220
Horner, J., 21, 23, 35, 98, 142, 146, 288, 296, 297
Horowitz, N., 250
Horsfall, G. H., 17, 30, 31, 32
Howard, D. V., 104
Howe, J., 218
Howell, R. J., 16
Hoyer, F. W., 53
Hoyer, W. J., 51, 53
Hubbard, D. J., 87
Huber, W., 149, 199
Hubler, V., 142
Huckman, M., 233
Hudson, A., 53
Hughes, C. P., 21
Hunziker, O., 85
Hurst, L. A., 234
Hutton, G. H., 43
Hyde, M. R., 138, 145

Iliesca, D., 245
Ingvar, D. H., 233, 234
Iqbal, K., (cq), 217
Irigaray, L., 210, 222, 223, 225, 227
Irving, M. H., 245
Issacs, W., 55
Ito, M., 85
Ivory, P., 58

Jacobs, L., 234
Jacobsen, S. A., 249

Author Index

Jacobson, G., 218
Jacoby, R. J., 80, 85
Jaffe, J., 4, 16
James, M., 184
Jarvis, L., 44
Jelinek, J. E., 6, 41, 180, 185, 188
Jellinger, K., 234
Jenkins, J. J., 8, 47, 93, 129, 133
Jennett, B., 256
Jimenz-Pabon, E., 47, 75, 93, 129, 133
Johanesson, G., 234
Johanson, M., 233
Johnson, G. O., 261
Johnson, J., 44
Johnson, M., 164
Johnson, R. C., 82
Jones, B., 187
Jones, L. V., 6, 11
Jones, P., 249
Jones, R., 57
Joynt, R. J., 5, 179
Just, M. A., 96

Kafer, R. A., 53
Kahn, R., 13
Kamin, L. J., 103
Kaplan, E., 9, 11, 17, 19, 20, 23, 81, 94, 101, 103, 106, 113, 118, 134, 137, 159, 192, 193, 225, 235, 291
Kaszniak, A. W., 222, 223, 233
Katz, R. C., 118, 287, 292
Katzman, R., 212
Kean, M. L., 135, 144, 147
Kearns, K., 142
Kearns, K. P., 135, 148
Keenan, J. S., 10, 14, 23, 47
Keet, J. P., 217
Keith, R., 14, 38, 93, 94
Kellar, E., 147
Kellar, L., 92, 138
Kelly, P. J., 246
Kelter, S., 17
Kent, R. D., 192
Kenyon, V. T., 57, 298
Kerschensteiner, M., 149, 199
Kertesz, A., 8, 9, 10, 11, 21, 23, 35, 37, 46, 47, 82, 92, 134, 136, 141, 147
Kety, S. S., 233
Kidd, M., 215
Kim, Y., 186
Kimbarow, M. L., 252

Kimura, D., 166, 186, 291
King, F. A., 180
King, F. L., 186
King, P., 200
Kinkel, W. R., 234
Kinsella, G., 139
Kirk, S. A., 260, 265
Kirk, W. D., 260, 265
Kirshner, H., 287, 289, 296
Kitselman, K., 8, 12, 19, 22, 29, 33, 47, 48, 60, 192
Klawans, H. L., 215
Kleefield, J., 164
Klein, D., 187
Klein, D. F., 43
Kleist, K., 29
Klonoff, H., 43
Knowles, J., 82
Knox, A. W., 87
Knudson, A. B. C., 288, 297
Kocel, K. M., 82
Kogan, N., 91
Kohl, F., 288
Koller, J., 294
Korein, J., 215
Kraepelin, E., 209
Kramer, L., 190
Kricheff, I. I., 233
Krishman, S. S., 217
Kryzer, K. M., 119
Kubota, K., 85
Kuhl, P., 180
Kupersmith, M., 215
Kushner-Vogel, D., 59

Labouvice-Vief, G., 51
Lachman, J. L., 90, 95
Lachman, R., 90, 95
Laird, F. I., 233
Lambrecht, K. J., 123
Landis, J., 169
LaPointe, L. L., 23, 50, 56, 64, 98, 118, 133, 142, 180, 185, 287, 292
Larsson, T., 218
Lascoe, D., 58
Lassen, N. A., 213, 219
Laughlin, S., 167
Lawson, J. S., 222
LeDoux, J. E., 179
Ledwon-Robinson, E., 252

Leehey, S. C., 187
Lehner, L., 142
Leland, B., 20, 260, 261, 265
Lemme, M. L., 133
Lemmo, M. A., 292
Leonard, L. B., 114, 149, 200
Lesser, R., 149
Levenstein, D. S. W., 43
Levin, H. S., 246, 249
Levine, H., 167
Levita, E., 47
Levy, R., 80, 85
Lewin, W., 245, 249, 256
Ley, R. G., 188
Lezak, M. D., 252
L'Hermitte, F., 46, 165
Lieberman, A., 215
Liepmann, H., 164
Light, L. L., 88, 90
Ligne, M. E., 252
Lillyquist, T. D., 87
Lindberg, R., 251
Lindholm, J. M., 86, 87
Linebaugh, C. W., 19, 119, 127, 128, 142, 184, 192, 197, 199
Linge, F. R., 62
Lloyd, L. L., 294
Loban, W., 126
Loewenson, R. B., 214
Logue, R. D., 127
Lomas, J., 47
Lorant, G., 165
Lorenze, E., 44
Love, R. J., 194, 197
Lo Verme, S. R., 9
Loverso, F. L., 145
Lubert, B., 291
Lubin, A., 43
Lubinski, R., 3, 13, 51, 150
Lucas, R., 14, 52
Lucchese, D., 92
Ludlow, C. L., 22
Luria, A. R., 11, 46, 137
Luzzatti, C., 179, 180

Macaluso-Haynes, S. M., 117, 118, 125
MacDonald, M. L., 51
Mace, L., 236
Mack, J. L., 145
Madden, D. J., 87

Magurs, G., 33
Mahoney, A. J. F., 216
Mahowald, M. W., 251
Malamud, N., 212, 213, 216, 218, 220
Malkmus, D., 256
Mandleberg, I. A., 249
Mandler, G., 234
Marcie, P., 6
Margerison, J. H., 234
Marin, O. S. M., 21, 58, 136, 144, 222, 224
Marinelli, R., 51, 52
Markel, N. N., 118, 287, 292
Markham, C. H., 213
Marshall, J., 215, 218
Marshall, R. C. 123, 126, 162, 296
Marshall, T. D., 139
Martin, A. D., 133, 134
Martin, J. R., 16
Martin, L. M., 12, 27, 28, 34, 53
Martin, R. L., 21
Martin, W. E., 213
Marzi, C. A., 187
Masani, P. A., 234
Mastri, A., 251
Mastri, A. R., 218
Masullo, C., 194
Mathieson, G., 214
Matsuzana, T., 85
Maurer, J. F., 84
McCabe, P., 8, 46, 47, 82
McCarthy, J., 260, 265
McDermott, J. R., 217
McDowell, H., 214
McFarling, D., 144
McKeever, W., 187
McNeel, M. L., 41
McNeil, M. R., 11, 20, 122, 193
Meehl, P. E., 48
Meirowsky, A. M., 41
Mercaitis, P. A., 293
Mesulam, M., 190
Metter, E. J., 193
Metzler, N. G., 6, 180, 185, 188
Meyer, J. S., 6, 250
Meyers, C. A., 246
Miceli, G., 194
Michalewski, H. J., 85
Milberg, W., 138
Milby, J. B., 249
Mildworf, B., 225, 235

Millac, P., 245
Miller, B., 180
Miller, E., 57, 249
Miller, G. A., 234
Miller, H., 249
Miller, L., 44
Miller, R., 180
Mills, L., 194
Mills, R. H., 15, 139
Milner, B., 33, 193, 194
Mitsuda, P. M., 298
Mitzutani, T., 214, 220
Mohr, J. P., 142
Monroe, P., 46
Montague, W. E., 104
Morrison, E. B., 13, 51, 103
Morrison, E. M., 150
Morrow, L., 186
Moses, J., 196
Mosher, L. R., 64
Moss, C. S., 39
Motti, F., 291
Mueller, D., 58
Mueller, P. B., 13
Muller, H. F., 234
Mundy-Castel, A. C., 234
Muscovitch, J., 187
Muscovitch, M., 187
Myers, P. S., 5, 6, 12, 19, 20, 24, 33, 56, 119, 178, 180, 183, 184, 185, 192, 193, 195, 197, 199, 200
Myerson, R., 135, 139, 141

Nachson, I., 186, 194
Naeser, M., 166, 167
Narin, F., 215
Nash, M., 87
Nasti, A., 51, 52
Nebes, R. D., 87, 96, 105
Nelson, H. E., 21
Neophytides, A., 220
Newcombe, F., 162, 184
Nichelli, P., 184, 291
Nicholas, L. E., 96, 135
Nikaido, A. M., 82
Noll, J. D., 97, 141, 294
Norman, D. A., 86
North, A. J., 117, 118, 125
Nuttall, K., 218

Obler, L. K., 3, 53, 84, 92, 210, 221, 222, 225, 227, 231, 235
Obrist, W. D., 234
O'Connell, A., 21
O'Connell, E., 53
O'Connell, P., 53, 147
O'Connell, P. F., 147
Oden, S. E., 119
Ojemann, G. A., 9
Orgass, B., 97
Ornstein, R., 184, 202
Orzeck, A. Z., 11
Osgood, C., 198
Osler, W., 1
Ostwald, P. F., 16
Overman, C. A., 222

Paivio, A., 182, 183
Panagos, J. M., 287
Parkinson, A. M., 186
Parkinson, S. R., 86, 87
Parsons, O., 12
Patrick, J. W., 82
Patterson, K., 202
Pear, B. L., 233
Pearl, R., 234
Pease, D. M., 139
Peck, M., 13
Perani, D., 179, 180
Perceman, E., 92, 138
Perl, D. P., 217
Perry, E. K., 217
Perry, R. H., 217
Peters, T. J., 13
Peterson, L., 287, 289, 296
Phillips, D. S., 123
Piaget, J., 224
Pickett, L., 293, 294
Pieczuro, A., 164
Pillon, B., 165
Poblette, M., 306
Podraza, B. L., 93, 94, 139
Poeck, K., 97, 149, 199
Pollack, M., 13, 43
Pollock, M., 213, 220
Poon, L. W., 103
Porch, B. E., 10, 11, 14, 17, 19, 21, 23, 37, 48, 93, 113, 123, 134, 161, 192, 293
Porec, J., 19, 37
Prather, P., 306

Author Index

Premack, D., 296
Prescott, T. E., 11, 17, 20, 122, 145, 193
Preston, J., 300
Previdi, 116
Primavera, L. H., 51, 52
Prins, R., 47
Prinsloo, T., 234
Prinz, P. M., 149, 150
Priozollo, F. J., 187
Purisch, A. D., 11
Pylyshn, Z., 183
Pyrek, J., 13

Quittkat, S., 217

Rabbitt, P., 235
Rabins, P. V., 236
Randolph, S. R., 97
Rao, P. R., 116, 288, 296, 297
Rapaczynski, W., 187
Rasmussen, T., 33
Ratcliff, G., 182
Rathbone-McCuan, E., 53
Ratusnik, D. L., 58, 222, 223
Rau, M. T., 123, 126
Rausch, M. A., 17
Raven, J., 82
Raven, J. C., 23, 82
Rebok, G. W., 51
Records, L. E., 21, 37, 38, 39
Reichstein, M. B., 17
Reisberg, B., 213, 218, 227, 233, 237
Reisine, T. D., 217
Reitan, R. M., 11
Rekart, D. M., 139
Remier, A., 33
Resch, J. A., 214
Ribancourt, B., 46, 67
Richardson, S. M., 149
Riege, W., 193
Riegel, K. F., 89
Rigrodsky, S., 13, 51, 103, 128, 150
Rioch, M. J., 43
Risberg, J., 233
Rivers, D. L., 194, 197
Rizvi, S., 249
Rizzolatti, C., 187
Rizzoli, H. V., 250
Roberts, M. A., 233
Robinson, J. H., 287
Rochester, S. R., 16

Rochford, G., 35, 222
Roch Lecours, A., 147
Roessmann, V., 214, 220
Roger, S. N., 235
Rollman, G., 194
Rose, J. E., 14, 52, 246, 249
Rose, P., 52
Rosen, M. J., 306
Rosenbek, J. C., 8, 9, 23, 65, 67, 133, 142, 190, 285, 288, 296
Ross, C. M., 261
Ross, E. D., 190
Ross, J. D., 261
Roth, M., 234
Rothi, L. J., 144, 172
Rouillon, F., 147
Rowan, A. J., 234
Rowbotham, G. F., 251
Rowher, W. D., 182
Rubens, A., 159, 164, 167
Rubens, A. B., 46, 251
Rudd, S. M., 45
Rupp, R. R., 84
Russell, D. S., 250
Russell, R. W., 245, 249, 250, 251
Russell, W. R., 184, 249
Russo, M., 182

Sabadel, 165
Sadowsky, D., 234
Saffran, E. M., 21, 58, 136, 144, 222, 224
Safron, A., 246
Sahoske, P., 164
Salzman, C., 80
Sanders, S. B., 142
Sarno, M. T., 6, 11, 47, 97, 246
Sarwar, M., 246
Saul, R. E., 85
Saxon, S. A., 249
Schachter, J., 149
Schaeffer, J. N., 56
Schaie, K. W., 81, 82, 83
Schaier, A. H., 98, 100
Scheerer, M., 261, 265
Scheinberg, P., 219
Schilder, P., 189, 249
Schinsky, L., 288, 296, 297
Schlanger, B., 296
Schlanger, B. B., 189
Schlanger, P., 189, 294, 296
Schlanger, P. H., 296, 297

Author Index

Scholes, R. J., 144, 189
Schuell, H., 8, 11, 12, 21, 47, 93, 129, 133, 198
Schulz, U., 85
Schwartz, G., 234
Schwartz, H. D., 186
Schwartz, M. F., 21, 58, 136, 144, 222, 224,
Scott, D. F., 234
Searle, J. R., 149
Selby, G., 214
Selinger, M., 145
Semenza, C., 92
Semmes, J., 178
Serby, M., 215
Seron, X., 145
Shafer, N., 142
Shane, H., 93, 94
Shane, H. C., 305
Shane, H. D., 288
Shapiro, B., 194
Shaughnessy, A., 142
Sheppard, A., 92
Sherman, J. A., 55
Shewan, C. M., 94, 122, 147
Short, M. J., 234
Sidman, R. L., 250
Sidtis, J., 194
Signoret, J., 165
Silfverskiold, P., 233
Silverman, F. H., 286, 296
Silverman, J., 200
Simmons, N., 288, 296
Simon, G. A., 41
Simpson, S. C., 53
Sinatra, K. S., 252
Sjorgren, T., 218
Skelly, M., 287, 288, 296, 297
Sklar, M., 11
Slater, E., 218
Smith, A., 86, 87, 88, 89, 90, 249
Smith, A. J., 217
Smith, C., 180
Smith, E., 249
Smith, K. C., 13
Smith, R. W., 288, 296, 297
Snow, C., 47
Snyder, L. H., 13
Sobel, L., 46
Solomon, K., 51
Sparf, B., 217

Sparks, R., 59, 171, 190, 297
Sperry, R. W., 184
Spiers, P. A., 11
Spink, J. M., 235
Spinnler, H., 182, 184
Spokes, E., 217
Sprafkin, J. N., 51, 52
Spreen, O., 11, 18, 20, 23, 121, 193, 225
Spring, C., 21, 35, 37
Stachowiak, F. F., 199
Stachowiak, F. J., 149
Stanton, K. M., 57, 180, 181, 185, 252
Steinhauer, M. B., 53
Stengel, E., 222
Stern, G., 249
Stone, C. P., 261
Stones, M. J., 104
Storandt, M., 81, 83, 87, 235
Strauss, E., 187
Stritch, S. J., 250, 251
Strohner, H., 17
Suberi, M., 187
Sutherland, B., 92
Sweet, R. D., 214
Swinney, D. A., 87, 144
Swisher, L. P., 6, 97

Talley-Kenyon, V. T., 180, 181, 185
Taub, H., 98, 99
Taylor, M. A., 17
Taylor, M. M., 56
Taylor, O. L., 87
Teasdale, G., 256
Teasdale, J., 246, 249
Terry, R. D., 216, 220
Thomas, J. C., 55, 102
Thompson, C. K., 142
Thompson, L. W., 85
Thomsen, I. V., 246, 249
Thorpe, P., 126
Thronesbery, C., 90, 95
Thurston, S., 16
Till, R. E., 95
Tillman, D., 89
Tissot, R., 223, 227
Todt, E. H., 16
Tomlinson, B. E., 213, 216, 217, 234, 250
Tomoeda, C. K., 222, 223, 225, 227
Tompkins, C., 123, 126
Tompkins, C. A., 296

Author Index 323

Tonkovich, J. D., 135, 145
Toone, B., 234
Treciokas, L. J., 213
Tucker, D. M., 189, 190

Ulatowska, H. K., 117, 118, 125, 135, 149, 152
Umilita, C., 187
Urell, T., 86, 87

Valenstein, E., 84, 85, 180, 189
Van Allen, M. W., 18, 184
Vanderheiden, G., 300
Vanderheiden, G. C., 284, 306
Van Eeckhout, P., 165
Varney, N. R., 182
Vaughn, G. R., 288, 297
Vigna, C., 187
Vignolo, L., 47, 60, 164
Vignolo, L. A., 11, 17, 18, 47, 97, 121, 148, 182
Voke, J., 84
von Stockert, T. R., 135, 144
Vrtunsk, P. B., 186

Wagenaar, E., 47
Wales, R., 139
Walker, E., 249, 250
Wallace, G., 187
Waller, M. R., 115
Walsh, D. A., 90, 95, 96
Walton, J. N., 250, 251
Wang, H. S., 212
Wang, M., 217
Wapner, W., 173, 188, 196, 198, 200, 293
Warren, R. L., 11, 87, 299
Warrington, E. K., 184, 222
Watson, J. M., 21, 37, 38, 39
Watson, R. T., 35, 179, 180, 186, 188, 189, 190
Waugh, N. C., 102
Waugh, P. F., 295
Webb, W., 296
Weber, R. J., 183
Wechsler, D., 226, 231, 260, 261, 265
Weigl, E., 133, 136, 139
Weigle, E., 261
Weinberg, J., 56, 181
Weingartner, H., 55
Weinstein, E. A., 6
Weinstein, S., 182

Weintraub, S., 20, 101, 137, 190, 193
Weisbroth, S., 44
Weiss, G. H., 41
Welford, A. T., 235
Wells, C. E., 33, 34, 36
Wepman, J. M., 6, 11, 33, 87, 133
Wertz, R. T., 8, 10, 12, 19, 21, 22, 23, 33, 35, 37, 46, 47, 48, 54, 60, 61, 65, 114, 133, 142, 283, 288, 296
West, J., 183
West, J. F., 6, 56
West, R., 81, 83
Whitaker, H. A., 223, 227
White, P., 217
Wilbur, R. B., 288
Wilcox, J. M., 59, 114, 135, 149, 150, 200, 289
Williams, C. D., 27
Williams, G. D., 218
Williams, I. E., 217
Williams, S. E., 139
Wilson, R. S., 222, 223
Wilson, W. P., 234
Wilson, W. R., 302
Winner, E., 199
Wisniewski, H. M., 216, 217, 218, 220
Wisniewski, K., 218
Wolfe, V., 58
Wolfson, S., 172
Woliver, R. E., 82
Woll, G., 17
Woodcock, R. W., 261
Woodford, R. B., 233
Wright, E. A., 234
Wright, V., 44

Yairi, E., 235
Yamamura, H. I., 217
Yamaura, H., 85
Yarnell, P., 46
Yavin, E., 217
Yorkston, K. M., 19, 56, 57, 105, 124, 125, 126, 127, 180, 181, 185, 197, 252, 295, 298, 299, 305, 306

Zaidel, E., 184, 202
Zimmerman, H. M., 215
Zorthian, A., 288, 296, 297
Zuger, R. R., 44
Zurif, E. B., 139, 141, 144, 173, 186, 293

SUBJECT INDEX

A

Acetylocholinesterase (ACT), 216–217
Aging (*see also* Aging/normal language, Alzheimer's disease, Aphasia, Dementia)
   & prognosis, 106–108
   & staff interaction, 51–53
   assessment, 13–14, 81–83
   environmental influence, 2–4, 12–14
   environmental modification, 51–54
   foster care, geriatric, 53
   group therapy, 52–53
   hearing loss (presbycusis), 2–3, 84
   institutionalization, depression, 27
   normal, 2–4, 12–14, 26–27, 43, 51–55, 80–81
   normal vs. pathological, 79–82, 234–235
Aging/normal language, 2–3, 79–108
   central nervous system (CNS), 84–85, 107
   classic aging pattern, 82–83, 235
   cognitive functions, 80–82
   CT scans, 85
   dichotic listening, 82, 86
   function studies, 92–101
   hearing loss (presbycusis), 2–3, 84
   language comprehension, 83–84, 86, 94, 96–100
   linguistic function, 83–108
   memory, 85–92
   right-hemisphere (RH) function, 82–83
   sentence production, 105
   vocabulary performance, 83–84
   vs. aphasia, 79–82
   word retrieval, 101–104
Agnosia, 17, 189
Agrammatism, 144, 174
Alphabet boards, 299

Alzheimer's disease (*see also* Dementia)
   cerebral blood flow abnormalities, 233
   characteristics, 215
   diagnosis, 230–231
   etiology, 213–218
   Family Handbook, 236
   genetics, 218–219
   Huntington's disease, 215
   language, 210–217, 219–220, 223, 225–227
   morphology, 215–216
   national organizations, 238
   Parkinson's disease, 213–215
   prognosis, 46
   treatment, 58, 237
American Indian Sign Language (Amerind), 287–288, 296
American Sign Language (Ameslan), 287, 296
Amnesia, 249
Amygdala, 85, 216
Anagram, 144
Analysis, discriminant function, 22
Anomia, 17, 141–142, 249
   aging, 104
   anaphora, indefinite, 105
   classification, 137–138
   treatment, 142–143
Anosognosia, 179, 192
Aphasia (*see also* Aphasia mild, Aphasia moderate, Aphasia severe, Broca's aphasia, Wernicke's aphasia)
   adults, 89
   amnestic, 246
   & aging deficits, 79–82
   & apraxia, 7–9
   anomic, 105

326   Subject Index

anterior, 92, 185
appraisal tools selection, 22-25
assessment, 22-25, 79, 82, 113-114, 121, 133-134, 159-166
auditory comprehension, 8, 162-163
closed head trauma, 46
co-existing disorders, 8-9, 37-39
cognitive systems, 79
coping deficits, 60-61
"crossed," 33
definition, 7-9, 36, 160, 284
diagnosis, 25, 36-39, 79, 133
dissociation of functions, 136-137
dysarthria, 9, 246
etiology, 47, 285
eye contact, 119
fluent, 148, 248
gestural deficits, 291-294
global, 160, 165-171
hearing loss, 107
intellectual impairment, 9, 37
language disruption, 135
language of confusion, 9
lesion impairment, 143
lexical-semantic abilities, 141
Melodic Intonation Therapy, 59
non-fluent, 248, 297
percentage of neurogenic disorders, 9
population, 93
posterior, 92
prognosis, 46-48, 107-108
Promoting Aphasics' Communicative Effectiveness (PACE), 59
semantic memory, 89, 91, 92
sentence production, 105
short-term memory, 87
subclinical, 246
test norms, 93
tests, 10-12, 17 (see also Tests)
treatment, 59-61, 127-129, 146, 166, 168-175
vs. dementia, 37-38
vs. schizophrenia, 17-18, 24-30
Visual Action Therapy, 59
Voluntary Control of Involuntary Utterances, 59
Aphasia, mild, 113-129
assessment, 121-127, 134
auditory comprehension, 114-116, 121-124
communicative burden, 119

coverbal behavior, 118-119, 149
discourse, connected, 117-118
distractor tasks, 115-116, 120
dysfluency, 116-117, 120
language reduction, 117
spoken vs. written, 118
treatment, 127-129
verbal expression, 116-118, 124-126
word retrieval, 116-117
Aphasia, moderate, 133-152
assessment, 133-134
dissociation of functions, 136-137
lexical-semantic disruption, 137-142
morphosyntactic disruption, 143-146
phonological disruption, 146-148
pragmatic disruption, 148-151
prosaic-phonologic factors, 144-145
psycholinguistics, 135
treatment, 137, 143, 145-146, 151
Aphasia, severe, 134, 159-175
assessment, 159-166, 175
auditory comprehension, 162-163
Broca's, 160 (see also Broca's aphasia)
classification, 160, 175
definition, 159
global, 160, 166-168
informal assessment, 164-165
mixed transcortical aphasia, 160
neurobehavioral features spared, 160
nonstandardized testing, 162-165
patient verbal strategies, 165
qualitative assessment, 160-166, 175
reading, 163
severity rating, 159-160
standardized testing, 159-161 (see also Tests)
treatment, 166, 168-175
unclassifiable, 168-171
Wernicke's, 160, 171-175 (see also Wernicke's aphasia)
writing, 163
Aphasiology, 107, 129
Aphemia, 159-160
Appraisal (see Assessment
Apraxia, 9
& aphasia, 164, 167, 297
constructional, 179, 184
definition, 285
limb, 164
oral/facial, 164
speech, 288

Subject Index

Apraxic motor theory, in gestural deficits, 291
Aprosodia, 190
Assessment (*see also* Tests)
   aging, 13-14
   aphasia, 22-25, 36-39, 79
   aphasia, mild, 121
   aphasia, moderate, 133
   aphasia, severe, 159-168
   aphasia vs. apraxia, 164, 167
   appraisal of tests, 10-12
   auditory comprehension, 121-124
   closed head injury (CHI), 254-255, 263-265
   co-existing disorders, 9-10, 40
   cognitive function, 80-81, 260-263
   communicative efficiency, 126-127
   comprehension, 115
   computerized tomography scan (CT scan), 12, 45, 166-167, 169-172
   cross-sectional design, 81
   definition, 10
   dementia, 20-22, 33-36
   evaluation methods, 255
   gestures, 294-295
   informal tests, 164-165
   language of confusion, 14-15, 28-29
   lesion localization, 166
   neuropsychological tests, 11-12
   normal aging, 12-14
   pseudodementia, 20
   psycholinguistic, 134
   purposes of, 64-65
   right-hemisphere involvement, 18-20, 30, 33
   schizophrenia, 15-18, 29-30
   semantic disruption, 140
   unclassifiable severe aphasia, 168-171
   Wernicke's severe aphasia, 173-174
   whole body commands, 164
   "window writing" technique, 163
Atrophy, 85
Auditory comprehension (*see* Comprehension, auditory)

B

Behavioral characteristics, post CHI, 255-256
Behavioral rating scale, post CHI, 256-260
Behavioral therapy, 58
Bilateral brain injury, 29, 34
Biostatisticians, 66
Body image disorders, 5
Body schema, 180
Boston Diagnostic Aphasia Examination (BDAE), 11
   aging, 81
   aphasia, 23-24, 36-37, 39, 118
   aphasia, mild, 113
   aphasia, moderate, 134
   aphasia, severe, 160-165, 167, 169-174
   cookie theft picture, 124-126, 167, 197, 235
   disadvantages, 161-162
   global aphasia, 167
   nonstandardized administration, 162-164
   normal adult performance, 94
   reading, 163-164
   right-hemisphere (RH) impairment, 19-20, 192-197
   stroke, 162-163
   word retrieval, 102
   writing, 163
Brain injury, bilateral, 9-10, 29
Broca's aphasia
   aging, 92
   aphasia, moderate, 139-142, 144-147
   aphasia, severe, 160
   gestures, 293

C

Canon Communicator, 303, 308
Central nervous system, 4, 7, 84-85, 107
Cerebral blood flow, regional (rCBF), 233
Cerebral cortex, 85
   hemisphere specialization, 202
Cerebral edema, post CHI, 250
Cerebral paralysis, post CHI, 251
Cerebral vascular accident (CVA), 9 (*see also* Aphasia, right-hemisphere)
   & prognosis, 46-47
   bilateral, 9-10
   language restoration, 39
   left-hemisphere, 65, 167-173
   nonstandardized testing, 162-164
   right hemiplegia, 165
   treatment, 166-175

Subject Index

Cholinergic system, 216-217
Chronic brain syndrome, 210
Classic aging pattern, 82-83, 235
Closed head injury (CHI), 245-277
  & aphasia, 46
  assessment, 254, 260, 263-265
  behavior characteristics, 255
  cerebral edema, 250
  cognitive dysfunction, 248, 258-263
  confused language, 246
  definition, 250
  environmental manipulation, 266-267
  language dysfunction, 148, 246-248
  left temporal, 173-175
  molecular commotion, 250
  neurological dysfunction, 250-251
  treatment, 174-175, 265-277
Cognitive disorganization, 195, 248, 252-254, 261
Cognitive function, 80-82
  assessment, 260
  cross-sectional design, 81
  language behavior, 276
  levels, 258-259, 267-274
  processes, 83, 252
Cognitive/language impairment, 251-254, 274-276
Cohort effect, 81
Combinatorial operation, 143
Committee on Organic Mental Disorders, 210
Communicative Abilities in Daily Living (CADL), 11
  aging, 105-106
  aphasia, mild, 113, 120
  effects of institutionalization on, 3
  performance categories, 150
Communication augmentation systems, aided, 283, 297-308
  components, 300-305
  future trends, 306-307
  needs assessment, 307-309
  schematic, 304
  service delivery systems, 305
  systems processes, 301-303
  systems output, 303-305
  users of communicative devices, 298-300
Communication augmentation systems, unaided (*see also* Gestural deficits, Gestures), 283, 286-297

American Indian Sign Language (Amerind), 287, 296
American Sign Language (Ameslan), 287, 296
  clinical application, 294-297
  communicative function, 288
  components, 286
  schematic, 290
Comprehension, auditory, 94-101
  accuracy, 97
  aging, 97-100
  context, 114
  depressed abilities, 115
  distractions, 115-116
  facilitation, 115
  inference detecting, 98
  mild aphasia assessment, 121-124
  paragraph, 98-100, 106, 115
  reduction, age-related, 99-100
  sentences, 96-98, 101, 115 (*see also* Morphosyntactic disruption)
  verbal-pictorial verification tasks, 96
Computerized tomography scan (CT scan), 12, 64, 85, 231
  correlation of lesion sites and deficits, 148
  dementia, 46, 233
  left-hemisphere lesions, 166-167, 169-170, 172
  normal aging data, 85
Confabulation, 5, 14-15, 19, 28-29, 54
Confrontation naming, 102, 104
Confusion, language of, 4, 14-15, 28-29, 43-44, 54
Conservation tasks, 128
Corpus striatum, 85
Cortical areas
  specialization of two hemispheres, 202
  symbolic motor sequences, 291
Corticobulbar disease, bilateral, 219
Corticospinal tract disease, 219
Coverbal behaviors, 118-119, 289, 292
Creutzfeldt-Jacob disease, 7, 211, 213, 217-218
Cross-sectional design, cognitive function, 81
CT scan (*see* Computerized tomography scan)

Subject Index

D

Deblocking procedures, 137
Deficits
    aphasic syntactive, 145
    configuration, site of lesion, 133, 148
    environmentally caused, 26-27
    gestural, 289-297
    linguistic, RH, 191-195
    perceptual, RH, 56, 178-185
    transcoding, 136
Dementia (*see also* Alzheimer's disease), 209-238
    age, education, IQ table, 226
    & family, 58-59
    assessment, 20-22, 230-235
    cerebral blood flow, 85
    characteristics, 215-221
    classification, 211-212
    cortical vs. subcortical, 212, 225
    definition, 7, 209
    discriminant function analysis, 22
    distribution, types by age, 213
    Down's syndrome, 218
    etiology, 216, 224
    Family Handbook, 236
    Huntington's disease, 215
    intellectual impairment, 224
    Korsakoff's disease, 221
    language deficits by stages, 227-229
    language profiles, 224
    literature review, 221-230
    morphological changes, 215
    multi-infarct (MID), 213, 219
    naming deficits, research, 222
    national organizations, 238
    Parkinson's disease, 213-214
    Pick's disease, 219
    presenile (Alzheimer's) disease, 209, 215
    primary degenerative, 210
    primary degenerative, 210
    prognosis, 45-46, 49
    secondary degenerative, 210
    senile brain disease (SBD), 215
    severe, 230
    treatable, 7, 45
    treatment, 57-60, 235-238
    vs. aphasia, 20-22, 35-36, 210
    vs. confused language, 34
    vs. depression, 27
    vs. normal aging, 234-235
    vs. pseudodementia, 20, 27-28, 46
    vs. schizophrenia, 35
Depression, vs. dementia, 27
Diagnosis (*see* Assessment, Tests)
Dichotic listening, 82, 86
Discriminant Function Equation, 232
Disinhibition, 227
Disorders, co-existing, 9, 37-38, 63-64
Distractor task, 115
Dual Coding Theory, 183
Dysarthria, 190, 246, 297
Dysfluency, 116-117, 120
Dyslexia, 162-164

E

Echolalia, 223
Electroencephalogram (EEG), 85, 234
Electroencephalography, 231
Encephalopathy, hemptic, 45
Encoding, 88, 108, 302
Environmental influence, communication deficit, 2-4, 26-27, 42-43, 51
Environmental modification, 51-54
Environmental stimuli management, 268
Extralinguistic cues, 115

F

Facial recognition, 179, 184, 188
Foley's taxonomy, 211
Frontal leucotomy, 188

G

Galvanic skin response (GSR), 186
Geriatric (*see* Aging)
Gestural communication systems (*see* Communication augmentation systems, unaided)
Gestural deficits, 289-297
    aphasia, 291-293
    apraxic motor theory, 291-292
    language based theory, 292-294
    left-hemisphere (LH) damage, 289
    pantomime, 293-294
Gestural imitation ability, 292

Subject Index

Gestures (*see also* Communication augmentation systems, unaided), 286-297
   American Indian Sign Language (Amerind), 287, 296
   American Sign Language (Ameslan), 287, 296
   coverbal, 287, 289, 292
   deblocking, 289
   iconic, 287, 296-297
   nonpropositional behavior, 292
   pantomime, 295-297
   propositional, 292
   subpropositional, 292, 297
   referential, 287
Glasgow Coma Scale, 256
Gliosis, progressive subcortical, 211
Global aphasia
   aphasia, severe, 160, 166-168
   artificial language, 296
   neurobehavioral characteristics, 167
Granuvacuolar degeneration (GVD), 215-216, 218
Group therapy, 51-53

H

Handivoice, 299, 302
Harmonic information, 194
Head trauma (*see* Closed head injury)
Hearing loss, 2-3, 84, 107
Hematoma, subdural, 7, 46
Hemi-inattention, 57
Hemispheres, specialization of, 202 (*see also* Right hemisphere)
Homonymous hemianopsia, 179
Homophones, 224
Huntington's chorea, 211
Huntington's disease, 7, 212, 225-227, 237
   definition, 220
   dementia, 215
   morphological changes, 221
   national organizations, 238
Hydrocephalus, occult, 7
Hypothalamus, 221

I

Ideographic reconstructions, 183
Idiomatic expressions, 199

Idiosyncratic responses, 89
Indifference reaction, 186
Inferencing, 98, 188
Intelligence quotient (IQ) (*see also* Tests)
   & aging, 82, 235
   dementia, 225
   language function, 84
   verbal, 196

K

Korsakoff's disease (KD), 7, 211, 221
Kuru disease, 217-218

L

Language
   & aging, 2-4, 79-84, 86, 93, 106, 235
   assessment, 263-265
   auditory comprehension, 84, 86-87
   cognitive organization, 272-273
   confused-agitated, 269-273
   confusion, language of, 4, 14, 28, 42-43
   decline, 80
   disorders of, table, 41
   disorganization, 265
   dysfunction, post CHI, 252
   environmental stimulation, 266-267
   gestures, 288
   patterns of errors, 263
   pragmatics, 149
   schizophrenia, deficit, 63
   systems, nonspeech, 283-309
Latency, naming, 102
L-dopa, 51
Left ear advantage, 186
Lexical focus, 128
Lexical-semantic disruption, 137-143
Lexical-syntactic dissociations, 143-144
Linguistic involvement
   behaviors, 149
   competence, 264
   deficits, 191, 289
   dysfunction, 247
   mechanisms, 84
   performance accuracy, 84
   right-hemisphere (RH), 195-203

M

Management (*see* Treatment)
Masking theory, 147
Melodic Intonation Therapy (MIT), 59, 166, 171, 190, 297
Memory (*see also* Memory, semantic)
    & aging, 85–92
    attention, 86
    episodic, 88, 96
    long-term, 87–90
    neurology, 166
    retrieval, 90, 302
    sensory, 86
    short-term, 86–87, 89, 93, 107
    storage, 89, 302
    studies, 95–96
Memory, semantic (*see also* Memory), 88–92, 95, 107
    acquisition, 90
    analytic-descriptive, 91
    & aging, 89, 104
    & aphasia, 89, 91–92
    & word fluency, 104
    categorical-inferential, 91–92
    conceptual style, 90–92
    disorganization, 92
    paradigmatic relationship, 91
    relation-thematic, 91–92
    retention, 90
    retrieval, 90
    syntagmatic relationship, 91
MENSA, 95
Minor-hemisphere mediation, 146
Mnemonic devices, 88
Molecular commotion, 250
Morphosyntactic disruption, 143–146
Morse Code, 300, 302
Mutism, 26, 55

N

Neglect, left-sided, 179–181, 185
Neologisms, 17, 147–148
Neuroanatomical data, 202
Neurobehavioral dichotomies, 257
Neurofibrillary tangles (NFT), 215–216
Neurological factors
    deterioration, progressive, 284
    disease, 299
    dysfunction, 250
    etiology categories, 247
Neuronal capacity, 202
Neuropsychologists, 11–12
Noncanonical elements, 196
Nonlinguistic symbols, 188
Nonvocal adults (*see also* Communicative augmentative systems), 284
Normal aging (*see* Aging, Aging/Normal language)

O

Occult hydrocephalus, 211
Oral-graphic dissociation, 142

P

Paired-associate learing (PAL), 182–183
Palsy, 211, 219
Paradigmatic responses, 89
Paralinguistic behaviors, 149
Paraphasia, 148
    semantic, 139, 228
    verbal, 128
Parkinson's disease
    co-occurring/dementia, 213–215
    dysarthria, 190
    idiopathic, 7, 220
    language tasks, 225–227
    morphological changes, 220
    national organizations, 238
    nonvascular dementia, 211
    postencephalitic, 220
    semantic association, 223
    spontaneous expression, 189–190
    subcortical changes, 212
    treatment, 51
Perceptual impairment hypothesis, 222
Perceptual motor processing, 102
Perseveration, 173, 185
Phonemic involvement, 126, 147–148, 194
Phonetic error, 126, 147
Phonological-articulatory process, 147–148
Phonologic disruption, 144, 146–148
Pick's disease, 7, 211, 213, 219–220
Pneumoencephalography, 233

Porch Index of Communicative Ability
(PICA)
    aphasia, 37-40, 49-50, 113, 161, 192
    case histories, 167, 171
    dementia, 21, 34, 40
    gestural deficits, 293
    language, 21, 134
    normal adults, 93
    normal aged, 4
    right-hemisphere (RH), 12, 19, 33, 192
    schizophrenia, 17, 30
    vs. Advance Auditory Battery (AAB), 123
Positron emission tomograph (PET), 12, 65
Pragmatic disruption, 148-151
Presbycusis (see Hearing loss)
Presenile brain disease (see Alzheimer's disease)
Prognosis
    & etiology, 45
    & lesion site, 46
    aphasia, 46-48
    confused language, 42-43
    dementia, 45-46
    environmental influence, normal aged, 42
    prognostic groupings, 47-48
    prognostic variables, 47
    right-hemisphere, 44-46
    schizophrenia, 43
    statistical prediction, 48
Promoting Aphasics' Communicative Efficiency (PACE), 59, 150-151, 289
Prosodic deficits
    right-hemisphere, 178, 185-191
    schizophrenia, 5, 16
Prosodic-phonological factors, 144-145
Prosopagnosia, 179, 184, 188
Pseudobulbar palsy, 219
Psuedodementia, 20, 27-28
Psycholinguistics
    & aging, 79, 101, 107
    & aphasia, 134
    definition, 135
Pure word deafness, 159-160

R

Reality orientation, 51-54, 237
Rehabilitation (see Treatment)

Response dominance, 104
Response latency, 99
Retrieval, word (see also Memory, semantic), 101-104, 116-117
Right-hemisphere (RH), 5-6, 177-203
    affect/prosody, 185-191
    & aging, 82
    appraisal, 18-20, 30, 33
    auditory comprehension, 122
    auditory perception, 6, 193
    auditory processing, 189
    cognitive impairment, 195-201
    confabulation, 19
    contextual clues, 188
    ear advantage, 186-187
    emotional response, 185-186, 188-191
    hemi-inattention, 56
    idioms, 199-200
    left-sided neglect, 179-182
    linguistic deficits, 191-195
    paired associate learning (PAL), 184
    phonemic discrimination, 194
    prognosis, 44-45, 49
    reading deficits, 57, 185
    symbols, nonlinguistic, 198-199
    treatment, 44-45, 56-57
    vs. aphasia, 19
    vs. left-hemisphere, 45, 126, 186, 188-189, 194, 197-200, 202
    visual processing, 197-198
    writing deficits, 183-186

S

Schizophrenia
    assessment, 15-18
    intelligence, 43-44
    mutism, 55
    prognosis, 43-44, 49
    speech characteristics, 5, 16, 56
    speech treatment, 55-56
    vs. aphasia, 17-18, 29-32, 35
    vs. dementia, 35
    vs. right-hemisphere, 29-30
Semantic deficits, 97, 102, 138-140, 149
Semantic features model, 140
Semantic Oppositional Rhyming Retrieval Training (SORRT), 127
Senile brain atrophy, 211
Senile brain disease (see Dementia)

Subject Index 333

Sensory functions, 84
Sensory memory, 86
Sentence disambiguation, 226
Sentence production, 105
Sentence verification, 96, 115
Sequence of Phonemes for Efficient English Communication (SPEEC), 306
Service delivery systems, 305
Simultagnosia, 184
Somatosensory speech, 6
Story Completion Task, 145
Stress-saliency hypothesis, 144
Stroke (*see* Cerebral vascular accident)
Stuttering, 116–117, 120
Subdural hematoma, 211
Subintimal hyperplasia, 219
Substantia nigra, 220
Supraspan word lists, 87
Syllable structure process, 148
Synonymy, superior, 95
Syntactical disruption, 125, 143–146
Syntagmatic responses, 89
Syntax Stimulation Program (SSP), 145
Systems, nonspeech communciation (*see* Communication augmentation systems)

T

Tachistoscopic studies, 189
Teletypewriter (TTY), 303
Testing, 162–165
    battery assessment, 10–12
    norms, aphasia, 93–94
    of comprehension, 94–101
Tests
    Advance Auditory Battery (AAB), 123
    Aphasia Language Performance Scales (ALPS), 10
    Appraisal of Language Disturbance, 10
    Auditory Attention-span for Unrelated Words and Related Syllables, 260
    Auditory Comprehension Test for Sentences (ACTS), 122
    Benton Revised Visual Retention Test, 261
    Boston Diagnostic Aphasia Exam (BDAE), 11, 16–17, 19–20, 23–24, 94, 102, 106, 113, 118, 124, 160–165, 167, 169–174, 192–197
    Boston Naming Test, 20, 193
    Clinical Dementia Rating (CDR), 21–22
    Color Form Sorting Test, 263
    Communicative Abilities in Daily Living (CADL), 3
    Detroit Test of Learning Aptitude (DTLA), 20, 265
    Developmental Test of Visual Perception, 260
    Diagnostic and Statistical Manual (DSM II), 210, 215
    Diagnostic and Statistical Manual on Mental Disorders (DSM I), 210
    Examination for Aphasia, 11
    Functional Communication Profile, 11
    G-F-W Auditory Memory Test, 261
    G-F-W Sound-Symbol Test, 261
    Goldstein-Scheerer Stick Test, 261
    Halstead Aphasia Test, Form M, 11
    Halstead-Reitan Battery, 44
    Helm-Elicited Language Program for Syntax Stimulation (HELPSS), 174
    Hooper Visual Organization Test, 19–20, 184, 192
    Illinois Test of Psycholinguistic Abilities (ITPA), 265
    informal, 164
    Language Modalities Test, 6
    Language Modalities Test for Aphasia (LMTA), 6, 11
    Lorr Feeling & Mood Scale, 190
    Luria-Nebraska Neuropsychological Battery, 11–12
    Luria's Mnestic Test, 261
    Mental Status Questionnaire, 13–14, 226
    Minnesota Test for Differential Diagnosis of Aphasia (MTDDA), 8, 11, 24, 48
    Neurosensory Center Comprehensive Exam for Aphasia (NCCEA), 11
    New Adult Reading Test, 21
    Nonverbal Test of Cognitive Skills, 261
    Nonvocal Communication Scale, 164–165
    Orzeck Aphasia Evaluation, 11
parietal, 94

Subject Index

Peabody Picture Vocabulary Test (PPVT), 226, 231-232
Porch Index of Communicative Abilities (PICA), 11-12, 14, 17, 19, 21, 93, 113, 123, 134, 161, 167, 171, 192, 293, 297
Raven's Progressive Matrices Test, 82, 297
Reading Comprehension Battery for Aphasia, 98
Reporter's Test, 124
Revised Token Test, 11, 20, 122, 193
Schuell's Diagnostic Battery, 93
Sklar Aphasia Scale, 11
Temporal Orientation Test, 18
Temporal Spatial Orientation Test, 15
Token Test, 17-18, 39, 97, 116, 121-122, 124
Wechsler Adult Intelligence Scale (WAIS), 82, 100, 169-170, 172, 196, 226, 231-232, 260-261, 265
Wechsler Memory Scale, 261
Western Aphasia Battery (WAB), 11, 21, 23-24, 35-36
Word Fluency Measure, 18, 20, 39, 121
Visual Attention Span for Objects and Letters, 260
Thalamus, 221
Topological orientation, 160
Trauma, head (see Closed head injury)
Treatment
    aged, environmental deficits, 51-53
    & prognosis, 42
    aphasia, 59-60, 127, 146, 166
    aphasia, mild, 121, 127-129
    aphasia, moderate, 137, 143, 145-146, 151
    aphasia, severe, 146, 166-171
    aphasia, Wernicke's, 146, 172-175
    closed head injury (CHI), 174-175, 266-277
    cognitive-linguistic disorganization, 274-276
    deblocking, 137
    dementia, 57-59, 235-238
    diagnostic, 14
    environmental manipulation, 266-268
    generalization, 142
    graphic communication, 165
    group therapy, 51-53
    institutional, 51-54
    intonational contour, 190
    language disorganization, 274-276
    language of confusion, 54
    left-hemisphere, 168, 170-173
    Lexical focus, 128
    manipulation of stimuli, 277
    Melodic Intonation Therapy (MIT), 59, 166, 171, 190, 197
    psycholinguistics, life-span, 106
    reading/writing, 185
    reality orientation, 52-53, 58-67
    refusal by patient, 174-175
    right-hemisphere, 56-57
    schizophrenic speech, 54-55
    semantic disruption, 140
    semantic oppositional and rhyming training, 127-128
    Story Completion Task, 145
    Syntax Stimulation Program, 145
    Verbing strategy, 145
T-unit, 118
Type token ratio analysis, 16

U

Unilateral neglect syndrome, 180
Utterances, 119

V

Verbal cues strategy, 181
Verbal expression, 116, 124
Verbing strategy, 145
Visual Action Therapy (VAT), 59-60, 164-166, 168, 171, 173
Visual imagery, 182
Visual processing tasks, 197
Visuoconstructive deficits, 179, 181
Visuospatial disorders (see Right-hemisphere)
Visuospatial thinking, 82
Voluntary Control of Involuntary Utterances (VCIU), 60, 165, 168-170, 173

W

Wechsler Adult Intelligence Scale (WAIS)
    age-related reduction, 100
    Alzheimer's patients, 226
    case histories, 169–170, 172, 196
    cognitive functions, 82
    digit span subtest, 260–261
    discriminant function equation, 232
    language integrity, 265
    neuropsychological evaluation, 231
Wernicke's aphasia
    aphasia, moderate, 139
    aphasia, severe, 160, 171–173
    language deficit, 293
    neurobehavioral characteristics, 172–173
    schizophrenia, 4
    semantic memory, 92
    sentence construction, 144
    treatment, 146, 172–175
    vs. normal aging, 92
    word finding, 139
White noise, 116
Word production anomia, 137
Word retrieval, 101, 105